Clinical Neuroanatomy and Neuroscience

Sixth Edition

Cover picture kindly provided by Dr. Alexander Leemans, Image Sciences Institute, University Medical Center, Utrecht, The Netherlands, via Dr. Dara Cannon, Co-Director, Clinical Neuroimaging Laboratory, Department of Psychiatry, National University of Ireland, Galway.

Commissioning Editor: Madelene Hyde
Development Editor: Joanne Scott
Editorial Assistant: Rachael Harrison
Project Manager: Alan Nicholson
Design: Charles Gray
Illustration Manager: Gillian Richards
Marketing Manager (US, ROW): Jason Oberacker/Ian Jordan

SIXTH EDITION

Clinical Neuroanatomy and Neuroscience

M J Turlough FitzGerald, MD, PhD, DSc, MRIA

Emeritus Professor of Anatomy
Department of Anatomy
National University of Ireland
Galway, Ireland

Gregory Gruener, MD, MBA

Director, Leischner Institute for Medical Education
Leischner Professor of Medical Education
Senior Associate Dean, Stritch School of Medicine
Professor of Neurology, Associate Chair of Neurology
Loyola University Chicago
Maywood, IL, USA

Estomih Mtui, MD

Associate Professor of Clinical Anatomy in Neurology and Neuroscience
Director, Program in Anatomy and Visualization
Weill Cornell Medical College
New York, NY, USA

SAUNDERS

ELSEVIER

SAUNDERS
ELSEVIER

SAUNDERS an imprint of Elsevier Limited
© 2012, Elsevier Limited. All rights reserved.

First edition 1985
Second edition 1992
Third edition 1996
Fourth edition 2002 (Reprinted 2002, 2003)
Fifth edition 2007
Sixth edition 2012

Notices

Knowledge and best practice in this field are constantly changing. As new research and experience broaden our understanding, changes in research methods, professional practices, or medical treatment may become necessary. Practitioners and researchers must always rely on their own experience and knowledge in evaluating and using any information, methods, compounds, or experiments described herein. In using such information or methods they should be mindful of their own safety and the safety of others, including parties for whom they have a professional responsibility.

With respect to any drug or pharmaceutical products identified, readers are advised to check the most current information provided (i) on procedures featured or (ii) by the manufacturer of each product to be administered, to verify the recommended dose or formula, the method and duration of administration, and contraindications. It is the responsibility of practitioners, relying on their own experience and knowledge of their patients, to make diagnoses, to determine dosages and the best treatment for each individual patient, and to take all appropriate safety precautions.

To the fullest extent of the law, neither the Publisher nor the authors, contributors, or editors, assume any liability for any injury and/or damage to persons or property as a matter of products liability, negligence or otherwise, or from any use or operation of any methods, products, instructions, or ideas contained in the material herein.

Main Edition
ISBN: 978-0-7020-3738-2

International Edition
ISBN: 978-0-7020-4042-9

British Library Cataloguing in Publication Data
A catalogue record for this book is available from the British Library

Fitzgerald, M. J. T.
  Clinical neuroanatomy and neuroscience. – 6th ed.
  1. Neuroanatomy. 2. Neurosciences. 3. Nervous system-Diseases. 4. Nervous system-Pathophysiology.
  I. Title II. Gruener, Gregory. III. Mtui, Estomih.
  611.8-dc22

Library of Congress Cataloging in Publication Data
A catalog record for this book is available from the Library of Congress

Printed in China
Last digit is the print number: 9 8 7 6 5 4 3 2 1

Contents

CONTENTS

Preface

This textbook is designed as a *vade mecum* ('go with me') for medical students. While based on campus, the gross and microscopic structures of the nervous system take precedence, along with their great diversity of functions. A strong stimulus to understand normal structure and function is provided by clinical examples of the consequences of breakdowns of diverse kinds. While hospital-based, consultation of the book in a clinical setting recalls the functional anatomy studied on campus. Sequential fusion of descriptive structure, function, and malfunction is known as *vertical integration* and is highly recommended owing to its manifest logic.

Chapters and Pages

Following a brief account of nervous system development in Chapter 1, the topography of the brain and spinal cord and their meningeal surrounds occupies Chapters 2–4. Next (Ch. 5) comes the clinically very important *blood supply*. Microscopic and ultramicroscopic anatomy of neurons (nerve cells) and neuroglia (their surrounding 'nerve glue') come to the fore in Chapter 6, along with some compression effects of expanding neuroglial tumors.

Chapter 7 changes the context by describing electrical events underlying the impulses that are triggered at the point of origin of axons and speed along the axons and their branches to liberate excitatory or inhibitory molecules onto target neurons. These molecules, pillars of the science of neuropharmacology, are examined in Chapter 8. Chapters 9–11 explore the structure and distribution of the peripheral nerves attached to the spinal cord and innervating the muscles and skin of the trunk and limbs. Electrical activity returns in Chapter 12 in the form of *electromyography*, a technique widely used in the detection of neuromuscular disorders of various kinds.

The *autonomic nervous system* (Ch. 13) controls the smooth musculature of the vascular system and of the alimentary, urinary, and reproductive tracts. The *spinal nerves* (Ch. 14) attached to the whole length of the spinal cord, are 'mixed' (both motor and sensory) and innervate all of the voluntary muscles and skin in the trunk and limbs. Description of the contents of the spinal cord itself occupies Chapters 15 and 16.

The *brainstem* (medulla oblongata, pons, and midbrain) connects the spinal cord to the cerebral hemispheres, as described by means of transverse sections in Chapter 17. The cranial nerves attached to it (nerves III to XII) are described in Chapters 19–23. Chapter 24 is devoted to the *reticular formation* of the brainstem which, *inter alia*, links cranial nerves to one another.

The *cerebellum* (Ch. 25) occupies the posterior cranial fossa. Its afferent (*L.* 'carry to') connections from voluntary muscles and its *efferent* ('carry out') connections with the motor cortex in the brain are vital for control the smoothness of all voluntary movements.

The *hypothalamus* (Ch. 26) can be traced back in nature as far as the reptiles. It still operates basic survival controls, including food and fluid intake, temperature control, and sleep. Above it are the thalamus and epithalamus (Ch. 27), the former having numerous vital connections to cerebral cortex and spinal cord.

The *Visual pathways* chapter (Ch. 28) lays out the largest v all horizontal pathways, stretching from the very front end of the brain – the retina – to the very back – the occipital cortex. Its clinical significance is obvious.

Chapter 29 examines the histological structure of the *cerebral cortex*, and provides a summary functional account of the different cortical areas. Electrical activities are examined by means of *electroencephalography* (Ch. 30) and *evoked potentials* (Ch. 31). Functional inequalities between the left and right sides of the brain are the subject of Chapter 32, *hemispherical asymmetries*.

The *basal ganglia* (Ch. 33) are a group of nuclei at the base of the brain primarily involved in the control of movement. The most frequent failure of control takes the form of *Parkinson's disease*.

The final anatomic structures, analyzed in Chapter 34, are the *olfactory* (smell) *system* and the *limbic system*, the latter being of major emotional significance.

Chapter 35 is about *cerebrovascular disease*. The main purpose of this chapter is to highlight the functional defects that follow cerebral hemorrhage or thrombosis.

Chapter title pages feature:

Chapter Summary A list of the items to be dealt with in the chapter.

Boxes Contain titles of structures/functions to be examined in detail.

Clinical Panels Functional disorders related to this material.

Study Guidelines A running commentary on the subject matter, stressing features of clinical importance.

Website features

Tutorials Each chapter contains a 'Web tutoria' notification at an appropriate point. Clicking the appropriate button will deliver a slide show on the relevant topic, with a script and optional voiceover commentary. Particular attention is drawn to 'Nuclear magnetic resonance (Web tutorial 2)' in Chapter 2 (55 slides) and 'Arterial supply of the forebrain (Web tutorial 5)' in Chapter 5 (27 slides).

MCQs Website MCQs are available for each chapter. All 200 are in USML Step 1 format. Half contain an illustration, half are text only.

Case studies 30 case studies (127 slides) demonstrating the clinical consequences of physical or inflammatory damage to nervous tissues.

Faculty resources

An image bank is available to help you prepare lectures via our Evolve website. Contact your local sales representative for more information, or go directly to the Evolve website to request access: http://evolve.elsevier.com

TF, GG, EM
2010

The table below lists the main clinical perspectives covered in the book

CLINICAL PERSPECTIVES

Chapters		Perspectives
1	Embryology	(Explanatory layout)
2	Cerebral topography	(Explanatory layout)
3	Midbrain, hindbrain, spinal cord	(Explanatory layout)
4	Meninges	Extradural hematoma. Subdural hematoma. Hydrocephalus. Meningitis. Spinal tap.
		Epidural analgesia. Caudal analgesia.
5	Blood supply of the brain	Blood–brain barrier pathology.
6	Neurons and neuroglia: overview	Brain tumors. Multiple sclerosis. Neuronal transport disorders.
7	Electrical events	(Explanatory layout)
8	Transmitters and receptors	Some general clinical applications concerning malfunctions and pharmacology.
9	Peripheral nerves	Degeneration and regeneration.
10	Innervation of muscles and joints	(Explanatory layout)
11	Innervation of skin	Neurogenic inflammation. Leprosy.
12	Electrodiagnostic examination	Peripheral neuropathies, including entrapment syndromes.
		Myasthenia gravis.
13	Autonomic nervous system and visceral afferents	Horner's syndrome. Raynaud syndrome. Stellate block. Lumbar sympathectomy. Visceral pain. Drug actions on the sympathetic and parasympathetic systems.
14	Nerve roots	Spina bifida. Cervical spondylosis. Prolapsed intervertebral disc.
15	Spinal cord: ascending pathways	Syringomyelia
16	Spinal cord: descending pathways	Upper motor neuron disease. Lower motor neuron disease. Spinal cord injury.
17	Brainstem	(Explanatory layout)
18	The lowest four cranial nerves	Supranuclear, nuclear, infranuclear lesions.
19	Vestibular nerve	Vestibular disorders. Lateral medullary syndrome.
20	Cochlear nerve	Conduction deafness. Sensorineural deafness.
21	Trigeminal nerve	Trigeminal neuralgia. Referred pain in diseases of the head and neck.
22	Facial nerve	Lesions of the facial nerve.
23	Ocular motor nerves	Several well-known ocular palsies.
24	Reticular formation	Cardiovascular, respiratory, urinary, locomotor controls. Spinal and supraspinal antinociception.
25	Cerebellum	Characteristic clinical pictures associated with lesions of vermis, of anterior lobe and of neocerebellum. Cerebellar cognitive affective syndrome.
26	Hypothalamus	Hypothalamic disorders, including major depression.
27	Thalamus, epithalamus	(Explanatory layout)
28	Visual pathways	Detection of lesions of the visual pathways, segment by segment.
29	Cerebral cortex	(Explanatory layout)
30	Electroencephalography	Narcolepsy. Seizures of several kinds and their EEG detection.
31	Evoked potentials	Use of visual, auditory, somatosensory and motor evoked potentials in disease detection. Clinical neurophysiology in relation to acupuncture.
32	Hemispheric asymmetries	The aphasias. Developmental dyslexia. Frontal lobe dysfunction. Parietal lobe dysfunction.
33	Basal ganglia	Parkinson's disease. Cerebral palsy. Huntington's disease. Hemiballism.
34	Olfactory and limbic systems	Alzheimer's disease. Schizophrenia. Drug addiction.
35	Cerebrovascular disease	Eight Clinical Panels about strokes of various kinds.

Panel of Consultants

Kamal Asaad MBBCH, MSc, PhD
Professor of Anatomy and Embryology
Department of Anatomy
Faculty of Medicine
Ain Shams University
Cairo, Egypt

Nadir E Bharucha MD, FAMS, FRCP
Professor and Head
Department of Neurology
Bombay Hospital Institute of Medical Sciences;
Head, Department of Neuroepidemiology, MRC, Bombay
Hospital
Mumbai, India

Jagjit S Chopra FRCP, Phd, FAMS, FIAN
Professor Emeritis
Postgraduate Institute of Medical Education and Research
Chandigarh, India

Timothy J Counihan MD, FRCPI
Honorary Senior Lecturer in Medicine (Neurology)
National University of Ireland
Galway, Ireland

Brian E Leonard PhD, DSc
Emeritus Professor of Pharmacology, National University
of Ireland,
Galway, Ireland;
Honorary Professor, Department of Psychiatry and
Psychotherapy
Ludwig Maximilian University
Munich, Germany

Richard Knight BA, BM BCh, MRCP, FRCP(E)
Professor of Clinical Neurology
Department of Neurology
University of Edinburgh
Edinburgh, UK

Pearse Morris MB, BCh
Professor of Radiology
Wake Forest University School of Medicine,
Winston-Salem, NC, USA

Masao Norita MD, PhD
Professor and Chair
Division of Neurobiology and Anatomy
Department of Sensory and Integrative Medicine
Niigata University Graduate School of Medical
and Dental Sciences
Asahimachi, Niigata, Japan

Wei-Yi Ong BDS, PhD
Associate Professor
Department of Anatomy and
Aging
Neurobiology Research Programme
National University of Singapore
Singapore

Hugh Staunton BSc, FRCPI, FRCP, PhD
Senior Lecturer
Department of Clinical Neurological Sciences
Royal College of Surgeons in Ireland
Dublin, Ireland

Mario Rende MD
Professor of Human Anatomy
Section of Anatomy,
Department of Experimental Medicine and
   Biochemical Sciences,
University of Perugia School of Medicine,
Perugia, Italy

David T Yew PhD, DSc, Dr med (habil)
Professor of Anatomy,
School of Biomedical Sciences,
Chinese University of Hong Kong,
Hong Kong, SAR

Student Consultants

Jarva Chow
Georgetown University School of Medicine
Year of Graduation 2010

Rebecca Colleran
National University of Ireland, Galway
MSc in Regenerative Medicine
Year of Graduation 2010

Daniel Crook
University of East Anglia School of Medicine, Health
Policy and Practice
Year of Graduation 2012

Helen R Levey, M.P.H.
Philadelphia College of Osteopathic Medicine, Georgia
Campus
Year of Graduation 2010

Yin Li
University of Pennsylvania School of Medicine
Year of Graduation 2016

Clement Loh Chee Hoou
University of New South Wales Medical School
Year of Graduation 2014

Acknowledgements

It is a pleasure to acknowledge the continued support of the Panel of Consultants, and the welcome input of students from several different countries. Particularly helpful has been Professor Kamal Asaad, Cairo, who has contributed valuably to each of the six chapters on the cranial nerves. Many thanks are also due to Editors Madelene Hyde (Philadelphia) and Joanne Scott (London) for their able assistance.

Embryology

STUDY GUIDELINES

This chapter aims to give you sufficient insight into development to account for the arrangement of structures in the mature nervous system. If not already familiar with adult brain anatomy, we suggest you read this chapter again following study of Chapters 2 and 3.

For descriptive purposes, the embryo is in the prone (face-down) position, whereby the terms *ventral* and *dorsal* correspond to the adult *anterior* and *posterior*, and *rostral* and *caudal* correspond to *superior* and *inferior*.

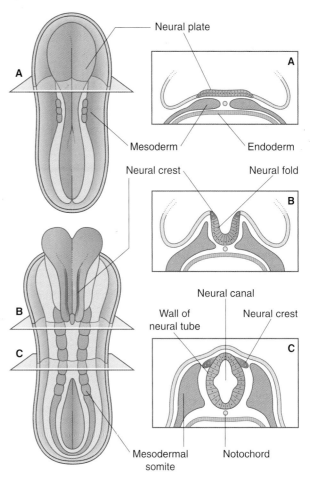

Figure 1.1 Cross-section **(A)** is from a 3-somite (20-day) embryo. Cross-sections **(B)** and **(C)** are from an 8-somite (22-day) embryo.

SPINAL CORD

Neurulation

The entire nervous system originates from the **neural plate**, an ectodermal thickening in the floor of the amniotic sac (Figure 1.1). During the third week after fertilization, the plate forms paired **neural folds**, which unite to create the **neural tube** and **neural canal**. Union of the folds commences in the future neck region of the embryo and proceeds rostrally and caudally from there. The open ends of the tube, the **neuropores**, are closed off before the end of the fourth week. The process of formation of the neural tube from the ectoderm is known as *neurulation*.

Cells at the edge of each neural fold escape from the line of union and form the **neural crest** alongside the tube. Cell types derived from the neural crest include spinal and autonomic ganglion cells and the Schwann cells of peripheral nerves.

Spinal nerves

The dorsal part of the neural tube is called the **alar plate**; the ventral part is the **basal plate** (Figure 1.2). Neurons developing in the alar plate are predominantly sensory in function and receive dorsal nerve roots growing in from the spinal ganglia. Neurons in the basal plate are predominantly motor and give rise to ventral nerve roots. At appropriate levels of the spinal cord, the ventral roots also contain autonomic fibers. The dorsal and ventral roots unite to form the spinal nerves, which emerge from the vertebral canal in the interval between the neural arches being formed by the mesenchymal vertebrae.

The cells of the spinal (dorsal root) ganglia are initially bipolar. They become unipolar by the coalescence of their two processes at one side of the parent cells.

BRAIN

Brain parts

Late in the fourth week, the rostral part of the neural tube undergoes flexion at the level of the future midbrain (Figure 1.3A). This region is the **mesencephalon**; slight constrictions

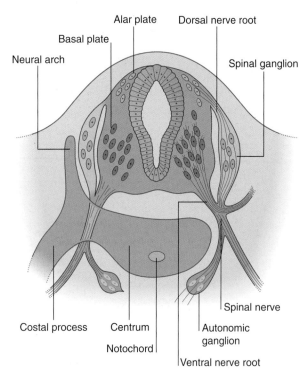

Figure 1.2 Neural tube, spinal nerve, and mesenchymal vertebra of an embryo at 6 weeks.

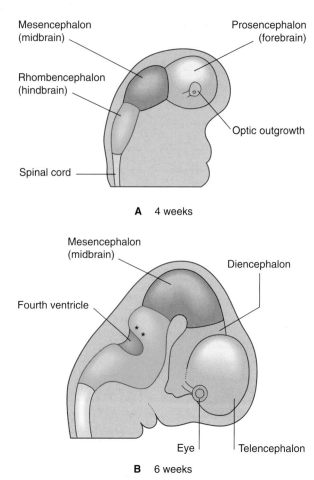

A 4 weeks

B 6 weeks

Figure 1.3 (A and B) Brain vesicles, seen from the right side. Asterisks indicate the site of initial development of the cerebellum.

mark its junction with the **prosencephalon** (future forebrain) and **rhombencephalon** (future hindbrain).

The alar plate of the prosencephalon expands on each side (Figure 1.3A) to form the **telencephalon** (cerebral hemispheres). The basal plate remains in place here as the **diencephalon**. Finally, an **optic outgrowth** from the diencephalon is the forerunner of the retina and optic nerve.

The diencephalon, mesencephalon, and rhombencephalon constitute the embryonic brainstem.

The brainstem buckles as development proceeds. As a result, the mesencephalon is carried to the summit of the brain. The rhombencephalon folds on itself, causing the alar plates to flare and creating the rhomboid (diamond-shaped) fourth ventricle of the brain. The rostral part of the rhombencephalon gives rise to the pons and cerebellum. The caudal part gives rise to the medulla oblongata (Figure 1.4).

Ventricular system and choroid plexuses

The neural canal dilates within the cerebral hemispheres, forming the lateral ventricles; these communicate with the third ventricle contained within the diencephalon. The third and fourth ventricles communicate through the aqueduct of the midbrain (Figure 1.5).

The thin roofs of the forebrain and hindbrain are invaginated by tufts of capillaries, which form the choroid plexuses of the four ventricles. The choroid plexuses secrete cerebrospinal fluid (CSF), which flows through the ventricular system. The fluid leaves the fourth ventricle through three apertures in its roof (Figure 1.6).

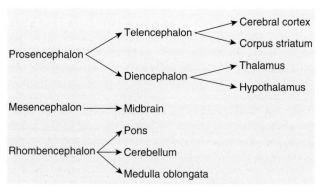

Figure 1.4 Some derivatives of the brain vesicles.

Cranial nerves

Figure 1.7 illustrates the state of development of the cranial nerves during the sixth week after fertilization.

- The olfactory nerve (I) forms from bipolar neurons developing in the epithelium lining the olfactory pit.

Figure 1.5 The developing ventricular system. Choroid plexuses are shown in red.

A 8 weeks

B 12 weeks

Figure 1.6 Dorsal views of the developing hindbrain (see arrow in inset). **(A)** At 8 weeks, the cerebellum is emerging from the fourth ventricle. **(B)** At 12 weeks, the ventricle is becoming hidden by the cerebellum, and three apertures have appeared in the roof plate.

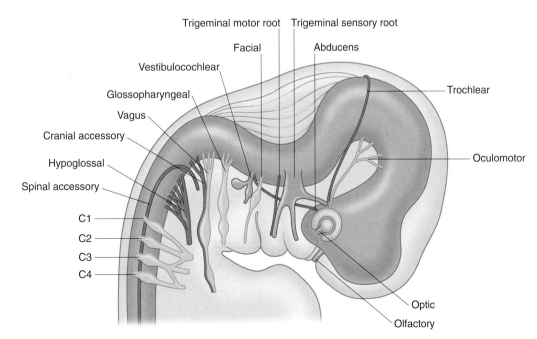

Figure 1.7 Cranial nerves of a 6-week-old embryo. (After Bossy et al. 1990, with permission of Springer-Verlag.)

- The optic nerve (II) is growing centrally from the retina.
- The oculomotor (III) and trochlear (IV) nerves arise from the midbrain, and the abducens (VI) nerve arises from the pons; all three will supply extrinsic muscles of the eye.
- The three divisions of the trigeminal (V) nerve will be sensory to the skin of the face and scalp, to the mucous membranes of the oronasal cavity, and to the teeth. A motor root will supply the muscles of mastication (chewing).
- The facial (VII) nerve will supply the muscles of facial expression. The vestibulocochlear (VIII) nerve will supply the organs of hearing and balance, which develop from the otocyst.
- The glossopharyngeal (IX) nerve is composite. Most of its fibers will be sensory to the oropharynx.
- The vagus (X) nerve too is composite. It contains a large sensory element for the supply of the mucous membranes of the digestive system, and a large motor (parasympathetic) element for the supply of the heart, lungs, and gastrointestinal tract.
- The cranial accessory (XIc) nerve will be distributed by the vagus to the muscles of the larynx and pharynx.
- The spinal accessory (XIs) nerve will supply the sternomastoid and trapezius muscles. The hypoglossal (XII) nerve will supply the muscles of the tongue.

Cerebral hemispheres

In the telencephalon, mitotic activity takes place in the **ventricular zone**, just outside the lateral ventricle. Daughter cells migrate to the outer surface of the expanding hemisphere and form the cerebral cortex.

Expansion of the cerebral hemispheres is not uniform. A region on the lateral surface, the **insula** (*L.* 'island'), is relatively quiescent and forms a pivot around which the expanding hemisphere rotates. Frontal, parietal, occipital, and temporal lobes can be identified at 14 weeks' gestational age (Figure 1.8).

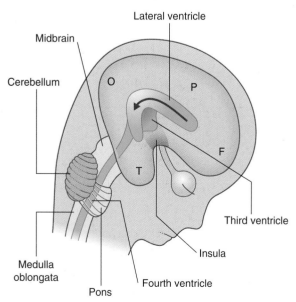

Figure 1.8 Fetal brain at 14 weeks. The arrow indicates the C-shaped growth of the hemisphere around the insula. F, P, O, T; frontal, parietal, occipital, temporal lobes.

On the medial surface of the hemisphere, a patch of cerebral cortex, the **hippocampus**, belongs to a fifth, **limbic lobe** of the brain. The hippocampus is drawn into the temporal lobe, leaving in its wake a strand of fibers called the **fornix**. Within the concavity of this arc is the **choroid fissure**, through which the choroid plexus invaginates into the lateral ventricle (Figure 1.9).

The anterior commissure develops as a connection linking olfactory (smell) regions of the left and right sides. Above this, a much larger commissure, the **corpus callosum**, links

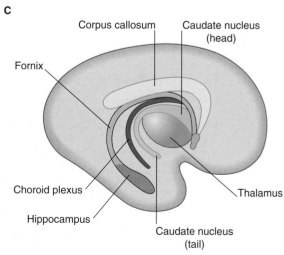

Figure 1.9 Medial aspect of the developing left hemisphere. The hippocampus, initially dorsal to the thalamus, migrates into the temporal lobe (arrows in **A** and **B**), leaving the fornix in its wake. The concavity of the arc so formed contains the choroid fissure (the line of insertion of the choroid plexus into the ventricle) and the tail of the caudate nucleus.

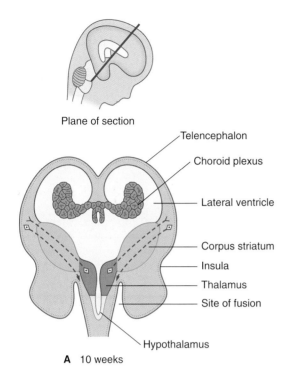

Plane of section

Telencephalon
Choroid plexus
Lateral ventricle
Corpus striatum
Insula
Thalamus
Site of fusion
Hypothalamus

A 10 weeks

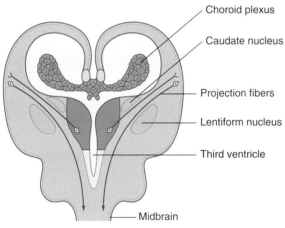

Choroid plexus
Caudate nucleus
Projection fibers
Lentiform nucleus
Third ventricle
Midbrain

B 17 weeks

Figure 1.10 Coronal sections of the developing cerebrum. In **A,** the corpus striatum is traversed by fibers projecting from thalamus to cerebral cortex and from cerebral cortex to spinal cord. In **B,** the corpus striatum has been divided to form the caudate and lentiform nuclei (fusion persists at the anterior end, not shown here).

Calcarine sulcus
Central sulcus
Lateral sulcus

B

A

Figure 1.11 Three major cortical sulci in a fetus of 28 weeks. **(A)** Lateral surface of left hemisphere; **(B)** medial surface.

matching areas of the cerebral cortex of the two sides. It extends backward above the fornix.

Coronal sections of the telencephalon reveal a mass of gray matter in the base of each hemisphere, which is the forerunner of the **corpus striatum**. Beside the third ventricle, the diencephalon gives rise to the **thalamus** and **hypothalamus** (Figure 1.10).

The expanding cerebral hemispheres come into contact with the diencephalon, and they fuse with it (see 'site of fusion' in Figure 1.10A). One consequence is that the term 'brainstem' is restricted thereafter to the remaining, free parts: midbrain, pons, and medulla oblongata. A second consequence is that the cerebral cortex is able to project fibers direct to the brainstem. Together with fibers projecting from thalamus to cortex, they split the corpus striatum into **caudate** and **lentiform** nuclei (Figure 1.10B).

By the 28th week of development, several sulci (fissures) have appeared on the surface of the brain, notably the lateral, central, and calcarine sulci (Figure 1.11).

Core Information

The nervous system takes the initial form of a cellular neural tube derived from the ectoderm and enclosing a neural canal. A ribbon of cells escapes along each side of the tube to form the neural crest. The more caudal part of the tube forms the spinal cord. The neural crest forms spinal ganglion cells that send dorsal nerve roots into the sensory, alar plate of the cord. The basal plate of the cord contains motor neurons that emit ventral roots to complete the spinal nerves by joining the dorsal roots.

The more rostral part of the tube forms three brain vesicles. Of these, the prosencephalon (forebrain) gives rise to the cerebral hemispheres (telencephalon) dorsally and the diencephalon ventrally; the mesencephalon becomes the midbrain, and the rhombencephalon becomes the hindbrain (pons, medulla oblongata, and cerebellum).

The neural tube expands rostrally to create the ventricular system of the brain. CSF is secreted by a choroid capillary plexus that invaginates the roof plates of the ventricles.

The cerebral hemispheres develop frontal, parietal, temporal, occipital, and limbic lobes. The hemispheres are cross-linked by the corpus callosum and anterior commissure. Gray matter in the base of each hemisphere is the forerunner of the corpus striatum. The hemispheres fuse with the side walls of the diencephalon, whereupon the mesencephalon and rhombencephalon are all that remain of the embryonic brainstem.

REFERENCES

Bossy J, O'Rahilly R, Müller F: Ontogenese du systeme nerveux. In Bossy J, editor: *Anatomie clinique: neuroanatomie*, Paris, 1990, Springer-Verlag, pp 357–388.

Dubois J, Benders M, Borradori-Tolsa, et al: Primary cortical folding in the human newborn: an early marker of later functional development, *Brain* 131:2028–4041, 2008.

Le Douarin, Britto JM, Creuzer S: Role of the neural crest in face and brain development, *Brain Res Dev* 55:237–247, 2007.

O'Rahilly R, Muller F: Significant features in the early prenatal development of the human brain, *Ann Anat* 104:105–118, 2008.

Cerebral topography

STUDY GUIDELINES

1 The most important objective is that you become able to recite **all** the central nervous system items identified in the MRI pictures without looking at the labels.
2 Try to get the nomenclature of the component parts of the basal ganglia into long-term memory. Not easily done!
3 Because of its clinical importance, you **must** be able to pop up a mental image of the position and named parts of the internal capsule, and to appreciate continuity of corona radiata, internal capsule, crus cerebri.

SURFACE FEATURES

Lobes

The surfaces of the two cerebral hemispheres are furrowed by **sulci**, the intervening ridges being called **gyri**. Most of the cerebral cortex is concealed from view in the walls of the sulci. Although the patterns of the various sulci vary from brain to brain, some are sufficiently constant to serve as descriptive landmarks. Deepest sulci are the **lateral sulcus** (*Sylvian fissure*) and the **central sulcus** (*Rolandic fissure*) (Figure 2.1A). These two serve to divide the hemisphere (side view) into four **lobes**, with the aid of two imaginary lines, one extending back from the lateral sulcus, the other reaching from the upper end of the **parietooccipital sulcus** (Figure 2.1B) to a blunt **preoccipital notch** at the lower border of the hemisphere (the sulcus and notch are labeled in Figure 2.3). The lobes are called **frontal**, **parietal**, **occipital**, and **temporal**.

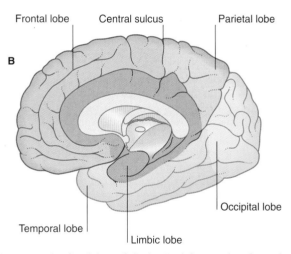

Figure 2.1 The five lobes of the brain. **(A)** Lateral surface of right cerebral hemisphere. **(B)** Medial surface of right hemisphere.

The blunt tips of the frontal, occipital, and temporal lobes are the respective **poles** of the hemispheres.

The **opercula** (lips) of the lateral sulcus can be pulled apart to expose the **insula** (Figure 2.2). The insula was mentioned in Chapter 1 as being relatively quiescent during prenatal expansion of the telencephalon.

The medial surface of the hemisphere is exposed by cutting the **corpus callosum**, a massive band of white matter connecting matching areas of the cortex of the two hemispheres. The corpus callosum consists of a main part or **trunk**, a posterior end or **splenium**, an anterior end or **genu** ('knee'), and a narrow **rostrum** reaching from the genu to the **anterior commissure** (Figure 2.3B). The frontal lobe lies anterior to a line drawn from the upper end of the central sulcus to the trunk of the corpus callosum (Figure 2.3B). The parietal lobe

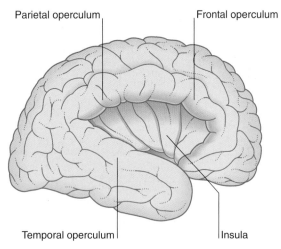

Parietal operculum   Frontal operculum

Temporal operculum   Insula

Figure 2.2 Insula, seen on retraction of the opercula.

lies behind this line, and it is separated from the occipital lobe by the parietooccipital sulcus. The temporal lobe lies in front of a line drawn from the preoccipital notch to the splenium.

Figures 2.3–2.6 should be consulted along with the following description of surface features of the lobes of the brain.

Frontal lobe

The lateral surface of the **frontal lobe** contains the **precentral gyrus** bounded in front by the **precentral sulcus**. Further forward, **superior, middle,** and **inferior frontal gyri** are separated by **superior** and **inferior frontal sulci**. On the medial surface, the superior frontal gyrus is separated from the **cingulate gyrus** by the **cingulate sulcus**. The inferior or orbital surface is marked by several **orbital gyri**. In contact with this surface are the **olfactory bulb** and **olfactory tract**.

Parietal lobe

The anterior part of the parietal lobe contains the postcentral gyrus bounded behind by the **postcentral sulcus**. The posterior parietal lobe is divided into superior and inferior parietal lobules by an **intraparietal sulcus**. The inferior parietal lobule shows a **supramarginal gyrus**, capping the upturned end of the lateral sulcus, and an **angular gyrus** capping the superior temporal sulcus.

The medial surface contains the posterior part of the **paracentral lobule** and, behind this, the **precuneus**. The paracentral lobule (partly contained in the frontal lobe) is so called because of its relationship to the central sulcus.

Occipital lobe

The lateral surface of the occipital lobe is marked by several **lateral occipital gyri**. The medial surface contains the **cuneus** ('wedge') between the **parietooccipital sulcus** and the important **calcarine sulcus**. The inferior surface shows three gyri and three sulci. The **lateral medial occipitotemporal gyri** are separated by the **occipitotemporal sulcus**. The **lingual gyrus** lies between the collateral sulcus and the anterior end of the calcarine sulcus.

Temporal lobe

The lateral surface of the temporal lobe displays **superior, middle,** and **inferior temporal gyri** separated by **superior** and **inferior temporal sulci**. The inferior surface shows the anterior parts of the **occipitotemporal gyri**. The **lingual gyrus** continues forward as the **parahippocampal gyrus**, which ends in a blunt medial projection, the **uncus**. As will be seen later in views of the sectioned brain, the parahippocampal gyrus underlies a rolled-in part of the cortex, the **hippocampus**.

Limbic lobe

A fifth, **limbic lobe** of the brain surrounds the medial margin of the hemisphere. Surface contributors to the limbic lobe include the cingulate and parahippocampal gyri. It is more usual to speak of the *limbic system*, which includes the hippocampus, fornix, amygdala, and other elements (Ch. 34).

Diencephalon

The largest components of the diencephalon are the **thalamus** and the **hypothalamus** (Figures 2.6 and 2.7). These nuclear groups form the side walls of the third ventricle. Between them is a shallow **hypothalamic sulcus**, which represents the rostral limit of the embryonic sulcus limitans.

Midline sagittal view of the brain

Figure 2.8 is taken from a midline sagittal section of the head of a cadaver, displaying the brain in relation to its surroundings.

INTERNAL ANATOMY OF THE CEREBRUM

The arrangement of the following structures will now be described: thalamus, caudate and lentiform nuclei, internal capsule; hippocampus and fornix; association and commissural fibers; lateral and third ventricles.

Thalamus, caudate and lentiform nuclei, internal capsule

The two thalami face one another across the slot-like third ventricle. More often than not, they kiss, creating an **interthalamic adhesion** (Figure 2.9). In Figure 2.10, the thalamus and related structures are assembled in a mediolateral sequence. In contact with the upper surface of the thalamus are the **head** and **body** of the **caudate nucleus**. The **tail** of the caudate nucleus passes forward below the thalamus but not in contact with it.

The thalamus is separated from the lentiform nucleus by the **internal capsule**, which is the most common site for a *stroke* resulting from local arterial embolism (blockage) or hemorrhage. The internal capsule contains fibers running from thalamus to cortex and from cortex to thalamus, brainstem, and spinal cord. In the interval between cortex and internal capsule, these ascending and descending fibers form the **corona radiata**. Below the internal capsule, the **crus** of the midbrain receives descending fibers continuing down the brainstem.

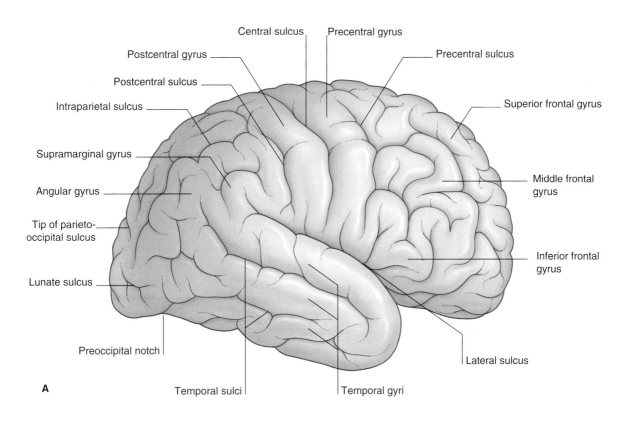

A

Central sulcus
Precentral gyrus
Postcentral gyrus
Precentral sulcus
Postcentral sulcus
Intraparietal sulcus
Superior frontal gyrus
Supramarginal gyrus
Angular gyrus
Middle frontal gyrus
Tip of parieto-occipital sulcus
Inferior frontal gyrus
Lunate sulcus
Preoccipital notch
Lateral sulcus
Temporal sulci
Temporal gyri

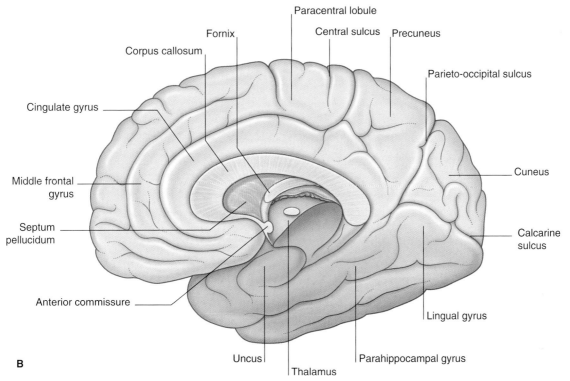

B

Paracentral lobule
Fornix
Central sulcus
Precuneus
Corpus callosum
Cingulate gyrus
Parieto-occipital sulcus
Middle frontal gyrus
Cuneus
Septum pellucidum
Calcarine sulcus
Anterior commissure
Lingual gyrus
Uncus
Parahippocampal gyrus
Thalamus

Figure 2.3 (A) Lateral and **(B)** medial views of the right cerebral hemisphere, depicting the main gyri and sulci.

Figure 2.4 'Thick slice' surface anatomy brain MRI scan from a healthy volunteer. (From Katada, 1990.)

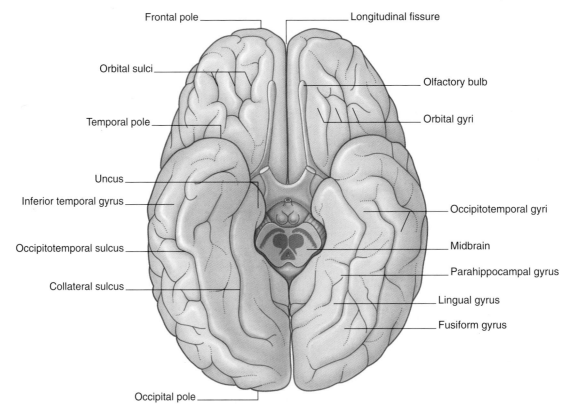

Figure 2.5 Cerebrum viewed from inferior aspect, depicting the main gyri and sulci.

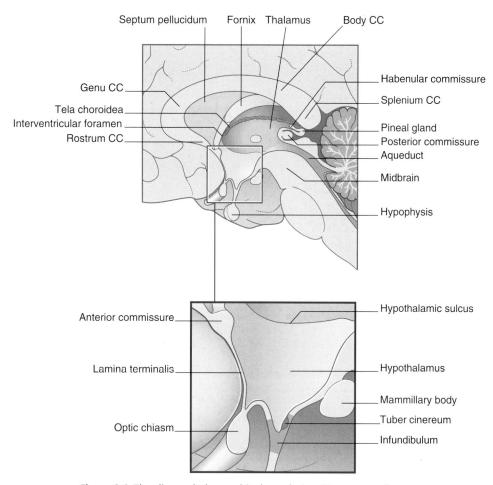

Figure 2.6 The diencephalon and its boundaries. CC, corpus callosum.

Figure 2.7 Sagittal MRI 'slice' of the living brain. (From a series kindly provided by Professor J. Paul Finn, Director, Magnetic Resonance Research, Department of Radiology, David Geffen School of Medicine at UCLA, California, USA.)

Figure 2.8 Sagittal section of fixed cadaver brain. (From Liu et al. 2003, with permission of Shantung Press of Science and Technology.)

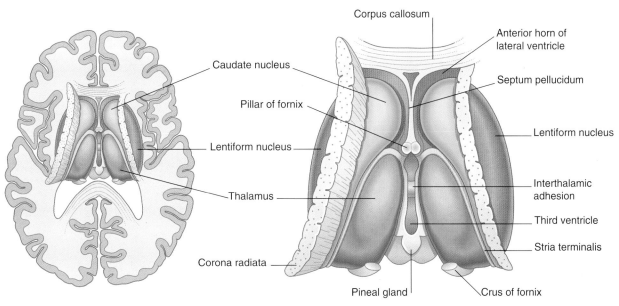

Figure 2.9 Thalamus and corpus striatum, seen on removal of the trunk of the corpus callosum and the trunk of the fornix.

Figure 2.10 Diagrammatic reconstruction of corpus striatum and related structures. The vertical lines on the left in **A** and **B** indicate the level of the coronal sections on the right. **(A)** Ventricular system. **(B)** Thalamus and caudate nucleus in place. **(C)** Addition of projections to and from cerebral cortex. **(D)** Lentiform nucleus in place.

The lens-shaped **lentiform nucleus** is composed of two parts: **putamen** and **globus pallidus**. The putamen and caudate nucleus are of similar structure, and their anterior ends are fused. Behind this, they are linked by strands of gray matter that traverse the internal capsule, hence the term **corpus striatum** (or, simply, **striatum**) used to include the putamen and caudate nucleus. The term **pallidum** refers to the globus pallidus.

The caudate and lentiform nuclei belong to the **basal ganglia**, a term originally applied to a half-dozen masses of gray matter located near the base of the hemisphere. In current usage, the term designates four nuclei known to be involved in motor control: the caudate and lentiform nuclei,

the subthalamic nucleus in the diencephalon, and the substantia nigra in the midbrain (Figure 2.11).

In horizontal section, the internal capsule has a dog-leg shape (see photograph of a fixed-brain section in Figure 2.12, and the living-brain magnetic resonance image [MRI] 'slice' in Figure 2.13). The internal capsule has four named parts in horizontal sections:

1. **anterior limb**, between the lentiform nucleus and the head of the caudate nucleus;
2. **genu**;
3. **posterior limb**, between the lentiform nucleus and the thalamus;
4. **retrolentiform part**, behind the lentiform nucleus and lateral to the thalamus;
5. **sublentiform part** (auditory radiation).

The **corticospinal tract** (CST) descends in the posterior limb of the internal capsule. It is also called the **pyramidal tract**, a *tract* being a bundle of fibers serving a common function. The CST originates mainly from the cortex within the precentral gyrus. It descends through the corona radiata, internal capsule, and crus of midbrain and continues to the lower end of the brainstem before crossing to the opposite side of the spinal cord.

Caudate nucleus———————————Corpus striatum (striatum)
————————————Putamen
Lentiform nucleus ————————Globus pallidus (pallidum)

Subthalamic nucleus

Substantia nigra

Figure 2.11 Nomenclature of basal ganglia.

Figure 2.12 Horizontal section of fixed cadaver brain at the level indicated at top. IC, internal capsule. (From Liu et al. 2003, with permission of Shantung Press of Science and Technology.)

Fornix

Thalamus

Lateral fissure

Midbrain

Pons

Medulla oblongata

Cingulate gyrus

Corpus callosum

Lateral ventricle

Third ventricle

Middle cerebellar peduncle

Cerebellar hemisphere

Figure 2.17 Coronal MRI 'slice' **at the level of Figure 2.16.** (From a series kindly provided by Professor J. Paul Finn, Director, Magnetic Resonance Research, Department of Radiology, David Geffen School of Medicine at UCLA, California, USA).

Association and commissural fibers

Fibers leaving the cerebral cortex fall into three groups:

1 **association fibers**, which pass from one part of a single hemisphere to another;
2 **commissural fibers**, which link matching areas of the two hemispheres;
3 **projection fibers**, which run to subcortical nuclei in the cerebral hemisphere, brainstem, and spinal cord.

Association fibers (Figure 2.20)

Short association fibers pass from one gyrus to another within a lobe.

Long association fibers link one lobe with another. Bundles of long association fibers include:

- the **superior longitudinal fasciculus**, linking the frontal and occipital lobes;
- the **inferior longitudinal fasciculus**, linking the occipital and temporal lobes;
- the **arcuate fasciculus**, linking the frontal lobe with the occipitotemporal cortex;
- the **uncinate fasciculus**, linking the frontal and anterior temporal lobes;
- the **cingulum**, underlying the cortex of the cingulate gyrus.

Cerebral commissures

Corpus callosum

The **corpus callosum** is the largest of the commissures linking matching areas of the left and right cerebral cortex (Figure

2.21). From the **body**, some fibers pass laterally and upward, intersecting the corona radiata. Other fibers pass laterally and then bend downward as the **tapetum** to reach the lower parts of the temporal and occipital lobes. Fibers traveling to the medial wall of the occipital lobe emerge from the **splenium** on each side and form the **occipital (major) forceps**. The **frontal (minor) forceps** emerges from each side of the genu to reach the medial wall of the frontal lobe.

Minor commissures

The **anterior commissure** interconnects the anterior parts of the temporal lobes, as well as the two olfactory tracts.

The **posterior commissure** and the **habenular commissure** lie directly in front of the pineal gland.

The **commissure of the fornix** contains some fibers traveling from one hippocampus to the other by way of the two crura.

Lateral and third ventricles

The **lateral ventricle** consists of a **body** within the parietal lobe, and **anterior (frontal)**, **posterior (occipital)**, and **inferior (temporal) horns** (Figure 2.22). The anterior limit of the central part is the **interventricular foramen**, located between the thalamus and anterior pillar of the fornix, through which it communicates with the third ventricle. The central part joins the occipital and temporal horns at the **atrium** (Figures 2.23 and 2.24).

The relationships of the lateral ventricle are listed below.

- **Anterior horn**. Lies between head of caudate nucleus and septum pellucidum. Its other boundaries are formed by the corpus callosum: trunk above, genu in front, rostrum below.

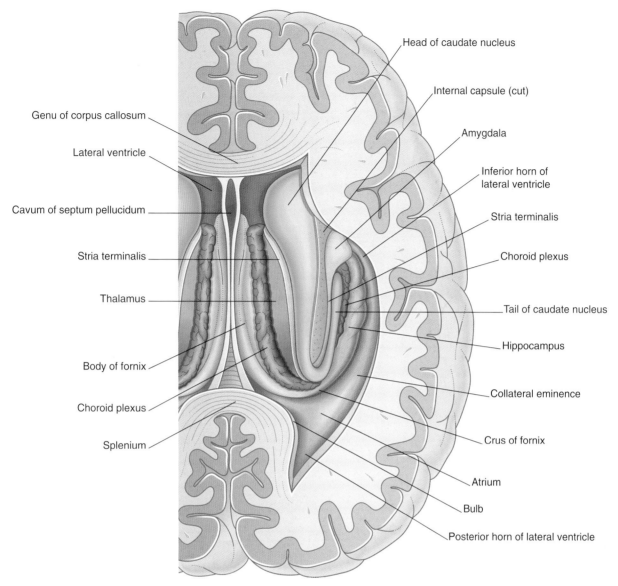

Figure 2.18 Tilted view of the ventricular system, showing the continuity of structures in the body and inferior horn of the lateral ventricle. *Note*: The amygdala, stria terminalis, and tail of caudate nucleus occupy the roof of the inferior horn; the hippocampus occupies the floor. (The choroid plexus is 'reduced' in order to show related structures.)

- **Body**. Lies below the trunk of the corpus callosum and above the thalamus and anterior part of the body of the fornix. Medially is the septum pellucidum, which tapers away posteriorly where the fornix rises to meet the corpus callosum. The **septum pellucidum** is formed of the thinned-out walls of the two cerebral hemispheres. Its bilateral origin may be indicated by a central cavity **(cavum)**.
- **Posterior horn**. Lies below the splenium and medial to the tapetum of the corpus callosum. On the medial side, the forceps major forms the **bulb** of the posterior horn.
- **Inferior horn**. Lies below the tail of the caudate nucleus and, at the anterior end, the **amygdala** (*Gr.* 'almond') (Figure 2.18), a nucleus belonging to the limbic system. The hippocampus and its associated structures occupy the full length of the floor.
- Outside these is the **collateral eminence**, created by the collateral sulcus.

The **third ventricle** is the cavity of the diencephalon. Its boundaries are shown in Figure 2.6. A **choroid plexus** hangs from its roof, which is formed of a double layer of pia mater called the **tela choroidea**. Above this are the fornix and corpus callosum. In the side walls are the thalamus and hypothalamus. The anterior wall is formed by the anterior commissure, the **lamina terminalis**, and the **optic chiasm**. In the floor are the **infundibulum**, the **tuber cinereum**, the **mammillary bodies** (also spelt 'mamillary'), and the upper end of the midbrain. The **pineal gland** and adjacent commissures form the posterior wall. The pineal gland is often calcified, and the **habenular commissure** is sometimes calcified, as early as the second decade of life, thereby becoming detectable even on plain radiographs of the skull. The pineal gland is sometimes displaced to one side by a tumor, hematoma, or other mass (space-occupying lesion) within the cranial cavity.

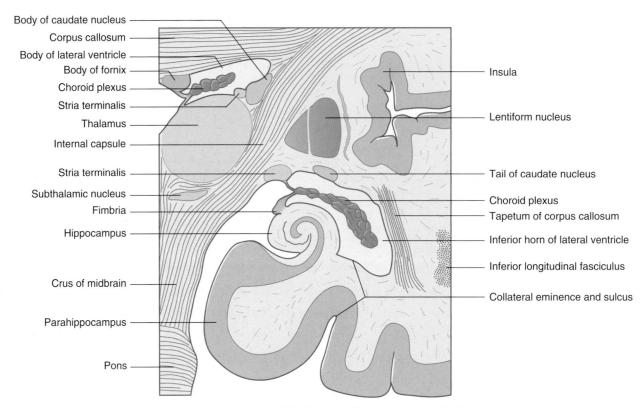

Body of caudate nucleus
Corpus callosum
Body of lateral ventricle
Body of fornix
Choroid plexus
Stria terminalis
Thalamus
Internal capsule
Stria terminalis
Subthalamic nucleus
Fimbria
Hippocampus
Crus of midbrain
Parahippocampus
Pons

Insula
Lentiform nucleus
Tail of caudate nucleus
Choroid plexus
Tapetum of corpus callosum
Inferior horn of lateral ventricle
Inferior longitudinal fasciculus
Collateral eminence and sulcus

Figure 2.19 Coronal section through the body and inferior horn of the lateral ventricle.

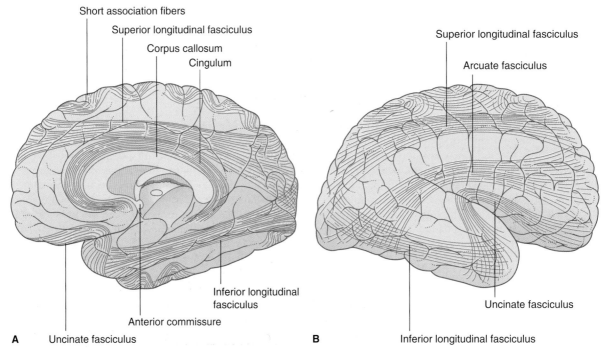

Short association fibers
Superior longitudinal fasciculus
Corpus callosum
Cingulum

Superior longitudinal fasciculus
Arcuate fasciculus

Inferior longitudinal
fasciculus

Uncinate fasciculus

Anterior commissure

Inferior longitudinal fasciculus

A Uncinate fasciculus

B

Figure 2.20 (A) Medial view of 'transparent' right cerebral hemisphere. **(B)** Lateral view of 'transparent' left hemisphere.

Figure 2.21 Horizontal section through genu and splenium of corpus callosum. Fibers passing laterally from the trunk intersect the corona radiata.

Figure 2.20 (*Cont'd*) **(C)** Coronal section, showing position of short and long association fiber bundles.

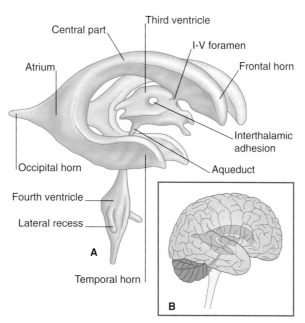

Figure 2.22 Ventricular system. **(A)** Isolated cast. **(B)** Ventricular system in situ.

Figure 2.23 Coronal section of fixed cadaver brain at the level indicated at top. (From Liu et al. 2003, with permission of Shantung Press of Science and Technology.)

Figure 2.24 Coronal MRI 'slice' at the level indicated at top. (From a series kindly provided by Professor J. Paul Finn, Director, Magnetic Resonance Research, Department of Radiology, David Geffen School of Medicine at UCLA, California, USA.)

Box 2.1 Brain planes

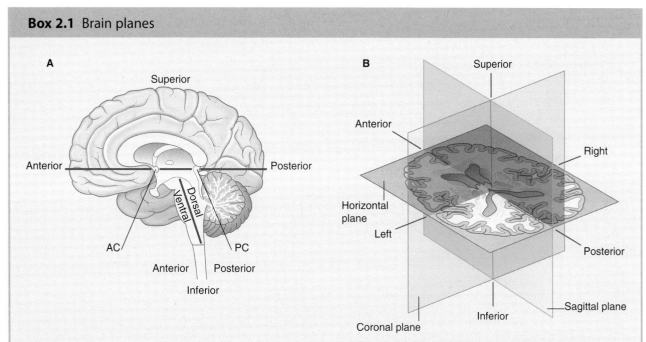

Figure Box 2.1.1 (A) Planes of reference for the central nervous system as a whole. In this presentation, only the brainstem (owing to its obliquity) differs from the standard for gross anatomy. However, some authors use the terms *ventral* and *dorsal* instead of *anterior* and *posterior* with respect to the spinal cord, and some use the terms *rostral* and *caudal* to signify *superior* and *anterior* with respect to spinal cord and/or brainstem. The horizontal line represents the bicommissural plane. AC, PC, anterior and posterior commissures. **(B)** The brain sectioned in the bicommissural plane. (Adapted from Kretschmann and Weinrich 1998, with permission of Thieme and the authors.)

Box 2.2 Magnetic resonance imaging

Magnetic resonance imaging of the CNS is immensely useful for detection of tumors and other space-occupying lesions (masses). When properly used, it is quite safe, even for young children and pregnant women. As will be shown later on, it can be adapted to the study of normal brain physiology in healthy volunteers.

The original name for the technique is *nuclear MRI*, because it is based on the behavior of atomic nuclei in applied magnetic fields. The simplest atomic nucleus is that of the element hydrogen, consisting of a single proton, and this is prevalent in many substances (e.g. water) throughout the body.

Nuclei possess a property known as *spin* (Figure Box 2.2.1), and it may be helpful to visualize this as akin to a spinning gyroscope. Normally, the direction of the spin (the axis of the gyroscope in our analogy) for any given nucleus is random. Spin produces a magnetic

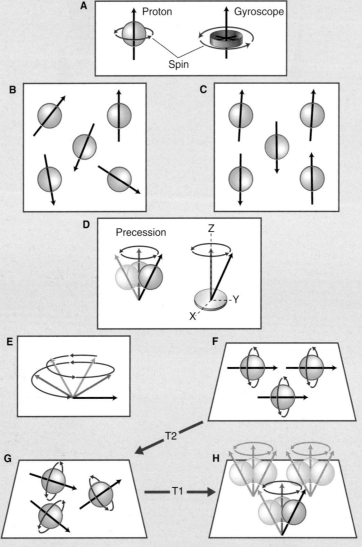

Figure Box 2.2.1 Basis of nuclear magnetic resonance and its manipulation by radio waves. **(A)** The proton of the hydrogen nucleus is in a constant state of spin analogous to that of a gyroscope. **(B)** At rest, the orientation of the axes of the spinning protons is random. **(C)** When the external magnet is switched on, all the axes become oriented along its longitudinal, z axis. The great majority are parallel, with a small minority antiparallel, as indicated. **(D)** At the same time, the magnetic moments immediately precess around the axis like a wobbling gyroscope, being oriented in an intermediate state between the z axis of the magnetic field and the x–y axis at right angles to it. **(E)** An excitatory radio-frequency pulse at right angles to the axis of the external magnetic field tips the net magnetic moment along a 'snail shell' spiral into the x–y plane. **(F)** While the radio-frequency transceiver pulse is 'on', the nuclei are precessing in phase. **(G)** Switching off the radio frequency allows the nuclei to dephase immediately, with a brief T2 time constant. **(H)** Conical precession is resumed under the influence of the external magnet with a longer, T1 time constant. (The assistance of Professor Hugh Garavan, Department of Psychology, Trinity College, Dublin, is gratefully appreciated.)

Box 2.2 *Continued*

moment (vector) that makes it behave like a tiny dipole (north and south) magnet. In the absence of any external magnetic field, the dipoles are randomly arranged.

In the presence of a magnetic field, however, the dipoles will orient themselves along the direction of the magnetic field z (vertical) line.

The cylindric external magnet of an MRI machine (Figure Box 2.2.2) is immensely powerful, capable of lifting the weight of several cars at one time. When the magnet is switched on, individual nuclear magnetic moments undergo a process called – *precession* analogous to the wobbling of a gyroscope – whereby they adopt a cone-shaped spin around the z axis of the external magnetic field.

Excitatory pulses are transmitted from radio-frequency coils set at right angles to the z axis of the external magnetic field. The effect is to tilt the net nuclear magnetic moment into the x–y axis, with all the nuclei precessing 'in phase'. When the radio-frequency coils are switched off, the nuclei '*dephase*' while still in the x–y axis, and then *relax* back to vertical alignment. The time constant involved is called *T2*. The external

Figure Box 2.2.2 The MRI machine. Outermost is the magnet. Innermost is the radio-frequency transceiver. In between are the gradient coils.

magnet then restores the conical precession around the z axis; the time constant here is much slower and is called *T1*.

Because the spinning, precessing nuclei behave like little magnets, if they are surrounded by a coil of wire, they will induce a current in that coil that can then be measured. As it happens, the radiotransmitter coil is able to receive and measure this current, hence term *transceiver* in the diagram.

This is the basic principle of nuclear magnetic resonance. However, to be able to construct an actual image, we require to *spatially* resolve the detected signal. This can be achieved by introducing *gradient coils*. Superimposition of a second magnetic field, set at right angles to that of the main magnet, causes the resonant frequency to be disturbed along the axis of the new field, the proton spin being highest at one end and lowest at the other end. The magnetic resonance machine in fact contains three gradient coils, one being set in each of the three planes of space. The three coils are activated sequentially, allowing three-dimensional localization of tissue signals. In this way, it is possible to 'slice' through the patient, detecting the signal emitted from different components in each selected plane of the patient, and building up an image piece by piece.

The varying densities within the magnetic resonance images reflect the varying rates of dephasing and of relaxation of protons in different locations. The protons of the cerebrospinal fluid, for example, are free to resonate at maximum frequency, whereas in the white matter they are largely bound to lipid molecules. The gray matter has intermediate values, some protons being protein-bound. The radio-frequency pulses can be varied to exploit these differences. Almost all the images shown in textbooks (including this one) are T1-weighted, favoring the very weak signal provided by free protons during the relaxation period. This accounts for the different densities of CSF, gray matter, and white matter, the last being strongest. The reverse is true for T2-weighted images. T2-weighted images are especially useful in detection of lesions in the white matter. For example, they can indicate an increase in free protons resulting from patchy loss of myelin sheath lipid in multiple sclerosis (see Ch. 6), or local edema of brain tissue resulting from a vascular stroke.

The standard orientation of coronal and axial slices is shown in Figure Box 2.2.3.

Box 2.2 *Continued*

Coronal view

Coronal slices are viewed 'face on'

Axial slices are viewed from below

Axial view

Figure Box 2.2.3 Standard orientation of magnetic resonance images. Coronal sections are viewed from in front. Axial sections are viewed from below.

REFERENCES

Jones DK: Fundamentals of diffusion MRI imaging. In Gillard JH, Waldman AD, Barker PB, editors. *Fundamentals of neuroimaging.* Cambridge, 2005, Cambridge University Press, pp 54–85.

Mitchell DG, Cohen MS: *MRI principles*, ed 3. Philadelphia, 2004, Saunders.

Saper CB, Iversen S, Frackoviak R: In Kandel ER, Schwarz JH, Jessell TJ, editors. *Principles of neural science*, ed 4. New York, 2000, McGraw-Hill, pp 370–375.

Box 2.3 Diffusion tensor imaging

Terms

- *Diffusion tensor imaging* is a technique developed in the mid-1990s that uses MRI to measure diffusion constants of water molecules along many (>6) directions and that characterizes diffusion anisotropy.
- An *isotropic* liquid has uniform diffusion properties on all sides, e.g. a drop of milk diffuses uniformly all around when released in water. *Isotropy* is uniformity in all directions and can be represented by a sphere.
- An *anisotropic* (*Gr.* 'not isotropic') liquid diffuses along a preferred axis and can be represented graphically as an ellipsoid.

- A *tensor* describes the shape of the ellipsoid. Diffusion tensors are second-order tensors (special cases of tensors are scalar [zero order or single digits] and vectors [first order or {1 × n} matrices]). A tensor can be reduced to its component axes (eigenvalues), termed lambda 1, 2 and 3, that describe the relative rate of diffusion along the length, breadth and width of the ellipsoid (eigenvectors).
- *Fractional anisotropy* (FA) describes the relationship between lambda 1, 2 and 3 as a fraction. The value of FA therefore ranges from 0 to 1.

Figure Box 2.3.1 Deterministic tractography across the entire brain performed using *ExploreDTI software. This image uses the common convention in diffusion tensor and tractography images where tracts in the anterior–posterior orientation are represented in green, superior–inferior in blue and right–left in red. SCP, superior cerebellar peduncle.

Box 2.3 *Continued*

Axial slice Sagittal slice Coronal slice

Figure Box 2.3.2 Fractional anisotropy is shown in three planes of space, with the same color-coding as in Figure 2.3.1. c.c., corpus callosum; MCP, middle cerebral peduncle; TFP, transverse fibers of pons.

In the nervous system, diffusion of intracellular water in white matter is restricted by the cell membranes. Extracellular water circulating in the ventricles and subarachnoid space and water in gray matter diffuses in a more isotropic manner. The interstitial fluid among myelinated fiber bundles preferentially diffuses parallel to the long axis of the fibers. The higher the fractional anisotropy, the more compact and uniform the bundles of fibers. This is particularly useful when comparing the relative integrity of matching myelinated pathways on each side of the brain or spinal white matter. One can reconstruct the three-dimensional trajectories of white matter tracts using tractography together with color encoding to denote direction. The reconstruction algorithm is based on fiber orientation information obtained from diffusion tensor imaging. A more advanced method that addresses the limitations of the tensor model (i.e. that summarizes information to one principal direction as the basis of tractography) and results in more accurate reconstruction is constrained spherical deconvolution (CSD). CSD uses information in multiple directions for each voxel and has begun to address the problems for tractography that occur in regions where fiber bundles cross.

(The assistance of Dr. Dara M. Cannon, Co-Director, Clinical Neuroimaging Laboratory, Department of Psychiatry, National University of Ireland, Galway is gratefully acknowledged.)

REFERENCES

Hess CP, Mukherjee P: Visualizing white matter pathways in the living human brain: diffusion tensor imaging and beyond. *Neuroimag Clin N Am* 17:407–426, 2007.

Mori S: *Introduction to diffusion tensor imaging.* Amsterdam, 2007, Elsevier.

*ExploreDTI.com provided by Dr. Alexander Leemans, Image Sciences Institute, University Medical Center, Utrecht.

Core Information

On the lateral surface of the cerebrum, four lobes are defined by the lateral and central sulci and an imaginary T-shaped line. The frontal lobe has six named gyri, the parietal lobe has seven, the occipital lobe five, the temporal lobe four. The insula is in the floor of the lateral sulcus.

On the medial surface, the corpus callosum comprises splenium, trunk, genu, and rostrum. The septum pellucidum stretches from the corpus callosum to the trunk of the fornix. Separating fornix from thalamus is the choroidal fissure through which the choroid plexus is inserted into the lateral ventricle. The third ventricle has the fornix in its roof, thalamus and hypothalamus in its side walls, infundibulum, tuber cinereum, and mammillary bodies in its floor. Behind it is the pineal gland, often calcified.

The basal ganglia comprise the corpus striatum (caudate and lentiform nuclei), subthalamic nucleus, and substantia nigra. The lentiform nucleus comprises putamen and globus pallidus. The striatum is made up of caudate and putamen, the pallidum of globus pallidus alone.

The internal capsule is the white matter separating the lentiform nucleus from the thalamus and head of caudate nucleus. The CST descends through the corona radiata and internal capsule to reach the brainstem.

Association fibers (e.g. the longitudinal, arcuate, uncinate fasciculi) link different areas within a hemisphere. Commissural fibers (e.g. corpus callosum, anterior and posterior commissures) link matching areas across the midline. Projection fibers (e.g. corticothalamic, corticobulbar, corticospinal) travel to thalamus and brainstem. The lateral ventricles have a central part and frontal, occipital, and temporal horns. Structures determining ventricular shape include corpus callosum, caudate nucleus, thalamus, amygdala, and hippocampus.

REFERENCES

Clarke C, Howard R: Nervous system structure and function. In Clarke C, Howard R, Rossor M, Shorvon S, editors. *Neurology: A Queen Square Textbook*. London, 2009, Wiley-Blackwell, pp 13–74.

England MA, Wakely J: *A colour atlas of the brain and spinal cord*. St. Louis, 2005, Mosby.

Katada K: MR imaging of brain surface structures: surface anatomy scanning (SAS), *Neuroradiology* 3(5):439–448, 1990.

Kretschmann H-J, Weinrich W: *Cranial neuroimaging and clinical neuroanatomy*. Stuttgart, 1998, Thieme.

Liu S, et al, editors: *Atlas of human sectional anatomy*. Jinan, 2003, Shantung Press of Science and Technology.

Midbrain, hindbrain, spinal cord

STUDY GUIDELINES

1 Become familiar with the locations of the ascending and descending pathways in the horizontal diagrams of brainstem and spinal cord.
2 Box 3.1 deserves special attention, because it indicates why certain pathways cross the midline and others do not. The brainstem crossings are formally addressed in Chapters 15 and 16.
3 Get to grips with the nomenclature used for parts of the midbrain.
4 Become able to divide the 31 spinal nerves into five groups.
5 Relate the three cerebellar peduncles to the fourth ventricle as seen in cross-sections.

Figure 3.1 Ventral view of the brainstem in situ.

The midbrain connects the diencephalon to the hindbrain. As explained in Chapter 1, the hindbrain is made up of the pons, medulla oblongata, and cerebellum. The medulla oblongata joins the spinal cord within the foramen magnum of the skull.

In this chapter, the cerebellum (part of the hindbrain) is considered *after* the spinal cord, for the sake of continuity of motor and sensory pathway descriptions.

BRAINSTEM

Ventral view (Figures 3.1 and 3.2A)

Midbrain

The ventral surface of the midbrain shows two massive **cerebral peduncles** bordering the **interpeduncular fossa**. The **optic tracts** wind around the midbrain at its junction with the diencephalon. Lateral to the midbrain is the uncus of the temporal lobe. The **oculomotor nerve** (III) emerges from the medial surface of the peduncle. The **trochlear nerve** (IV) passes between the peduncle and the uncus.

Pons

The bulk of the pons is composed of **transverse fibers** that raise numerous surface ridges. On each side, the pons is marked off from the middle cerebellar peduncle by the attachment of the **trigeminal nerve** (V). The **middle cerebellar peduncle** plunges into the hemisphere of the cerebellum.

At the lower border of the pons are the attachments of the **abducens** (VI), **facial** (VII), and **vestibulocochlear** (VIII) **nerves** (see Table 3.1).

Medulla oblongata

The pyramids are alongside the anterior median fissure. Just above the spinomedullary junction, the fissure is invaded by the **decussation of the pyramids**, where fibers of the two pyramids intersect while crossing the midline. Lateral to the pyramid is the **olive**, and behind the olive is the **inferior cerebellar peduncle**. Attached between pyramid and olive is the **hypoglossal nerve** (XII). Attached between olive and

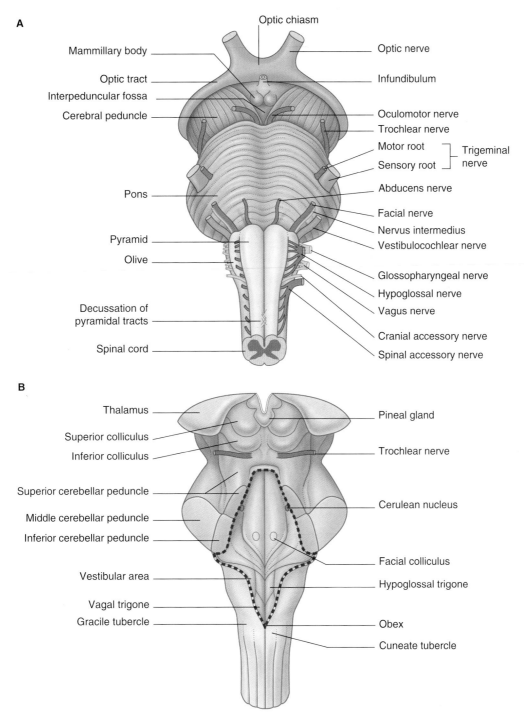

A

Optic chiasm

Mammillary body

Optic tract

Interpeduncular fossa

Cerebral peduncle

Pons

Pyramid

Olive

Decussation of
pyramidal tracts

Spinal cord

Optic nerve

Infundibulum

Oculomotor nerve

Trochlear nerve

Motor root

Sensory root

Trigeminal
nerve

Abducens nerve

Facial nerve

Nervus intermedius

Vestibulocochlear nerve

Glossopharyngeal nerve

Hypoglossal nerve

Vagus nerve

Cranial accessory nerve

Spinal accessory nerve

B

Thalamus

Superior colliculus

Inferior colliculus

Superior cerebellar peduncle

Middle cerebellar peduncle

Inferior cerebellar peduncle

Vestibular area

Vagal trigone

Gracile tubercle

Pineal gland

Trochlear nerve

Cerulean nucleus

Facial colliculus

Hypoglossal trigone

Obex

Cuneate tubercle

Figure 3.2 (A) Anterior and **(B)** posterior view of the brainstem.

inferior cerebellar peduncle are the **glossopharyngeal** (IX), **vagus** (X), and **cranial accessory** (XIc) **nerves**. The **spinal accessory nerve** (XIs) arises from the spinal cord and runs up through the foramen magnum to join the cranial accessory.

Dorsal view (Figure 3.2B)

The roof or **tectum** of the midbrain is composed of four *colliculi*. The **superior colliculi** belong to the visual system, and the **inferior colliculi** belong to the auditory system. The

trochlear nerve (IV) emerges below the inferior colliculus on each side.

The diamond-shaped **fourth ventricle** lies behind the pons and upper medulla oblongata, under cover of the cerebellum. The upper half of the diamond is bounded by the **superior cerebellar peduncles**, which are attached to the midbrain. The lower half is bounded by the **inferior cerebellar peduncles**, which are attached to the medulla oblongata. The middle cerebellar peduncles enter from the pons and overlap the other two.

Near the midline in the midregion of the ventricle is the **facial colliculus**, which is created by the facial nerve curving around the nucleus of the abducens nerve. The **vestibular area**, and the **vagal** and **hypoglossal trigones** overlie the corresponding cranial nerve nuclei. The **obex** is the **inferior** apex of the ventricle.

Below the fourth ventricle, the medulla oblongata shows a pair of **gracile tubercle**s flanked by a pair of **cuneate tubercles**.

Sectional views

In the midbrain, the central canal of the embryonic neural tube is represented by the **aqueduct**. Behind the pons and upper medulla oblongata (Figure 3.3), it is represented by

the fourth ventricle, which is tent-shaped in this view. The central canal resumes at midmedullary level; it is continuous with the central canal of the spinal cord, although movement of cerebrospinal fluid into the cord canal is negligible.

The intermediate region of the brainstem is called the **tegmentum**, which in the midbrain contains the paired **red nucleus**. Ventral to the tegmentum in the pons is the **basilar region**. Ventral to the tegmentum in the medulla oblongata are the pyramids.

The tegmentum of the entire brainstem is permeated by an important network of neurons, the **reticular formation**. The tegmentum also contains *ascending sensory pathways* carrying general sensory information from the trunk and limbs. Illustrated in Figures 3.4–3.6 are the *posterior column–medial lemniscal* (PCML) *pathways*, which inform the brain about the position of the limbs in space. At spinal cord level, the label **PCML** is used here because these pathways occupy the **posterior columns** of white matter in the cord. In the brainstem, the label **PCML** is used because they continue upward as the **medial lemnisci**.

The most important *motor pathways* from a clinical standpoint are the **corticospinal tracts** (CSTs), the pathways for execution of voluntary movements. The CSTs are placed ventrally, occupying the crura of the midbrain, the basilar pons, and the pyramids of the medulla oblongata.

Note that, in the medulla oblongata, the PCML and CST *decussate*: one of each pair intersects with the other to gain the contralateral (opposite) side of the neuraxis (brainstem–spinal cord). The four most important decussations are illustrated in Box 3.1.

In the following account of seven horizontal sections of the brainstem, the positions of the cranial nerve nuclei are not included.

Midbrain (Figure 3.4)

The main landmarks have already been identified. The medial lemniscal component of PCML occupies the lateral

Table 3.1 The cranial nerves	
Number	**Name**
I	Olfactory, enters the olfactory bulb from the nose
II	Optic
III	Oculomotor
IV	Trochlear
V	Trigeminal
VI	Abducens
VII	Facial
VIII	Vestibulocochlear
IX	Glossopharyngeal
X	Vagus
XI	Accessory
XII	Hypoglossal

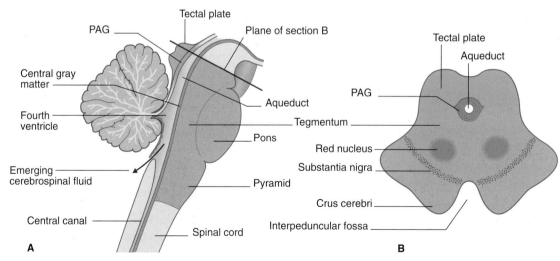

Figure 3.3 (A) Sagittal section of the brainstem. Cerebrospinal fluid descends along the aqueduct into the fourth ventricle and emerges into the subarachnoid space via three apertures including the median aperture containing the arrow. **(B)** Transverse section of midbrain at the level indicated in (A). The substantia nigra separates the tegmentum from the two crura cerebri. The interpeduncular fossa is so called because the entire midbrain is said to be made up of a pair of cerebral peduncles. PAG, periaqueductal gray matter.

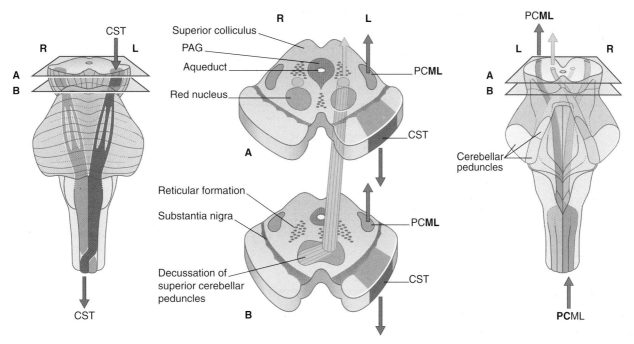

Figure 3.4 Transverse sections of midbrain. **(A)** At level of superior colliculi. **(B)** At level of inferior colliculi. In this and following diagrams, the corticospinal tract (CST) and posterior column–medial lemniscal (PCML) pathway connected to the *left* cerebral hemisphere are highlighted. PAG, periaqueductal gray matter.

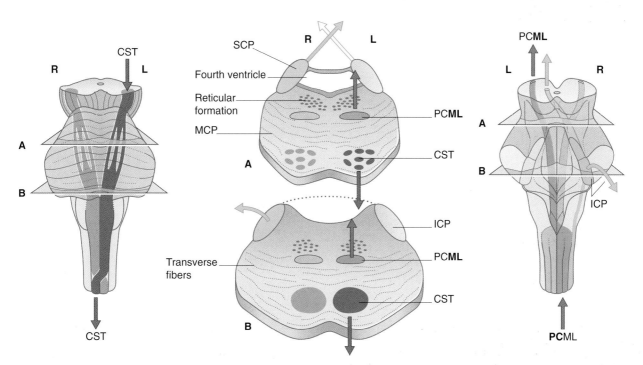

Figure 3.5 Transverse sections of pons. **(A)** Upper pons. **(B)** Lower pons. SCP, MCP, ICP, superior, middle, inferior cerebellar peduncles. CST, corticospinal tract; PCML, posterior column–medial lemniscal pathway.

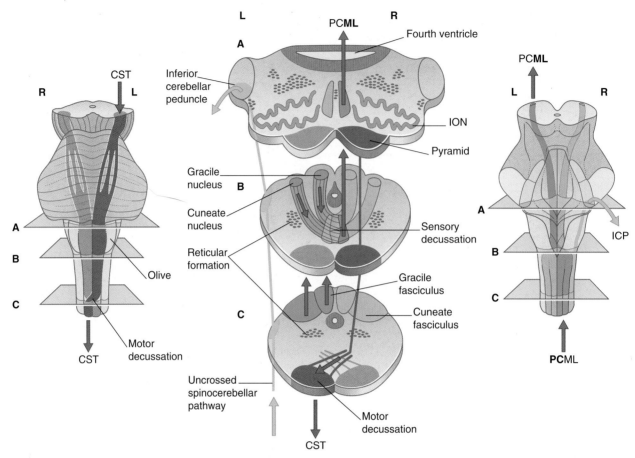

Figure 3.6 Transverse sections of medulla oblongata. **(A)** Level of inferior olivary nucleus (ION). **(B)** Level of sensory decussation. **(C)** Level of motor decussation. CST, Corticospinal tract; ICP, inferior cerebellar peduncle; PCML, posterior column–medial lemniscal pathways.

Box 3.1 Four decussations

Figure Box 3.1.1 (A) The stage is set. The subject's right hand is about to click a mouse while the eyes are directed elsewhere. The coronal section identifies key structures.

Box 3.1 *Continued*

Figure Box 3.1.1 (B) Afferents. The left parietal lobe constructs a map of the right hand in relation to the mouse, based on information sent to the left somatic sensory cortex (postcentral gyrus) from the skin and deep tissues. The information is relayed by three successive sets of neurons from the skin and by another set of three from the deep tissues. The first set in each case is composed of *first-order* or *primary afferent neurons.* These neurons are called *unipolar,* because each axon emerges from a single point (or pole) of the cell body and divides in a T-shaped manner to provide continuity of impulse conduction from tissue to central nervous system. The primary afferent neurons terminate by forming contacts known as *synapses* on the *multipolar* (more or less star-shaped) cells of the *second-order (secondary)* set. The axons of the second-order neurons project across the midline before turning up to terminate on *third-order (tertiary)* multipolar neurons projecting to the postcentral gyrus.

Primary afferents activated by contacts with the skin of the hand (S1) terminate in the posterior horn of the gray matter of the spinal cord. Second-order cutaneous afferents (S2) cross the midline in the anterior white commissure and ascend to the thalamus within the *spinothalamic tract* (STT), to be relayed by third-order neurons to the hand area of the sensory cortex.

The most significant deep tissue sensory organs are *neuromuscular spindles* (muscle spindles) contained within skeletal muscles. The primary afferents supplying the muscle spindles of the intrinsic muscles of the hand belong to large unipolar neurons whose axons (labeled M1) ascend ipsilaterally (on the same side of the spinal cord) within the posterior funiculus, as already seen in *Figure 3.5.* They synapse in the nucleus cuneatus in the medulla oblongata. The multipolar second-order neurons send their axons across the midline in the sensory decussation (seen in *Figure 3.6*).The axons ascend (M2) through pons and midbrain before synapsing on third-order neurons (M3) projecting from thalamus to sensory cortex.

PCML, posterior column–medial lemniscal pathway.

Box 3.1 *Continued*

C   Motor cortex hand area

R   L

C4

C3

Dentate nucleus

C2

C2

C1

M1

PCST

✕ = Decussation of dentatothalamic tracts

D   Motor cortex hand area

R   L

TFP   CST

Ghost of contra-lateral CST

CST

Decussation of pyramids

Lower motor neuron

✕ (upper) = decussation of TFPs

✕ (lower) = decussation of CSTs

Figure Box 3.1.1 (C) Cerebellar control. Before the brain sends an instruction to click the mouse, it requires information on the current state of contraction of the muscles. This information is constantly being sent from the muscles to the cerebellar hemisphere on the same side. As indicated in the diagram, M1 neurons are dual-purpose sensory neurons. At their point of entry to the posterior funiculus, they give off a branch, here labeled C1, to a *spinocerebellar* neuron that projects (C2) to the ipsilateral cerebellum. From here, a *cerebellothalamic* neuron (C3) is shown projecting across the midbrain to the contralateral thalamus, where a further neuron (C4) relays information to the hand area of the *motor* cortex in the precentral gyrus.

(D) Motor output. Multipolar neurons in the left motor cortex now fire impulses along the upper motor neurons that constitute the corticospinal tract (CST), which crosses to the opposite side in the motor decussation, as already noted in *Figure 3.6.* The CST synapses on *lower motor neurons* projecting from the anterior horn of the spinal gray matter to activate flexor muscles of the index finger and local stabilizing muscles.

Note that a copy of the outgoing message is sent to the right cerebellar hemisphere by way of *transverse fibers of the pons* (TFP) originating in multipolar neurons located on the left side of the pons.

Figure 3.7 Horizontal section of fixed cadaver, taken at level of the midbrain. The cerebellum is seen through the tentorial notch. (From Liu et al. 2003, with permission of Shantung Press of Science and Technology.)

part of the tegmentum *(upper section)*, on its way to a sensory nucleus of the thalamus immediately above this level. The CST has arisen in the cerebral cortex, and it is descending in the midregion of the cerebral crus on the same side.

The *decussation of the superior cerebellar peduncles* straddles the midline at the level of the inferior colliculi *(lower section)*.

Pons (Figure 3.5)

In the *upper section*, the cavity of the fourth ventricle is bordered laterally by the superior cerebellar peduncles, which are ascending (arrows) to decussate in the lower midbrain. In the floor of the ventricle is the central gray matter. The medial lemniscus occupies the ventral part of the tegmentum on each side. The basilar region contains millions of **transverse fibers**, some of which separate the CST into individual fascicles. The transverse fibers enter the cerebellum via the middle cerebellar peduncles and *appear* to form a bridge (hence, *pons*) connecting the cerebellar hemispheres. But the *individual* transverse fibers arise on one side of the pons and cross to enter the contralateral cerebellar

hemisphere. The transverse fibers belong to the giant *corticopontocerebellar pathway*, which travels from the cerebral cortex of one side to the contralateral cerebellar hemisphere, as depicted in Box 3.1.

The *lower section* contains the inferior cerebellar peduncle, about to plunge into the cerebellum. The CST bundles have reunited prior to entering the medulla oblongata.

Medulla oblongata (Figure 3.6)

Follow the CST from above down. It descends through sections A and B as the **pyramid**. In C, it intersects with its opposite number in the *motor decussation*, prior to entering the contralateral side of the spinal cord.

Follow the PCML pathway from below upward. In section C, it takes the form of the **gracile** and **cuneate fasciculi**, known in the spinal cord as the *posterior columns* of white matter. In section B, the posterior columns terminate in the **gracile** and **cuneate nuclei**. From these nuclei, fresh sets of fibers swing around the central gray matter and intersect with their opposite numbers in the *sensory decussation*. Having crossed the midline, the fibers turn upward. In section A, they form the medial lemniscal component of PCML.

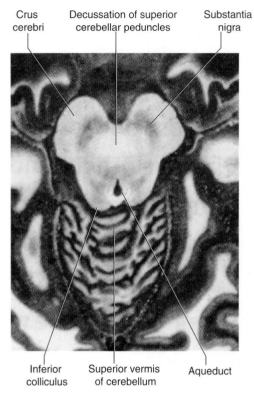

Crus cerebri   Decussation of superior cerebellar peduncles   Substantia nigra

Inferior colliculus   Superior vermis of cerebellum   Aqueduct

Figure 3.8 Enlargement from Figure 3.7.

On the left side of the medulla is shown the *posterior spinocerebellar tract*. Its function (non-conscious) is to inform the cerebellum of the state of activity of the ipsilateral (same side) skeletal muscles in the trunk and limbs.

The upper third of the medulla shows the wrinkled **inferior olivary nucleus**, which creates the olive of gross anatomy.

Sections of brainstem in situ are in Figures 3.7–3.11.

SPINAL CORD

General features

The spinal cord occupies the upper two-thirds of the vertebral canal. Thirty-one pairs of spinal nerves are attached to it by means of **anterior** and **posterior nerve roots** (Figure 3.12A). The cord shows **cervical** and **lumbar enlargements** that accommodate nerve cells supplying the upper and lower limbs.

Internal anatomy

In transverse sections, the cord shows butterfly-shaped gray matter surrounded by three columns or **funiculi** of white matter (Figure 3.12B): an **anterior funiculus** in the interval between the **anterior median fissure** and the emerging **anterior nerve roots**; a **lateral funiculus** between the anterior and **posterior nerve roots**; and a **posterior funiculus** between the posterior roots and the **posterior median septum**.

Temporalis muscle

Infundibulum

Oculomotor merae

Crest of petrous temporal bone

Dentate nucleus

Vermis

Vallecula

Optic tract

Basilar artery

Pons

Superior cerebellar peduncle

Commencement of sigmoid sinus

Fourth ventricle

Figure 3.9 Horizontal section taken at the level of upper pons. The fourth ventricle is slot-like at this level; on each side is a superior cerebellar peduncle traveling upward and medially from dentate nucleus toward the contralateral thalamus. (From Liu et al. 2003, with permission of Shantung Press of Science and Technology.)

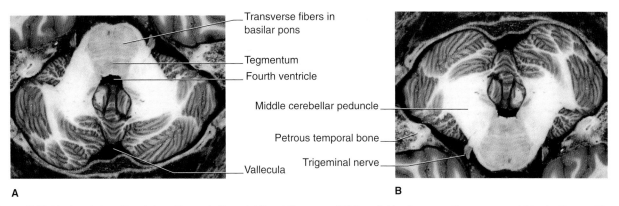

A

B

Figure 3.10 Horizontal section taken through the middle of the pons. **(A)** In axial brain scans, the pons would be in the position shown, i.e. in the roof of the fourth ventricle. **(B)** In standard anatomic descriptions including histologic sections (cf. Ch. 17), the pons occupies the floor of the fourth ventricle, as shown here. Note the massive size of the middle cerebellar peduncles. (From Liu et al. 2003, with permission of Shantung Press of Science and Technology.)

Image A labels: Transverse fibers in basilar pons; Tegmentum; Fourth ventricle; Middle cerebellar peduncle; Petrous temporal bone; Trigeminal nerve; Vallecula

Labels: Caudate nucleus; Fornix; Lateral fissure; Thalamus; Midbrain; Pons; Medulla oblongata; Cingulate gyrus; Corpus callosum; Third ventricle; Hippocampus; Middle cerebellar peduncle; Cerebellar hemisphere

Figure 3.11 Coronal section of brainstem and cerebellum at the level shown at top. Note that the section passes through the tegmentum of the midbrain. The spinal and trigeminal lemnisci are entering the posterior–posterolateral nuclei of thalamus. The periaqueductal gray matter is sectioned longitudinally; the aqueduct itself is seen below the third ventricle.

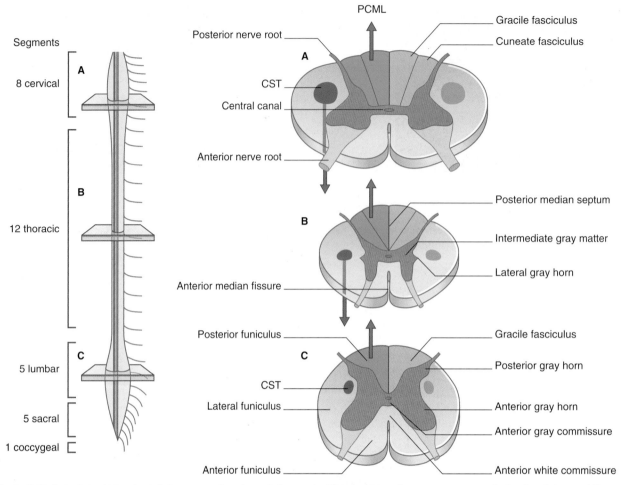

Figure 3.12 Spinal cord. On the left is an anterior view of the cord with nerve attachments enumerated. On the right are **(A)** cervical enlargement level, **(B)** thoracic level, and **(C)** lumbar enlargement level, showing the arrangement of the largest motor and sensory pathways in the white matter, namely the corticospinal tract (CST) and the posterior column–medial lemniscal pathway (PCML) comprising the gracile fasciculi.

The gray matter consists of **central gray matter** surrounding a minute central canal, and **anterior and posterior gray horns** on each side. At the levels of attachment of the 12 thoracic and upper two or three lumbar nerve roots, a **lateral gray horn** is present as well. Posterior nerve roots enter the posterior gray horn, and anterior nerve roots emerge from the anterior gray horn.

Axons pass from one side of the spinal cord to the other in the **anterior white** and **gray commissures** deep to the anterior median fissure.

The CST descends the cord within the lateral funiculus. Its principal targets are neurons in the anterior gray horn concerned with activation of skeletal muscles. *Special note:* In Chapter 16, it will be seen that a small, *anterior* CST separates from the main bundle and descends within the anterior funiculus. Accordingly, the proper name of the bundle depicted here is the *lateral* CST.

In the cord, the PCML pathway is represented by the **gracile** and **cuneate fasciculi**. The fasciculi are composed of the *central processes of peripheral sensory neurons* supplying muscles, joints, and skin. Processes entering from the lower part of the body form the gracile ('slender') fasciculus; those from the upper part form the cuneate ('wedge-shaped') fasciculus (Figures 3.13 and 3.14).

CEREBELLUM

The cerebellum is made up of two hemispheres connected by the **vermis** in the midline (Figure 3.15). The vermis is distinct only on the undersurface, where it occupies the floor of a deep groove, the **vallecula**. The hemispheres show numerous deep **fissures**, with **folia** between. About 80% of the cortex (surface gray matter) is hidden from view on the surfaces of the folia.

The oldest part of the cerebellum (present even in fishes) is the flocculonodular lobe consisting of the **nodule** of the vermis and the **flocculus** in the hemisphere on each side. More recent is the **anterior lobe**, which is bounded posteriorly by the **fissura prima** and contains the **pyramis** and the **uvula**. Most recent is the **posterior lobe**. A prominent feature of the posterior lobe is the **tonsil**. This tonsil lies directly above the foramen magnum of the skull; if the intracranial pressure is raised (e.g. by a brain tumor), one or both tonsils may descend into the foramen and pose a threat to life by compressing the medulla oblongata.

The white matter contains several deep nuclei. The largest of these is the **dentate nucleus** (Figure 3.16).

Liver

Transverse colon

Pancreas

Sigmoid colon

Thoracic spinal cord

Lumbar enlargement
of spinal cord

Conus medullaris

Cauda equina within
lumbar cistern

Vertebra L5

Figure 3.13 Midline sagittal section of fixed cadaver, displaying spinal cord and cauda equina in situ. It should be borne in mind that the cauda equina contains not only the motor and sensory nerve roots of the lumbosacral plexus supplying the lower limbs but also the autonomic motor nerves supplying smooth muscle of hindgut (sigmoid colon and rectum), bladder, uterus, and erectile tissues. (From Liu et al. 2003, with permission of Shantung Press of Science and Technology.)

Figure 3.14 Remarkable photograph of coronal section of fixed cadaver, confirming the high level of commencement of the cauda equina as viewed from in front. In clinical context, this photograph is a reminder of the hazard to somatic (notably sciatic) and parasympathetic (notably to bladder and rectum) nerves incurred by crush fractures of lumbar vertebrae. (From Liu et al. 2003, with permission of Shantung Press of Science and Technology.)

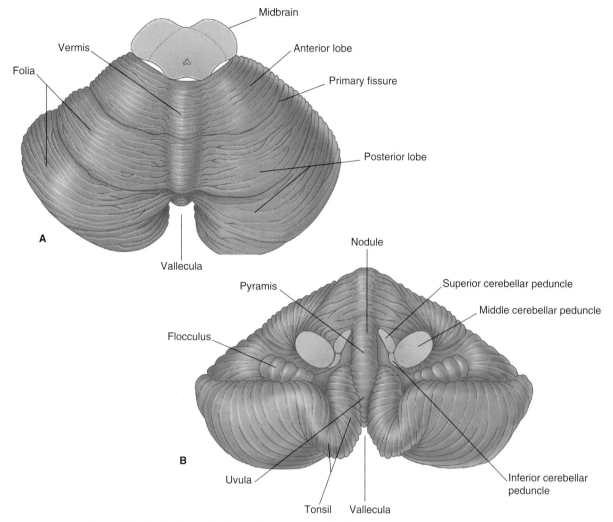

Figure 3.15 Cerebellum. **(A)** Viewed from above. **(B)** Viewed from the position of the pons.

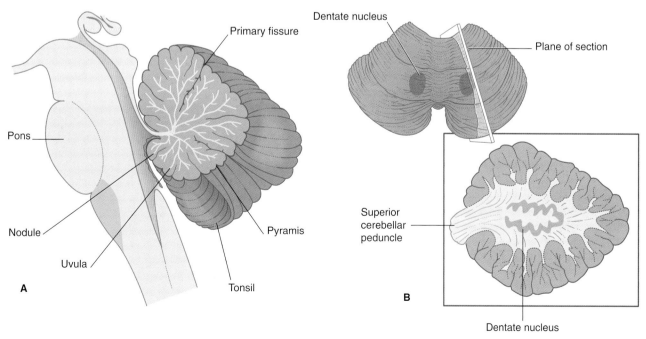

Figure 3.16 (A) Sagittal section of hindbrain. **(B)** Oblique section of cerebellum.

Core Information

Brainstem

The midbrain comprises tectum, tegmentum, and a crus cerebri on each side. The cerebral aqueduct is surrounded by periaqueductal gray matter. The tegmentum contains the red nucleus at the level of the upper part of the midbrain, and elements of the reticular formation at all levels of the brainstem. The largest component of the pons is the basilar region containing millions of transverse fibers belonging to the corticopontocerebellar pathways. The most prominent structure in the medulla oblongata is the inferior olivary nucleus.

The CST descends in the crus of midbrain, basilar pons, and medullary pyramid. Its principal component, the lateral CST, enters the pyramidal decussation and descends the spinal cord in the opposite lateral funiculus. Most of its fibers terminate in the anterior gray horn.

The posterior columns of the spinal cord comprise the gracile and cuneate fasciculi, which terminate in the lower medulla by synapsing upon neurons of the corresponding nuclei. A second set of fibers traverse the sensory decussation before ascending, as the medial lemniscus, to the contralateral sensory thalamus.

The posterior spinocerebellar tract carries information about ipsilateral muscular activity. It enters the inferior cerebellar peduncle. The cerebellum responds by sending signals through the superior cerebellar peduncle of that side to the contralateral motor thalamus via the decussation in the lower midbrain.

Spinal cord

The spinal cord occupies the upper two-thirds of the vertebral canal, the sacral nerve roots being attached to it at the level of the first lumbar vertebra. In all, 31 pairs of roots are attached. The gray matter is most abundant at the levels of attachment of the brachial and lumbosacral plexuses. Anterior and posterior horns are present at all levels, and lateral horns at the level of thoracic and upper lumbar root attachments. The white matter comprises anterior, lateral, and posterior funiculi. Axons cross the midline in the gray commissures and in the white commisure. In general, propriospinal pathways are innermost, motor pathways are intermediate, and sensory pathways are outermost.

Cerebellum

The hemispheres are deeply fissured and are linked by the vermis. The oldest part is the flocculonodular lobe. More recent is the anterior lobe. Most recent is the posterior lobe, which includes the tonsils. The white matter contains several nuclei, including the dentate nucleus.

REFERENCES

Clarke C, Howard R: Nervous system structure and function. In Clarke C, Howard R, Rossor M, Shorvon S, editors. *Neurology: A Queen Square Textbook*. London, 2009, Wiley-Blackwell, pp 13–74.

England MA, Wakely J: *A colour atlas of the brain and spinal cord*. St. Louis, 2005, Mosby.

Kretschmann H-J, Weinrich W: *Cranial neuroimaging and clinical neuroanatomy*. Stuttgart, 2004, Thieme.

Liu S, et al, editors: *Atlas of human sectional anatomy*. Jinan, 2003, Shantung Press of Science and Technology.

Meninges

STUDY GUIDELINES

1 Be able to compare the structure of the dura mater with that of the pia–arachnoid.
2 Be able to follow a drop of blood from the superior sagittal sinus to the internal jugular vein, and from an ophthalmic vein to the sigmoid sinus.
3 Name the nerves supplying (a) the supratentorial dura and (b) the infratentorial dura.
4 Identify the different vessels responsible for extradural, subdural, and subarachnoid bleeding.
5 Appreciate the mechanism of papilledema and why spinal tap (lumbar puncture) should not be undertaken in its presence.
6 Trace a drop of cerebrospinal fluid from a lateral ventricle to (a) its point of entry into the bloodstream, (b) to an in situ lumbar puncture needle.
7 Know about a major cause of hydrocephalus (a) in infancy, (b) in adults, and why both are examples of 'outlet obstruction'.

The meninges surround the central nervous system (CNS) and suspend it in the protective jacket provided by the cerebrospinal fluid (CSF). The meninges comprise the tough dura mater or **pachymeninx** (*Gr.* 'thick membrane'), and the **leptomeninges** (*Gr.* 'slender membranes') consisting of the **arachnoid mater** and **pia mater**. Between the arachnoid and the pia is the **subarachnoid space** filled with CSF.

CRANIAL MENINGES

Dura mater

The terminology used to describe the cranial dura mater varies among different authors. It seems best to regard it as a single, tough layer of fibrous tissue that is fused with the endosteum (inner periosteum) of the skull, except where it is reflected into the interior of the vault or is stretched across the skull base. Wherever it separates from the periosteum, the intervening space contains venous sinuses (Figure 4.1).

Two great dural folds extend into the cranial cavity and help to stabilize the brain. These are the **falx cerebri** and the **tentorium cerebelli**.

The falx cerebri occupies the longitudinal fissure between the cerebral hemispheres. Its attached border extends from the crista galli of the ethmoid bone to the upper surface of the tentorium cerebelli. Along the vault of the skull, it encloses the **superior sagittal sinus**. Its free border contains the **inferior sagittal sinus** that unites with the **great cerebral vein** to form the **straight sinus**. The straight sinus travels along the line of attachment of falx cerebri to tentorium cerebelli and meets the superior sagittal sinus at the **confluence of the sinuses**.

The crescentic **tentorium cerebelli** arches like a tent above the posterior cranial fossa, being lifted up by the falx cerebri in the midline. The attached margin of the tentorium encloses the **transverse sinuses** on the inner surface of the occipital bone and the **superior petrosal sinuses** along the upper border of the petrous temporal bone. The attached margin reaches to the posterior clinoid processes of the sphenoid bone. Most of the blood from the superior sagittal sinus usually empties into the right transverse sinus (Figure 4.2).

The free margin of the tentorium is U-shaped. The tips of the U are attached to the anterior clinoid processes. Just behind this, the two limbs of the U are linked by a sheet of dura, the **diaphragma sellae**, which is pierced by the pituitary stalk. Laterally, the dura falls away into the middle cranial fossae from the limbs of the U, creating the **cavernous sinus** on each side (Figure 4.3). Behind the sphenoid bone, the concavity of the U encloses the midbrain.

The cavernous sinus receives blood from the orbit via the ophthalmic veins. The superior petrosal sinus joins the transverse sinus at its junction with the **sigmoid sinus**. The sigmoid sinus descends along the occipital bone and discharges into the bulb of the internal jugular vein. The bulb receives the inferior petrosal sinus which descends along the edge of the occipital bone.

The tentorium cerebelli divides the cranial cavity into a **supratentorial compartment** containing the forebrain, and an **infratentorial compartment** containing the hindbrain. A small **falx cerebelli** is attached to the undersurface of the tentorium cerebelli and to the internal occipital crest of the occipital bone.

Innervation of the cranial dura mater

The dura mater lining the supratentorial compartment of the cranial cavity receives sensory innervation from the trigeminal nerve. That lining the anterior cranial fossa and anterior

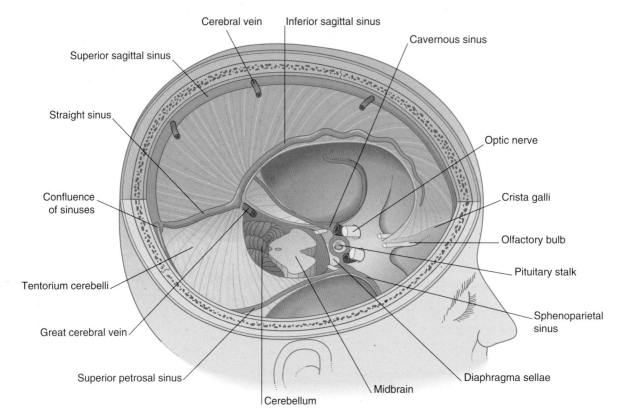

Figure 4.1 Dural reflections and venous sinuses. The midbrain occupies the tentorial notch.

part of the skull vault is supplied by its ophthalmic branch; that lining the middle cranial fossa and midregion of the vault is mainly supplied by the **nervus spinosus** (Figure 4.2). This nerve leaves the mandibular nerve outside the foramen ovale, to return via the foramen spinosum and accompany the **middle meningeal artery** and its branches. Stretching or inflammation of the supratentorial dura gives rise to frontal or parietal headache.

The dura mater lining the infratentorial compartment is supplied by branches of upper cervical spinal nerves entering the foramen magnum (Figure 4.2). Occipital and posterior neck pains accompany disturbance of the infratentorial dura. Acute meningitis involving posterior cranial fossa meninges is associated with *neck rigidity* and often with *head retraction* brought about by reflex contraction of the posterior nuchal muscles, which are supplied by cervical nerves. Violent occipital headache follows *subarachnoid hemorrhage* (Ch. 35), where free blood swirls around the hindbrain.

Meningeal arteries

Embedded in the endosteum of the skull are several **meningeal arteries** whose main function is to supply the diploë (bone marrow). Much the largest is the middle meningeal artery, which ramifies over the inner surface of the temporal and parietal bones. Tearing of this artery, with its accompanying vein, is the usual source of an *extradural hematoma* (Clinical Panel 4.1).

Arachnoid mater

The arachnoid (*Gr.* 'spidery') is a thin, fibrocellular layer in direct contact with the dura mater (Figure 4.4). The outermost cells of the arachnoid are bonded to one another by tight junctions that seal the **subarachnoid space**. Innumerable **arachnoid trabeculae** cross the space to reach the pia mater.

Pia mater

The pia mater invests the brain closely, following its contours and lining the various sulci (Figure 4.4). Like the arachnoid, it is fibrocellular. The cellular component of the pia is external and is permeable to CSF. The fibrous component occupies a narrow **subpial space** that is continuous with **perivascular spaces** around cerebral blood vessels penetrating the brain surface.

Note: Although the subarachnoid and subpial spaces are proven, there is no sign of any 'subdural space' in properly fixed material. Such a space can be created, however, by leakage of blood into the cellular layer of the dura mater following a tear of a cerebral vein at its point of anchorage to the fibrous layer. (See *Subdural hematoma* in Clinical Panel 4.1.)

Subarachnoid cisterns

Along the base of the brain and the sides of the brainstem, pools of CSF occupy subarachnoid cisterns (Figures 4.5 and 4.6). The largest of these is the **cisterna magna**, in the interval

Internal carotid artery leaving cavernous sinus

Diaphragma sellae

Meningeal branches of V

V3   V2   V1

Hypophysis

Optic nerve

Ophthalmic artery

Foramen rotundum

Middle meningeal
vessels and nervus
spinosus

Anterior
clinoid process

Superior
ophthalmic vein

Foramen ovale

Foramen
spinosum

VI

III

Midbrain

IV

Cerebellum

V

Petrosal sinuses

Sigmoid sinus

Pons

Tentorium cerebelli

Great cerebral
vein

Meningeal
branches of
C2 and 3

Straight sinus

Confluence of sinuses

Transverse sinus

Figure 4.2 Venous sinuses on the base of the skull. The dura mater has been removed on the right side. The inset indicates where grooves for sinuses are seen on the dry skull. On the left, the midbrain is seen at the level of the tentorial notch. On the right, a lower level section shows the trigeminal nerve attached to the pons.

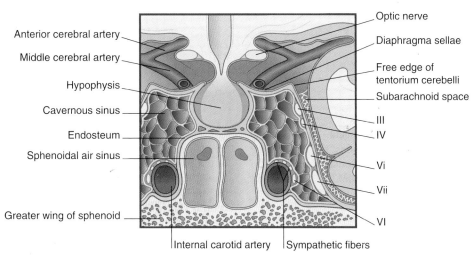

Anterior cerebral artery

Middle cerebral artery

Hypophysis

Cavernous sinus

Endosteum

Sphenoidal air sinus

Greater wing of sphenoid

Optic nerve

Diaphragma sellae

Free edge of
tentorium cerebelli

Subarachnoid space

III

IV

Vi

Vii

VI

Internal carotid artery   Sympathetic fibers

Figure 4.3 Coronal section of the cavernous sinus.

Clinical Panel 4.2 Lumbar puncture (Figure CP 4.2.1)

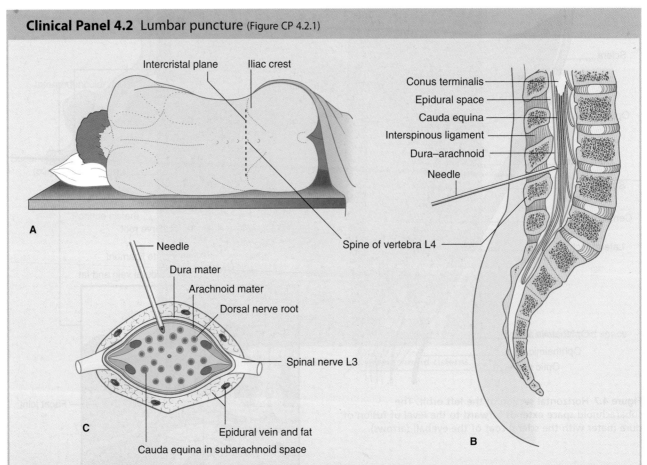

Figure CP 4.2.1 Lumbar puncture (spinal tap). **(A)** The patient lies on one side, curled forward to open the interspinous spaces of the lumbar region. The spine of vertebra L4 is identified in the intercristal (supracristal) plane at the level of the tops of the iliac crests. **(B)** Under aseptic conditions, a lumbar puncture needle is introduced obliquely above the spine of vertebra L4, parallel to the plane of the spine. The needle is passed through the interspinous ligament. A slight 'give' is perceived when the needle pierces the dura–arachnoid mater and enters the subarachnoid space. **(C)** Transverse section showing the cauda equina floating in the subarachnoid space. The anterior and posterior roots of spinal nerve L3 are coming together as they leave the lumbar cistern.

cistern may be tapped to procure samples of CSF for analysis (Clinical Panel 4.2) or to deliver a spinal anesthetic (Ch. 14).

The spinal dura mater (with its arachnoid lining) is sometimes referred to as the *thecal sac* (*Gr.* 'enclosing capsule')

CIRCULATION OF CEREBROSPINAL FLUID (Figure 4.10)

The principal source of the CSF is the secretion of the choroid plexuses into the ventricles of the brain. From the lateral ventricles, the CSF enters the third through the interventricular foramen. It descends to the fourth ventricle through the aqueduct and squirts into the subarachnoid space through the median and lateral apertures. (Flow within the central canal of the spinal cord is negligible.)

Within the subarachnoid space, some of the CSF descends through the foramen magnum, reaching the lumbar cistern in about 12 h. From the subarachnoid space at the base of the brain, the CSF ascends through the tentorial notch and bathes the surface of the cerebral hemispheres before being

returned to the blood through the **arachnoid granulations** (Figure 4.4). The arachnoid granulations are pinhead pouches of arachnoid mater projecting through the dural wall of the major venous sinuses – especially the superior sagittal sinus and the small venous **lacunae** that open into it. CSF is transported across the arachnoid epithelium in giant vacuoles.

As much as a quarter of the circulating CSF may not reach the superior sagittal sinus. Some enters small arachnoid villi projecting into spinal veins exiting intervertebral foramina, and some drains into lymphatics in the adventitia of arteries at the base of the brain and in the epineurium of cranial nerves. These lymphatics drain into cervical lymph nodes. Bimanual downward massage of the sides of the neck is sometimes used to enhance this drainage in patients suffering from cerebral edema.

About 300 mL of CSF is secreted by the choroid plexuses every 24 h. Another 200 mL is produced from other sources, as described in Chapter 5. Blockage of flow through the ventricular system or cranial subarachnoid space will cause back-up within the ventricular system: a state of *hydrocephalus* (Clinical Panel 4.3).

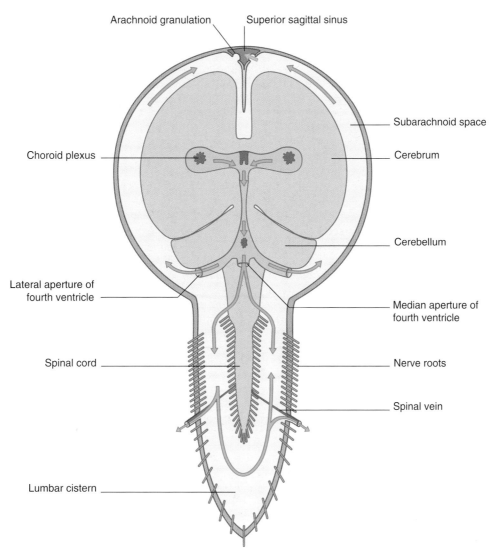

Arachnoid granulation

Superior sagittal sinus

Subarachnoid space

Choroid plexus

Cerebrum

Cerebellum

Lateral aperture of
fourth ventricle

Median aperture of
fourth ventricle

Spinal cord

Nerve roots

Spinal vein

Lumbar cistern

Figure 4.10 Circulation of cerebrospinal fluid.

Clinical Panel 4.3 Hydrocephalus

Hydrocephalus (*Gr.* 'water in the brain') denotes accumulation of CSF in the ventricular system. With the exception of overproduction of CSF by a rare papilloma of the choroid plexus, hydrocephalus results from obstruction of the normal CSF circulation, with consequent dilatation of the ventricles. (The term is not used to describe the accumulation of fluid in the ventricles and subarachnoid space in association with senile atrophy of the brain.)

In the great majority of cases, hydrocephalus is caused by obstruction of the foramina opening the fourth ventricle to the subarachnoid space. A major cause of outlet obstruction in *infancy* is the *Arnold–Chiari malformation,* where the cerebellum is partly extruded into the vertebral canal during fetal life because the posterior cranial fossa is underdeveloped. In untreated cases, the child's head may become as

large as a football and the cerebral hemispheres paper-thin. The condition is nearly always associated with spina bifida (Ch. 14). Early treatment is essential to prevent severe brain damage. The obstruction can be bypassed by means of a catheter having one end inserted into a lateral ventricle and the other inserted into the internal jugular vein.

A major cause of outlet obstruction is displacement of the cerebellum into the foramen magnum by a space-occupying lesion (mass) such as a tumor or hematoma (see Ch. 6).

Meningitis can cause hydrocephalus at any age. The development of leptomeningeal adhesions may compromise CSF circulation at the level of the ventricular outlets, the tentorial notch, and/or the arachnoid granulations.

Core Information

Meninges

The meninges comprise dura, arachnoid, and pia mater. The subarachnoid space contains CSF.

The cranial dura mater shows two large folds: the falx cerebri and tentorium cerebelli. The attached edge of the falx encloses the superior sagittal sinus, which usually enters the right transverse sinus. The free edge of the falx encloses the inferior sagittal sinus, which joins the great cerebral vein, forming the straight sinus that enters the confluence of the superior sagittal and transverse sinuses. The attached edge of the tentorium encloses the transverse sinus, which descends and continues as sigmoid sinus to join the internal jugular vein. The midbrain is partly enclosed by the free edge of the tentorium, which is attached to the anterior clinoid processes of the sphenoid bone and provides a U-shaped gap for passage of the midbrain. Dura drapes from each side of the U into the middle cranial fossa, creating the cavernous sinus. This sinus receives blood from the ophthalmic veins and drains via petrosal sinuses into each end of the sigmoid sinus.

The supratentorial dura mater is innervated by the trigeminal nerve, the infratentorial dura by upper cervical nerves. The meningeal vessels run extradurally to supply the diploë; if torn by skull fracture, they may form an extradural hematoma compressing the brain. A subdural hematoma may be caused by leakage from a cerebral vein in transit to the superior sagittal sinus.

Cerebrospinal fluid

Pools of CSF at the base of the brain include the cisterna magna, the cisterna pontis, the interpeduncular cistern, and the cisterna ambiens. CSF also extends along the meningeal sheath of the optic nerve, and raised intracranial pressure may compress the central vein of the retina, causing papilledema. The spinal dural sac extends down to S2 vertebral level. The lumbar cistern contains spinal nerve roots and is accessible for lumbar puncture (spinal tap). CSF secreted by the choroid plexuses escapes into the subarachnoid space through the three apertures of the fourth ventricle. Some descends to the lumbar cistern. The CSF ascends through the tentorial notch and the cerebral subarachnoid space to reach the superior sagittal sinus and its lacunae via the arachnoid granulations. Blockage of CSF flow anywhere along its course leads to hydrocephalus.

REFERENCES

Weller RO, Djuanda E, Yow HY, Carare RO: Lymphatic drainage of the brain and the pathophysiology of neurological disease, *Acta Neuropathol* 117:1–14, 2009.

Vandenabeele L, Creemers J, Lambrichts I: Ultrastructure of the human spinal arachnoid mater and dura mater, *J Anat* 189:417–430, 1996.

Blood supply of the brain

STUDY GUIDELINES

1. On simple outline drawings of the lateral, medial, and inferior surfaces of a cerebral hemisphere, learn to shade in the territories of the three cerebral arteries.
2. Identify the main sources of arterial supply to the internal capsule.
3. Become familiar with carotid and vertebral angiograms.
4. Be able to list the territories supplied by the vertebral and basilar arteries.
5. Identify the two blood–brain barriers. Be able to understand why, for example, shallow breathing following abdominal surgery may tip a patient into coma.

Because interpretation of the symptoms caused by cerebrovascular accidents requires prior understanding of brain function, Clinical Panels on this subject are placed in the final chapter.

A Clinical Panel on blood–brain barrier pathology is placed in the present chapter because the symptoms are of a general nature.

INTRODUCTION

The brain is absolutely dependent on a continuous supply of oxygenated blood. It controls the delivery of blood by sensing the momentary pressure changes in its main arteries of supply, the internal carotids. It controls the arterial oxygen tension by monitoring respiratory gas levels in the internal carotid artery and in the cerebrospinal fluid (CSF) beside the medulla oblongata. The control systems used by the brain are exquisitely sophisticated, but they can be brought to nothing if a distributing artery ruptures spontaneously or is rammed shut by an embolus.

ARTERIAL SUPPLY OF THE FOREBRAIN

The blood supply to the forebrain is derived from the two **internal carotid arteries** and from the **basilar artery** (Figure 5.1).

Each internal carotid artery enters the subarachnoid space by piercing the roof of the cavernous sinus. In the subarachnoid space, it gives off **ophthalmic, posterior communicating,** and **anterior choroidal arteries** before dividing into the **anterior** and **middle cerebral arteries**.

The basilar artery divides at the upper border of the pons into the two **posterior cerebral arteries.** The **cerebral arterial circle** (*circle of Willis*) is completed by a linkage of the posterior communicating artery with the posterior cerebral on each side, and by linkage of the two anterior cerebrals by the **anterior communicating artery**.

The choroid plexus of the lateral ventricle is supplied from the **anterior choroidal** branch of the internal carotid artery and by the **posterior choroidal branch** from the posterior cerebral artery.

Dozens of fine **central (perforating) branches** are given off by the constituent arteries of the circle of Willis. They enter the brain through the **anterior perforated substance** beside the optic chiasm and through the **posterior perforated substance** behind the mammillary bodies. They have been classified in various ways but can be conveniently grouped into short and long branches. **Short central branches** arise from all the constituent arteries and from the two choroidal arteries. They supply the optic nerve, chiasm, and tract, and the hypothalamus. **Long central branches** arise from the three cerebral arteries. They supply the thalamus, corpus striatum, and internal capsule. They include the **striate branches** of the anterior and middle cerebral arteries.

Anterior cerebral artery (Figure 5.2)

The anterior cerebral artery passes above the optic chiasm to gain the medial surface of the cerebral hemisphere. It forms an arch around the genu of the corpus callosum, making it easy to identify in a carotid angiogram (see later). Close to the anterior communicating artery, it gives off the **medial striate artery**, also known as the *recurrent artery of Heubner* (*pron.*'Hoibner'), which contributes to the blood supply of the internal capsule. Cortical branches of the anterior cerebral artery supply the medial surface of the hemisphere as far back as the parietooccipital sulcus (Table 5.1).

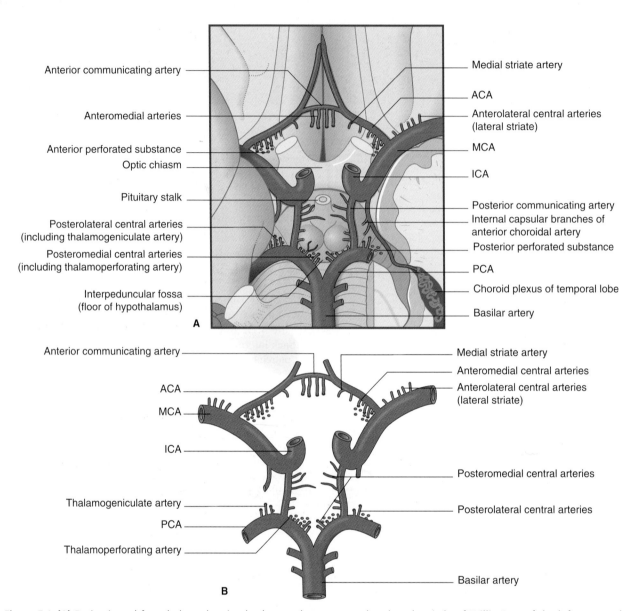

Anterior communicating artery

Anteromedial arteries

Anterior perforated substance

Optic chiasm

Pituitary stalk

Posterolateral central arteries
(including thalamogeniculate artery)

Posteromedial central arteries
(including thalamoperforating artery)

Interpeduncular fossa
(floor of hypothalamus)

Medial striate artery

ACA

Anterolateral central arteries
(lateral striate)

MCA

ICA

Posterior communicating artery
Internal capsular branches of
anterior choroidal artery
Posterior perforated substance

PCA

Choroid plexus of temporal lobe

Basilar artery

A

Anterior communicating artery

ACA

MCA

ICA

Thalamogeniculate artery

PCA

Thalamoperforating artery

Medial striate artery
Anteromedial central arteries
Anterolateral central arteries
(lateral striate)

Posteromedial central arteries

Posterolateral central arteries

Basilar artery

B

Figure 5.1 (A) Brain viewed from below, showing background structures related to the circle of Willis. Part of the left temporal lobe (to right of picture) has been removed to show the choroid plexus in the inferior horn of the lateral ventricle. **(B)** The arteries comprising the circle of Willis. The four groups of central branches are shown; the thalamoperforating artery belongs to the posteromedial group, and the thalamogeniculate artery belongs to the posterolateral group. ACA, MCA, PCA, anterior, middle, posterior cerebral arteries; ICA, internal carotid artery.

Table 5.1 Named cortical[a] branches of the anterior cerebral artery

Branch	Territory
Orbitofrontal	Orbital surface of frontal lobe
Polar frontal	Frontal pole
Callosomarginal	Cingulate and superior frontal gyri; paracentral lobule
Pericallosal	Corpus callosum

[a]*The term cortical is conventional. Terminal is better, because these arteries also supply the underlying white matter.*

The branches overlap on to the orbital and lateral surfaces of the hemisphere.

Middle cerebral artery (Figure 5.3)

The middle cerebral artery is the main continuation of the internal carotid, receiving 60–80% of the carotid blood flow. It immediately gives off important central branches, then passes along the depth of the lateral fissure to reach the surface of the insula. There it usually breaks into upper and lower divisions. The upper division supplies the frontal lobe, the lower division supplies the parietal and temporal lobes and the midregion of the optic radiation. Named branches

Figure 5.2 Medial view of the right hemisphere, showing the cortical branches and territories of the three cerebral arteries. ACA, PCA, anterior, posterior cerebral arteries.

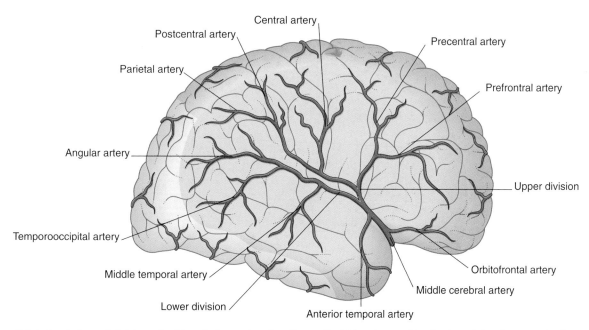

Figure 5.3 Lateral view of right cerebral hemisphere, showing the cortical branches and territories of the three cerebral arteries.

and their territories are listed in Table 5.2. Overall, the middle cerebral supplies two-thirds of the lateral surface of the brain.

The **central branches** of the middle cerebral include the **lateral striate arteries** (Figure 5.4). These arteries supply the corpus striatum, internal capsule, and thalamus. Occlusion of one of the lateral striate arteries is the chief cause of classic *stroke*, where damage to the pyramidal tract in the posterior limb of the internal capsule causes *hemiplegia*, a term denoting paralysis of the contralateral arm, leg, and lower part of face.

Note: Additional information on the blood supply of the internal capsule is provided in Chapter 35.

Posterior cerebral artery (Figures 5.2 and 5.5)

The two posterior cerebral arteries are the terminal branches of the basilar. However, in embryonic life they arise from the internal carotid, and in about 25% of individuals the internal carotid persists as the primary source of blood on one or both sides, by way of a large **posterior communicating artery**.

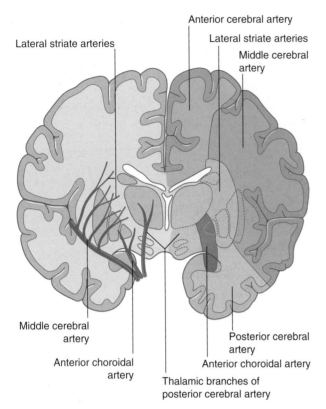

Figure 5.4 Distribution of perforating branches of the middle cerebral, anterior choroidal, and posterior cerebral arteries (schematic). The anterior choroidal artery arises from the internal carotid.

Close to its origin, each posterior cerebral artery gives branches to the midbrain and a **posterior choroidal artery** to the choroid plexus of the lateral ventricle. Additional, **central branches** are sent into the posterior perforated substance (Figure 5.1). The main artery winds around the midbrain in company with the optic tract. It supplies the splenium of the corpus callosum and the cortex of the occipital and temporal lobes. Named cortical branches and their territories are given in Table 5.3.

Table 5.2 Cortical branches of the middle cerebral artery

Origin	Branch(es)	Territory
Stem	Frontobasal	Orbital surface of frontal lobe
	Anterior temporal	Anterior temporal cortex
Upper division	Prefrontal	Prefrontal cortex
	Precentral	Premotor areas
	Central	Pre- and postcentral gyri
	Postcentral	Postcentral and anterior parietal cortex
	Parietal	Posterior parietal cortex
Lower division	Middle temporal	Midtemporal cortex
	Temporooccipital	Temporal and occipital cortex
	Angular	Angular and neighboring gyri

Figure 5.5 View from below the cerebral hemispheres, showing the cortical branches and territories of the three cerebral arteries. ACA, MCA, PCA, anterior, middle, posterior cerebral arteries; ICA, internal carotid artery.

The central branches, called **thalamoperforating** and **thalamogeniculate**, supply the thalamus, subthalamic nucleus, and optic radiation.

Note: Additional information on the central branches is provided in Chapter 35.

Neuroangiography

The cerebral arteries and veins can be displayed under general anesthesia by rapid injection of a radiopaque dye into the internal carotid or vertebral artery, followed by serial radiography every 2 s. The dye completes its journey through the arteries, brain capillaries, and veins in about 10 s. The *arterial phase* of the journey yields either a *carotid angiogram* or a *vertebrobasilar angiogram*. Improved vascular definition in radiographs of the arterial phase or of the *venous phase* can be procured by a process of *subtraction*, whereby positive and negative images of the overlying skull are superimposed on one another, thereby virtually deleting the skull image.

A relatively recent technique, *three-dimensional angiography*, is based on simultaneous angiography from two slightly separate perspectives.

Arterial phases of carotid angiograms are shown in Figures 5.6–5.8.

Figure 5.9 was taken at the *parenchymal phase*, when the dye is filling a web of minute terminal branches of the anterior and middle cerebral arteries, some of these anastomosing on the brain surface but most occupying the parenchyma, i.e cortex and subjacent white matter.

ARTERIAL SUPPLY TO HINDBRAIN

The brainstem and cerebellum are supplied by the vertebral and basilar arteries and their branches (Figure 5.10).

The two **vertebral arteries** arise from the subclavian arteries and ascend the neck in the foramina transversaria of the upper six cervical vertebrae. They enter the skull through the foramen magnum and unite at the lower border of the pons to form the **basilar artery**. The basilar artery ascends to the upper border of the pons and divides into two posterior cerebral arteries (Figures 5.11 and 5.12).

Table 5.3 Named cortical branches of the posterior cerebral artery

Branch	Artery	Territory
Lateral	Anterior temporal	Anterior temporal cortex
	Posterior temporal	Posterior temporal cortex
	Occipitotemporal	Posterior temporal and occipital cortex
Medial	Calcarine	Calcarine cortex
	Parietooccipital	Cuneus and precuneus
	Callosal	Splenium of corpus callosum

Callosomarginal branch of ACA

Pericallosal branch of ACA

Frontal branches of ACA

Heubner's artery

Stem of ACA

Ophthalmic artery

Divisions of MCA

Posterior cranial fossa

ICA in carotid canal

Figure 5.6 Arterial phase of a carotid angiogram, lateral view. Contrast medium injected into the left internal carotid artery is passing through the anterior and middle cerebral arteries (ACA, MCA). The base of the skull is shown in hatched outline. ICA, internal carotid artery. (From an original series kindly provided by Dr. Michael Modic, Department of Radiology, The Cleveland Clinic Foundation.)

Coiled MCA branches
within lateral sulcus

MCA

ICA

In cavernous
sinus

In carotid
canal

In neck

Pericallosal branch
of right ACA

Pericallosal branch
of left ACA

Anterior communicating
artery

ACA

Outline of orbit
and nasal cavity

Figure 5.7 Arterial phase of a right carotid angiogram, anteroposterior view. Note some perfusion of left anterior cerebral artery (ACA) territory (via the anterior communicating artery). ICA, internal carotid artery; MCA, middle cerebral artery. (Angiogram kindly provided by Dr. Pearse Morris, Director, Interventional Neuroradiology, Wake Forest University School of Medicine, Winston-Salem, North Carolina, USA.)

All primary branches of the vertebral and basilar arteries give branches to the brainstem.

Vertebral branches

The **posterior inferior cerebellar artery** supplies the side of the medulla before giving branches to the cerebellum. **Anterior** and **posterior spinal arteries** supply the ventral and dorsal medulla, respectively, before descending through the foramen magnum.

Basilar branches

The **anterior inferior cerebellar** and **superior cerebellar arteries** supply the side of the pons before giving branches to the cerebellum. The anterior inferior cerebellar usually gives off the **labyrinthine artery** to the inner ear.

About a dozen **pontine arteries** supply the full thickness of the medial part of the pons.

The midbrain is supplied by the **posterior cerebral artery**, and by the **posterior communicating artery** linking the posterior cerebral to the internal carotid.

VENOUS DRAINAGE OF THE BRAIN

The venous drainage of the brain is of great importance in relation to neurosurgical procedures. It is also important to

the professional neurologist, because a variety of clinical syndromes can be produced by venous obstruction, venous thrombosis, and congenital arteriovenous communications. In general medical practice, however, problems (other than subdural hematomas, Ch. 4) caused by cerebral veins are rare in comparison with arterial disease.

The cerebral hemispheres are drained by superficial and deep cerebral veins. Like the intracranial venous sinuses, they are devoid of valves.

Superficial veins

The **superficial cerebral veins** lie in the subarachnoid space overlying the hemispheres. They drain the cerebral cortex and underlying white matter, and empty into intracranial venous sinuses (Figures 5.13A, 5.14, and 5.15).

The upper part of each hemisphere drains into the superior sagittal sinus. The middle part drains into the cavernous sinus (as a rule) by way of the **superficial middle cerebral vein**. The lower part drains into the transverse sinus.

Deep veins (Figure 5.13B)

The deep cerebral veins drain the corpus striatum, thalamus, and choroid plexuses.

A **thalamostriate vein** drains the thalamus and caudate nucleus. Together with a **choroidal vein**, it forms the **internal**

A

ACA   ICA   MCA   Aneurysm

B

Figure 5.8 (A) Excerpt from a conventional carotid angiogram, anteroposterior view, showing an aneurysm attached to the middle cerebral artery. **(B)** Excerpt from a three-dimensional image of the same area. ACA, MCA, anterior and middle cerebral arteries; ICA, internal carotid artery. (Originals kindly provided by Dr. Pearse Morris, Director, Interventional Neuroradiology, Wake Forest University School of Medicine, Winston-Salem, North Carolina, USA.)

MCA   ACA

ICA

Figure 5.9 Parenchymal phase of a carotid angiogram, anteroposterior view. ACA, MCA, anterior and middle cerebral arteries; ICA, internal carotid artery. (Angiogram kindly provided by Dr. Pearse Morris, Director, Interventional Neuroradiology, Wake Forest University School of Medicine, Winston-Salem, North Carolina, USA.)

cerebral vein. The two internal cerebral veins unite beneath the corpus callosum to form the **great cerebral vein** (of Galen).

A **basal vein** is formed beneath the anterior perforated substance by the union of **anterior** and **deep middle cerebral veins**. The basal vein runs around the crus cerebri and empties into the great cerebral vein.

Finally, the great cerebral vein enters the midpoint of the tentorium cerebelli. As it does so, it unites with the **inferior sagittal sinus** to form the **straight sinus**. The straight sinus empties in turn into the left (occasionally, right, as we shall see) **transverse sinus**.

REGULATION OF BLOOD FLOW

Under normal conditions, cerebral blood flow (perfusion) amounts to 700–850 mL per minute, accounting for 20% of the total cardiac output. The blood flow is primarily controlled by *autoregulation*, which is defined as the capacity of a tissue to regulate its own blood supply.

The most rapid source of autoregulation is the *intraluminal pressure* within the arterioles. Any increase in pressure elicits a direct, *myogenic* response. When other factors are controlled (in animal experiments), the myogenic response is sufficient to maintain steady-state perfusion of the brain within a systemic blood pressure range of 80–180 mmHg (11–24 kPa).

A second powerful source of autoregulation in the central nervous system (CNS) is the *H^+ ion concentration* in the extracellular fluid (ECF) surrounding the arterioles within the brain parenchyma. Generalized relaxation of arteriolar smooth muscle tone is produced by hypercapnia (excess plasma P_{CO_2}). On the other hand, hypocapnia leads to arteriolar constriction.

Local blood flow increases within cortical areas and deep nuclei involved in particular motor, sensory or cognitive

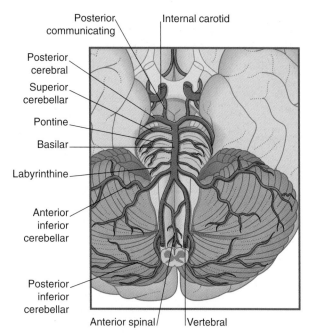

Posterior communicating
Internal carotid
Posterior cerebral
Superior cerebellar
Pontine
Basilar
Labyrinthine
Anterior inferior cerebellar
Posterior inferior cerebellar
Anterior spinal
Vertebral

Figure 5.10 Arterial supply of hindbrain.

tasks. Local arteriolar relaxation can be accounted for by a rise in K$^+$ levels caused by propagation of action potentials, and by a rise in H$^+$ caused by increased cell metabolism.

THE BLOOD–BRAIN BARRIER

The nervous system is isolated from the blood by a barrier system that provides a stable and chemically optimal environment for neuronal function. The neurons and neuroglia are bathed in *brain extracellular fluid (ECF)*, which accounts for 15% of total brain volume.

The extracellular compartments of the CNS are shown diagrammatically in Figure 5.16. As previously described (Ch. 4), CSF secreted by the choroid plexuses circulates through the ventricular system and the subarachnoid space before passing through the arachnoid villi into the dural venous sinuses. In addition, CSF diffuses passively through the ependyma–glial membrane lining the ventricles and enters the brain extracellular spaces. It adds to the ECF produced by the capillary bed and by cell metabolism, and it diffuses through the pia–glial membrane into the subarachnoid space. This 'sink' movement of fluid compensates for the absence of lymphatics in the CNS.

Metabolic water is the only component of the CSF that does not pass through the blood–brain barrier. It carries

Central branches
Stem of PCA
Top of basilar artery
Commencement of basilar artery
Parieto-occipital artery
Calcarine artery
Cerebellar arteries
PICA
Vertebral artery entering foramen magnum

Figure 5.11 Vertebrobasilar angiogram, lateral view. Contrast medium was injected into the left vertebral artery. Basilar supply to the upper half of the cerebellum is somewhat obscured by overlying posterior parietal branches of the posterior cerebral artery. PCA, posterior cerebral artery; PICA, posterior inferior cerebellar artery. (From an original series kindly provided by Dr. Michael Modic, Department of Radiology, The Cleveland Clinic Foundation.)

Figure 5.12 Vertebrobasilar angiogram, Townes's view (from above and in front), showing the vertebrobasilar arterial system. Note the large aneurysm arising from the bifurcation point of the basilar artery and accounting for the patient's persistent headache. AICA, anterior inferior cerebellar artery; PICA, posterior inferior cerebellar artery. (Angiogram kindly provided by Dr. Pearse Morris, Director, Interventional Neuroradiology, Wake Forest University School of Medicine, Winston-Salem, North Carolina, USA.)

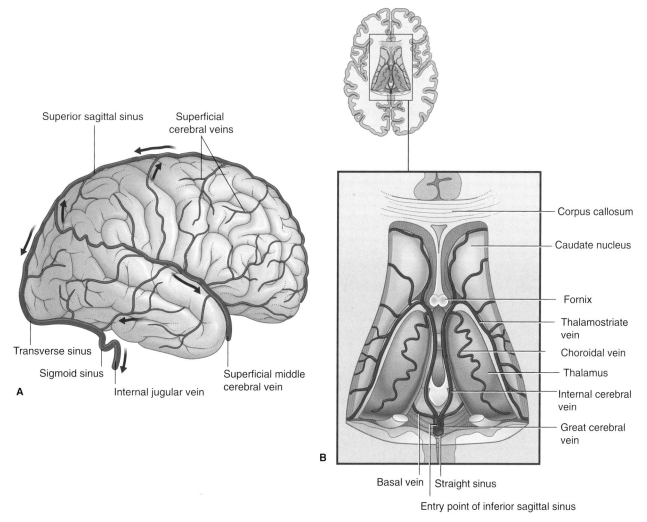

Figure 5.13 Cerebral veins. **(A)** Superficial veins viewed from the right side; arrows indicate direction of blood flow. **(B)** Deep veins viewed from above.

Superficial middle cerebral vein · Superficial cerebral veins · Superior sagittal sinus · Anastomotic vein · Inferior sagittal sinus · Great cerebral vein · Straight sinus · Transverse sinus · Anastomotic vein · Sigmoid sinus · Cavernous sinus · Internal jugular vein

Figure 5.14 Internal carotid angiogram, venous phase, lateral view. The dye is draining into the dural venous sinuses. (Photograph kindly provided by Dr. James Toland, Department of Radiology, Beaumont Hospital, Dublin, Ireland.)

Upper part, Lower part, of superior sagittal sinus · Superficial cerebral veins · Superficial middle cerebral vein · Transverse sinus · Sigmoid sinus · Internal jugular vein

Figure 5.15 Internal carotid angiogram, venous phase, anteroposterior view. Same patient as in Figure 5.6; this picture taken circa 8 s later. The vascular pattern is unusual, in that the left rather than the right transverse sinus is dominant. (Angiogram kindly provided by Dr. Pearse Morris, Director, Interventional Neuroradiology, Wake Forest University School of Medicine, Winston-Salem, North Carolina, USA.)

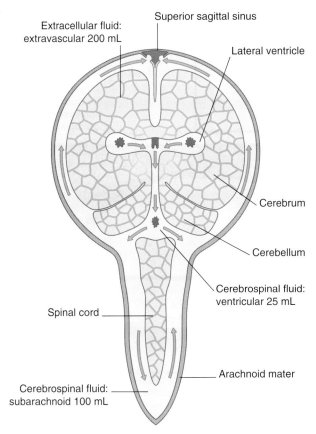

Figure 5.16 Extracellular compartments of the brain. *Arrows* indicate circulation of cerebrospinal fluid.

with it any neurotransmitter substances that have not been recaptured following liberation by neurons, and it accounts for the presence in the subarachnoid space of transmitters and transmitter metabolites that could not penetrate the blood–brain barrier.

Relative contributions to the CSF obtained from a spinal tap are approximately as follow:

- choroid plexuses, 60%
- capillary bed, 30%
- metabolic water, 10%.

The blood–brain barrier has two components. One is at the level of the choroid plexus, the other resides in the CNS capillary bed.

Blood–CSF barrier (Figure 5.17)

The blood–CSF barrier resides in the specialized ependymal lining of the choroid plexuses. This choroidal epithelium differs from the general ependymal epithelium in three ways.

1. Cilia are almost completely replaced by microvilli.
2. The cells are bonded by tight junctions. These pericellular belts of membrane fusion are the actual site of the blood–CSF barrier.
3. The epithelium contains numerous enzymes specifically involved in transport of ions and metabolites.

Figure 5.17 (A) Diagram of blood–cerebrospinal fluid barrier. **(B)** Ultrastructure of choroidal epithelium. The epithelial cells are rich in mitochondria and granular endoplasmic reticulum. Apical regions of adjacent cells are bonded by a tight junction (arrow). (From Pannese 1994, with permission of Thieme.)

Clinical Panel 5.2 Intracranial pressure curve

Figure CP 5.2.1 represents progressive ventricular expansion in an adult case of hydrocephalus. As noted in Clinical Panel 4.3, hydrocephalus can result from obstruction of the fourth ventricular outlets by leptomeningeal webs caused by meningitis. The same effect can be induced by accumulated blood around the base of the brain following spontaneous arterial hemorrhage into the subarachnoid space.

The lateral ventricles are expanding progressively (arrows). The rising intracranial pressure is being monitored by an intraparenchymal pressure monitor. The vascular perfusion pressure rises in parallel.

(1) The pressure–volume curve commences with a relatively flat part: interstitial fluid is displaced into the subarachnoid space; subarachnoid CSF is shifted into the spinal dural sac; and venous blood is squeezed through the intracranial sinuses into the internal jugular vein. (2) ICP rises with increasing speed during the steep part. (3) A critical pressure point is reached where *decompensation* takes place: the vascular circulation is completely blocked, the vital centers run out of oxygen, the patient loses consciousness and will die unless the CSF is urgently drained through a burr (drill) hole.

REFERENCE

Bodkin PA, Hassan MF, Kane PJ, Brady N, Whittle IR: 'Surgical' causes of benign intracranial hypertension, *J R Soc Med* 101: 250–261, 2008.

Figure CP 5.2.1 (A) Adult hydrocephalus. Arrows indicate compression of cerebral parenchyma by expanding lateral ventricles. IPM, intraparencymal pressure monitor. **(B)** Intracranial pressure–CSF volume curve. (Based on Steiner and Andrews 2006.)

Core Information

Arteries

The circle of Willis comprises the anterior communicating artery and two anterior cerebral arteries, the internal carotids, two posterior communicating arteries, and the two posterior cerebral arteries.

The anterior cerebral artery gives off Heubner's artery to the anteroinferior internal capsule, then arches around the corpus callosum and supplies the medial surface of the hemisphere as far back as the parietooccipital sulcus, with overlap on to the lateral surface.

The middle cerebral artery enters the lateral sulcus and supplies two-thirds of the lateral surface of the hemisphere. Its central branches include the leak-prone lateral striate supplying the upper part of the internal capsule.

The posterior cerebral artery arises from the basilar artery; it supplies the splenium of corpus callosum and the occipital and temporal cortex.

The vertebral arteries enter the foramen magnum. They supply spinal cord, posterior-inferior cerebellum and medulla oblongata before uniting to form the basilar artery. The basilar artery supplies the anterior-inferior and superior cerebellum, the pons and inner ear, before dividing into posterior cerebral arteries.

Veins

Superficial cerebral veins drain the cerebral cortex and empty into dural venous sinuses. The internal cerebral veins drain the thalami and unite as the great cerebral vein. The great veins drain the corpus striatum via the basal vein before entering the straight sinus.

Autoregulation

Hypercapnia causes arteriolar dilatation, hypocapnia causes constriction. A rise of intraluminal pressure produces a direct, myogenic response by arteriolar walls.

Blood–brain barrier

A blood–CSF barrier resides in the choroidal epithelium (modified ependyma) of the ventricles. A blood–ECF barrier resides in the endothelium of the brain capillary bed.

REFERENCES

Balabanonov B, Dore-Duffy P: Role of the microvascular pericyte in the blood–brain barrier, *J Neurosci Res* 53:637–644, 1998.

Duvernoy HM, Delon S, Vannson JL: Cortical blood vessels of the human brain, *Brain Res Bull* 7:519–530, 1981.

Pannese E: *Neurocytology. Fine structure of neurons, nerve processes and neuroglial cells.* New York, 1994, Thieme.

Popescu BO, Toescu EC, Popescu LM, et al: Blood–brain barrier alterations in ageing and dementia, *J Neurol Sci* 283:99–106, 2009.

Scremin IU: Cerebral vascular system. In Paxinos G, Mai JK, editors: *The human nervous system*, ed 2. Amsterdam, 2004, Elsevier.

Steiner LA, Andrews PJD: Monitoring the injured brain: ICP and CBF, *Br J Anaesth* 1:26–38, 2006.

STUDY GUIDELINES

1 Appreciate the challenge faced by many neurons in having to deliver and retrieve materials over enormous distances, and the economy of transmitter recycling at nerve endings.
2 Appreciate how a healthy transport system can spread disease in the nervous system.
3 Appreciate the lock and key analogy used in pharmacology.
4 Draw an axodendritic synapse, then add another axon dividing to exert both pre- and postsynaptic inhibition.
5 Understand why demyelinating disorders compromise conduction.
6 Draw up a structure–function list for neuroglial cells.
7 Gliomas will obviously interfere with brain function in the region they grow. Try to understand how they may exert 'distance effects'.

Figure 6.1 Profiles of neurons from the brain. **(1)** Pyramidal cell, cerebral cortex. **(2)** Neuroendocrine cell, hypothalamus. **(3)** Spiny neuron, corpus striatum. **(4)** Basket cell, cerebellum. Neurons 1 and 3 show dendritic spines. A, axon; AC, axon collateral; D, dendrites.

Nerve cells, or **neurons**, are the structural and functional units of the nervous system. They generate and conduct electrical changes in the form of nerve impulses. They communicate chemically with other neurons at points of contact called **synapses**. **Neuroglia** (literally, 'nerve glue') is the connective tissue of the nervous system.

Neuroglial cells outnumber neurons by about five to one. They have important nutritive and supportive functions.

NEURONS

Billions of neurons form a shell, or **cortex**, on the surface of the cerebral and cerebellar hemispheres. In this general context, **nuclei** are aggregates of neurons buried within the white matter.

In the central nervous system (CNS), almost all neurons are multipolar, their cell bodies or **somas** having multiple poles or angular points. At every pole but one, a **dendrite** emerges and divides repeatedly (Figure 6.1). On some neurons, the shafts of the dendrites are smooth. On others, the shafts show numerous short **spines** (Figure 6.2). The dendrites receive synaptic contacts from other neurons, from some on the spines and from others on the shafts.

The remaining pole of the soma gives rise to the **axon**, which conducts nerve impulses. Most axons give off *collateral* branches (Figure 6.3). *Terminal* branches synapse on target neurons.

Most synaptic contacts between neurons are either *axodendritic* or *axosomatic*. Axodendritic synapses are usually excitatory in their effect on target neurons, whereas most axosomatic synapses have an inhibitory effect.

Internal structure of neurons

All parts of neurons are permeated by **microtubules** and **neurofilaments** (Figure 6.4). The soma contains the nucleus and the cytoplasm or **perikaryon** (*Gr.*'around the nucleus').

Polyribosomes

A · A · S · S · A · S · A

Mitochondria · Smooth endoplasmic reticulum

Figure 6.2 Dendritic spines. This section is taken from the cerebellum, where the dendrites of the giant cells of Purkinje are studded with spines. In this field, three spines (S) are in receipt of synaptic contacts by axonic boutons (A). A fourth axon (top left) is synapsing on the shaft of the dendrite. (From Pannese 1994, with permission of Thieme.)

The perikaryon contains clumps of granular endoplasmic reticulum known as *Nissl bodies* (Figure 6.5), also Golgi complexes, free ribosomes, mitochondria, and smooth endoplasmic reticulum (Figure 6.4).

Intracellular transport

Turnover of membranous and skeletal materials takes place in all cells. In neurons, fresh components are continuously synthesized in the soma and moved into the axon and dendrites by a process of *anterograde transport*. At the same time, worn-out materials are returned to the soma by *retrograde transport* for degradation in lysosomes (see also *target recognition*, later).

Anterograde transport is of two kinds: *rapid* and *slow*. Included in rapid transport (at a speed of 300–400 mm/day) are free elements such as synaptic vesicles, transmitter substances (or their precursor molecules), and mitochondria.

Also included are lipid and protein molecules (including receptor proteins) for insertion into the plasma membrane. Included in slow transport (at 5–10 mm/day) are the skeletal elements, and soluble proteins including some of those involved in transmitter release at nerve endings. Microtubules seem to be largely constructed within the axon. They are exported from the soma in preassembled short sheaves that propel one another along the initial segment of the axon; further progress is mainly by a process of elongation (up to 1 mm apiece) performed by the addition of tubulin polymers at their distal ends, with some disassembly at their proximal ends. The bulk movement of neurofilaments slows down to almost zero distally; there, the filaments are refreshed by the insertion of filament polymers moving from the soma by slow transport.

Retrograde transport of worn-out mitochondria, SER, and plasma membrane (including receptors therein) is fairly rapid (150–200 mm/day). In addition to its function in waste

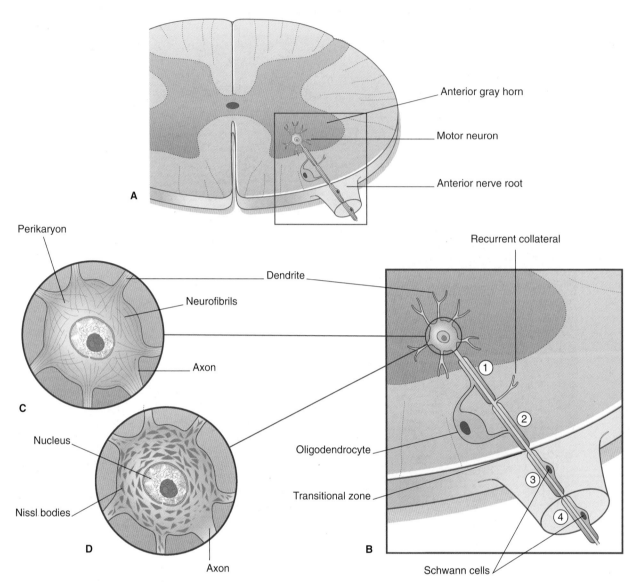

Figure 6.3 (A) Motor neuron in the anterior gray horn of the spinal cord. **(B)** Enlargement from (A). Myelin segments 1 and 2 occupy central nervous system white matter and have been laid down by an oligodendrocyte; a recurrent collateral branch of the axon originated from the node. Myelin segments 3 and 4 occupy peripheral nervous system and have been laid down by Schwann cells; the node at the transitional zone is bounded by an oligodendrocyte and a Schwann cell. **(C)** Neurofibrils (matted neurofilaments) are seen after staining with silver salts. **(D)** Nissl bodies (clumps of granular endoplasmic reticulum) are seen after staining with a cationic dye such as thionin.

disposal, retrograde transport is involved in *target cell recognition*. At synaptic contacts, axons constantly 'nibble' the plasma membrane of target neurons by means of endocytotic uptake of protein-containing *signaling endosomes*. These proteins are known as *neurotrophins* ('neuron foods'). They are brought to the soma and incorporated into Golgi complexes there. In addition, uptake of target cell 'marker' molecules is important for cell recognition during development. It may also be necessary for viability later on, because adult neurons shrink and may even die if their axons are severed proximal to their first branches.

The longest-known neurotrophin is *nerve growth factor*, on which the developing peripheral sensory and autonomic systems are especially dependent. Adult brain neurons synthesize *brain-derived neurotrophic factor (BDNF)* in the soma and send it to their nerve endings by anterograde transport. Animal studies have shown that BDNF maintains the general health of neurons in terms of metabolic activity, impulse propagation, and synaptic transmission.

Transport mechanisms

Microtubules are the supporting structures for neuronal transport. Microtubule-binding proteins, in the form of ATPases, propel organelles and molecules along the outer surface of the microtubules. Distinct ATPases are used for anterograde and retrograde work. Retrograde transport of signaling endosomes is performed by the *dynein* ATPase.

Failure of dynein performance has been linked to motor neuron disease, described in Chapter 16.

Neurofilaments do not seem to be involved in the transport mechanism. They are rather evenly spaced, having side arms that keep them apart and provide skeletal stability by attachment to proteins beneath the axolemmal membrane. Neurofilament numbers are in direct proportion to axonal diameter, and the filaments may in truth *determine* axonal diameter.

Some points of clinical relevance are highlighted in Clinical Panel 6.1.

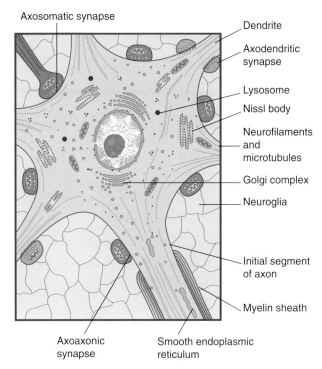

Axosomatic synapse

Dendrite

Axodendritic synapse

Lysosome

Nissl body

Neurofilaments and microtubules

Golgi complex

Neuroglia

Initial segment of axon

Myelin sheath

Axoaxonic synapse

Smooth endoplasmic reticulum

Figure 6.4 Ultrastructure of a motor neuron. Stems of five dendrites are included, also three excitatory synapses *(red)* and five inhibitory synapses.

SYNAPSES

Synapses are the points of contact between neurons.

Electrical synapses

Electrical synapses are scarce in the mammalian nervous system. They consist of gap junctions (nexuses) between dendrites or somas of contiguous neurons, where there is cytoplasmic continuity through 1.5-nm channels. No transmitter is involved, and there is no synaptic delay. They permit electrotonic changes to pass from one neuron to another. Being tightly coupled, modulation is not possible. Their function is to ensure synchronous activity of neurons having a common action. An example is the inspiratory center in the medulla oblongata, where all the cells exhibit synchronous discharge during inspiration. A second example is among neuronal circuits controlling *saccades*, where the gaze darts from one object of interest to another.

Chemical synapses

Conventional synapses are *chemical,* depending for their effect on the release of a *transmitter substance.* The typical chemical synapse comprises a **presynaptic membrane**, a **synaptic cleft**, and a **postsynaptic membrane** (Figure 6.6). The presynaptic membrane belongs to the terminal bouton, the postsynaptic membrane to the target neuron. Transmitter substance is released from the bouton by exocytosis, traverses the narrow synaptic cleft, and activates receptors in the postsynaptic membrane. Underlying the postsynaptic membrane is a **subsynaptic web**, in which numerous biochemical changes are initiated by receptor activation.

The bouton contains **synaptic vesicles** loaded with transmitter substance, together with numerous mitochondria and sacs of SER (Figure 6.7). Following conventional methods of fixation, *presynaptic dense projections* are visible, and microtubules seem to guide the synaptic vesicles to active zones in the intervals between the projections.

Clinical Panel 6.1 Clinical relevance of neuronal transport

Tetanus
Wounds contaminated by soil or street dust may contain *Clostridium tetani.* The toxin produced by this organism binds to the plasma membrane of nerve endings, is taken up by endocytosis, and is carried to the spinal cord by retrograde transport. Other neurons upstream take in the toxin by endocytosis – notably Renshaw cells (Ch. 15), which normally exert a braking action on motor neurons through the release of an inhibitory transmitter substance, *glycine.* Tetanus toxin prevents the release of glycine. As a result, motor neurons go out of control, particularly those supplying the muscles of the face, jaws, and spine. These muscles exhibit prolonged, agonizing spasms. About half of the patients who show these classic signs of tetanus die of exhaustion within a few days. Tetanus is entirely preventable by appropriate and timely immunization.

Viruses and toxic metals
Retrograde axonal transport has been blamed for the passage of viruses from the nasopharynx to the central nervous system, also for the uptake of toxic metals such as lead and aluminum. Viruses, in particular, may be spread widely through the brain by means of retrograde transneuronal uptake.

Peripheral neuropathies
Defective anterograde transport seems to be involved in certain 'dying back' neuropathies in which the distal parts of the longer peripheral nerves undergo progressive atrophy.

Cell membrane

Endoplasmic reticulum

Polyribosomes

Mitochondria

Figure 6.5 Nissl substance in the soma of a motor neuron. The endoplasmic reticulum has a characteristic stacked arrangement. Polyribosomes are studded along the outer surface of the cisternae; many others lie free in the cytoplasm. (*Note*: Faint color tones have been added here and later for ease of identification.) (From Pannese 1994, with permission of Thieme.)

Microtubule

Smooth endoplasmic reticulum

Axon

Mitochondrion in bouton

Active zone

Synaptic cleft

Subsynaptic web

Dendrite

Neuroglia

Synaptic vesicle

Presynaptic dense projection

Mitochondrion

Figure 6.6 Ultrastructure of an axodendritic synapse.

Mitochondria

Sac of smooth ER

Synaptic vesicles

Synaptic cleft

Postsynaptic density

Tubules of smooth ER

Microtubules

Neurofilaments

Figure 6.7 Axodendritic synapse. Section of spinal cord showing an axon terminal synapsing on the dendrite of a possible motor neuron. The spherical synaptic vesicles together with the asymmetric morphology (strong postsynaptic density) indicate an excitatory synapse. The dendrite is cut transversely, as are the numerous microtubules; some of the neurofilaments can also be seen. The synapse is invested by a protoplasmic astrocyte. (From Pannese 1994, with permission of Thieme.)

Receptor activation

Transmitter molecules cross the synaptic cleft and activate receptor proteins that straddle the postsynaptic membrane (Figure 6.8). The activated receptors initiate ionic events that either depolarize the postsynaptic membrane (excitatory postsynaptic effect) or hyperpolarize it (inhibitory postsynaptic effect). The voltage change passes over the soma in a decremental wave called *electrotonus*, and alters the resting potential of the first part or **initial segment** of the axon. (See Ch. 7 for details of the ionic events.) If excitatory postsynaptic potentials are dominant, the initial segment will be depolarized to threshold and generate action potentials.

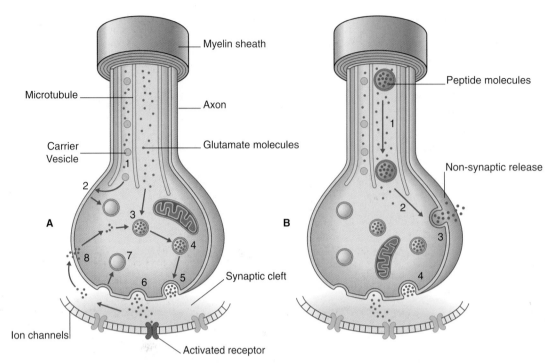

Figure 6.8 Dynamic events at two types of nerve terminal. **(A)** Small molecule transmitter, exemplified by a glutamatergic nerve ending. **(1)** Carrier vesicles containing synaptic vesicle membrane proteins are rapidly transported along microtubules and stored in the plasma membrane of the terminal bouton. At the same time, enzymes and glutamate molecules are conveyed by slow transport. **(2)** Vesicle membrane proteins are retrieved from the plasma membrane and form synaptic vesicles. **(3)** Glutamate is taken into the vesicles, where it is stored and concentrated. **(4)** Loaded vesicles approach the presynaptic membrane. **(5)** Following depolarization, the 'docked' vesicles undergo exocytosis. **(6)** Released transmitter diffuses across the synaptic cleft and activates specific receptors in the postsynaptic membrane. **(7)** Vesicular membranes are retrieved by means of endocytosis. **(8)** Some glutamate is actively transported back into the bouton for recycling. **(B)** Neuropeptide cotransmission. The example here is peptide *substance P* cotransmission with glutamate, a combination found at the central end of unipolar neurons serving pain sensation. **(1)** The vesicles and peptide precursors (propeptides) are synthesized in Golgi complexes in the perikaryon and taken to the terminal bouton by rapid transport. **(2)** As they enter the bouton, peptide formation is being completed, whereupon the vesicle approaches the plasma membrane. **(3)** Following membrane depolarization, the vesicular contents are sent into the intercellular space by means of exocytosis. **(4)** Glutamate is simultaneously released into the synaptic cleft.

In the CNS, the commonest excitatory transmitter is *glutamate;* the commonest inhibitory one is *gamma-aminobutyric acid* (GABA). In the peripheral nervous system, the transmitter for motor neurons supplying striated muscle is *acetylcholine;* the main transmitter for sensory neurons is *glutamate.*

The sequence of events involved in *glutamatergic* synaptic transmission is shown in Figure 6.8A. In the case of peptide *cotransmission* with glutamate, release of (one or more) peptides is *non-synaptic*, as shown in Figure 6.8B.

Many sensory neurons liberate one or more peptides in addition to glutamate; the peptides may be liberated from any part of the neuron, but their usual role is to *modulate* (raise or lower) the effectiveness of the transmitter.

A further kind of transmission is known as *volume* transmission. This kind is typical of *monoamine (biogenic amine) neurons*, which fall into two categories. One category synthesizes a *catecholamine*, namely *norepinephrine (noradrenaline)* or *dopamine*, both synthesized from the amino acid tyrosine. The other synthesizes *serotonin*, derived from tryptophan. As illustrated in Figure 6.9, for dopamine, the transmitter is liberated from *varicosities* (where they are also

synthesized) as well as from synaptic contacts. The transmitter enters the extracellular fluid of the CNS and activates specific receptors up to 100 μm away before being degraded. The monoamine neurons have enormous territorial distribution, and deviation from normal function is implicated in a variety of ailments including Parkinson disease, schizophrenia, and major depression.

Nitric oxide (a gaseous molecule) within glutamatergic neurons is also associated with volume transmission. Excess nitric oxide liberation is *cytotoxic*, notably in areas rendered avascular by cerebral arterial thrombosis. Glutamate itself is also potentially cytotoxic.

In the context of volume transmission, the conventional kind is called 'wiring' to indicate its relatively fixed nature.

Lock and key analogy for drug therapy

The receptor may be likened to a lock, the transmitter being the key that operates it. The transmitter output of certain neurons may falter as a consequence of age or disease, and a duplicate key can often be provided in the form of a drug that mimics the action of the transmitter. Such a drug is

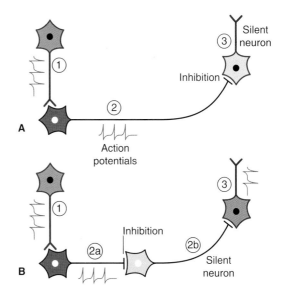

Figure 6.10 Disinhibition. **(A)** Excitatory neuron 1 is activating inhibitory neuron 2 with consequent silencing of neuron 3 by neuron 2. **(B)** Interpolation of a second inhibitory neuron (2b) has the opposite effect on neuron 3, because 2b is silenced. Neuron 3 (spontaneously active unless inhibited) is released.

Figure 6.9 Volume transmission in the brain. The axons of a glutamatergic neuron **(1)** and of a dopaminergic neuron **(2)** are making conventional synaptic contacts on the spine of a spiny stellate cell **(3)** in the striatum. Dopamine (DA) is also escaping from a varicosity and diffusing through the extracellular space (ECS) to activate dopamine receptors on the dendritic shaft and on the wall of a capillary pericyte (see Ch. 5).

called an *agonist*. On the other hand, excessive production of a transmitter may be countered by a *receptor blocker* – the equivalent of a dummy key that will occupy the lock without activating it.

Inhibition versus disinhibition

Spontaneously active neurons are often held in check by inhibitory neurons (usually GABAergic), as shown in Figure 6.10A. The inhibitory neurons may be silenced by others of the same kind, leading to *disinhibition* of the target cell (Figure 6.10B). Disinhibition is a major feature of neuronal activity in the basal ganglia (Ch. 33).

Less common chemical synapses

Two varieties of **axoaxonic** synapses are recognized. In both cases, the boutons belong to inhibitory neurons. One variety occurs on the initial segment of the axon, where it exercises a powerful veto on impulse generation (Figure 6.11). In the second kind, the boutons are applied to excitatory boutons of other neurons, and they inhibit transmitter release. The effect is called *presynaptic inhibition,* any conventional contact being *postsynaptic* in this context (Figure 6.12).

Dendrodendritic (D-D) synapses occur between dendritic spines of contiguous spiny neurons, and alter the electrotonus of the target neuron rather than generating nerve impulses. In *one-way* D-D synapses, one of the two spines

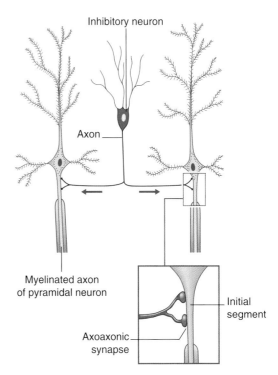

Figure 6.11 Axoaxonic synapses in the cerebral cortex. *Arrows* indicate direction of impulse conduction.

contains synaptic vesicles. In *reciprocal* synapses, both do. Excitatory D-D synapses are shown in Figure 6.13. Inhibitory D-D synapses are numerous in relay nuclei of the thalamus (Ch. 25).

Somatodendritic and **somatosomatic** synapses have also been identified, but they are scarce.

Clinical Panel 6.2 Gliomas

Brain tumors most commonly originate from neuroglial cells, especially astrocytes.

General symptoms produced by expanding brain tumors are indicative of *raised intracranial pressure*. They include headache, drowsiness, and vomiting. Radiologic investigation may reveal displacement of midline structures to the opposite side. Tumors below the tentorium (usually cerebellar) are likely to block the exit of cerebrospinal fluid from the fourth ventricle, in which case ballooning of the ventricular system will add to the intracranial pressure.

Local symptoms depend on the position of the tumor. For example, clumsiness of an arm or leg may be caused by a cerebellar tumor on the same side, and motor weakness of an arm or leg may be caused by a cerebral tumor on the opposite side.

Progression

Expansion of a tumor may cause one or more brain hernias to develop, as shown in Figure CP 6.2.1.

1. *Subfalcine herniation* (in the interval between falx cerebri and corpus callosum) seldom causes specific symptoms.
2. *Uncal herniation* is the term used to denote displacement of the uncus of the temporal lobe into the tentorial notch. Compression of the ipsilateral crus cerebri by the uncus (Figure CP 6.2.2) may give rise to contralateral motor weakness. Alternatively, compression of the contralateral crus against the sharp edge of the tentorium cerebelli may cause *ipsilateral* motor weakness.
3. *Pressure coning:* a cone of cerebellar tissue (the tonsil) may descend into the foramen magnum, squeezing the medulla oblongata and causing death from respiratory or cardiovascular failure by inactivation of *vital centers* in the reticular formation (Ch. 22).

Figure CP 6.2.1 Brain herniations. For numbers, see text.

Figure CP 6.2.2 Enlargement from *Figure 3.7* emphasizing the proximity of the uncus to the pyramidal tract (PT).

Clinical Panel 6.3 Multiple sclerosis

Multiple sclerosis (MS) is the commonest neurologic disorder of young adults in the temperate latitudes north and south of the equator. It is more prevalent in women, with a female:male ratio of 3:2. The peak age of onset is around 30 years, the range being 15–45.

Multiple sclerosis is a *primary demyelinating disease:* the initial feature is the development of plaques (patches) of demyelination in the white matter. The denuded axons also undergo large-scale degeneration, probably initiated by failure of the sodium pump, as described in Chapter 7. Impulse conduction in neighboring myelinated fibers is also compromised by edema (inflammatory exudate). Over time, the plaques are progressively replaced by glial scar tissue. Old plaques feel firm (sclerotic) in postmortem slices of the brain.

Common locations of early plaques are the cervical spinal cord, upper brainstem, optic nerve, and periventricular white matter (Figure CP 6.3.1) including that of the cerebellum. MS is not a systems disease: it is not anatomically selective, and a plaque may involve parts of adjacent motor and sensory pathways.

Presenting symptoms can be correlated with lesion sites as follows.

- *Motor weakness,* usually in one or both legs, signifies a lesion involving the corticospinal tract.
- *Clumsiness* in reaching and grasping usually accompanies a lesion in the cerebellar white matter.
- *Numbness or tingling,* often spreading up from the legs to the trunk, may be caused by a lesion in the posterior white matter of the spinal cord. Tingling ('pins and needles') is attributed to spontaneous firing of partially demyelinated sensory fibers.
- *Diplopia* (double vision) may be produced by a plaque within the pons or midbrain affecting the function of one of the ocular motor nerves.
- A *scotoma* (patch of blindness in the visual field of one eye) is produced by a plaque within the optic nerve.
- *Urinary retention* (failure of the bladder to empty) can be caused by interruption of the central autonomic pathway descending from the brainstem to the lower part of the cord.

The usual course of the disease is one of remissions and relapses, with an overall slow progression and development of multiple disabilities.

Figure CP 6.3.1 An MRI scan of a 28-year-old man with multifocal demyelination secondary to multiple sclerosis. Axial T$_2$-weighted image showing multiple lesions of high signal intensity in the white matter. On the left side of the brain, at least five of these plaques are periventricular. (Kindly provided by Dr. Joe Walsh, Department of Radiology, University College Hospital, Galway, Ireland.)

Note: Recent research in several laboratories has elicited frequent additional evidence of gray matter degeneration, mainly in the cerebral cortex, leading in many cases to cognitive deficiencies. Several putative causes are under investigation.

REFERENCE
Geurts JGG, Barkhof F: Grey matter pathology in multiple sclerosis, *Lancet Neurol* 7:841–851, 2008.

Core Information

Neurons

The multipolar neuron of the central nervous system (CNS) comprises soma, dendrites, and axon; the axon gives off collateral and terminal branches. The soma contains rough and smooth endoplasmic reticulum, Golgi complexes, neurofilaments, and microtubules. Microtubules pervade the entire neuron; they are involved in anterograde transport of synaptic vesicles, mitochondria, and membranous replacement material, and in retrograde transport of marker molecules and degraded organelles.

The three kinds of chemical neuronal interaction are synaptic (e.g. glutamatergic), non-synaptic (e.g. peptidergic), and volume (e.g. monoaminergic, serotonergic).

Anatomic varieties of chemical synapse include axodendritic, axosomatic, axoaxonic, and dendrodendritic. Structure includes pre- and postsynaptic membranes, synaptic cleft, and subsynaptic web.

Electrical synapses via gap junctions render some neuronal groups electrically coupled, for synchronous activation.

Neuroglia

Astrocytes have supportive, nutritive, and retrieval functions. They are the main source of brain tumors. Oligodendrocytes form CNS myelin sheaths, which are subject to destruction in demyelinating diseases. Microglia are potential phagocytes.

REFERENCES

Gage FH, Kempermann G, Song H, editors: *Adult neurogenesis*, Cold Spring Harbor, New York, 2008, Cold Spring Harbor Laboratory Press.

Hirokawa N, Reiko T: Molecular motors in neuronal development, intracellular transport and diseases, *Curr Opin Neurobiol* 14:564–573, 2004.

Howe CH, Mobley WC: Long-distance retrograde neurotrophic signaling, *Curr Opin Neurobiol* 15:40–48, 2005.

Jessen KR: Glial cells, *Int J Biochem Cell Biol* 36:1861–1867, 2004.

Koehler RC, Roman RJ, Harder GR: Astrocytes and the regulation of cerebral blood flow, *Trends Neurosci* 32:160–169, 2009.

Pannese E: *Neurocytology. Fine structure of neurons, nerve processes and neuroglial cells*, New York, 1994, Thieme.

Stys PK: General mechanisms of axonal damage and its repair, *J Neurol Sci* 233:3–13, 2005.

Sykova E, Nicholson C: Diffusion in brain extracellular space, *Physiol Rev* 88:1277–1340, 2008.

Torrealba F, Carrasco MA: A review on electron microscopy and neurotransmitter systems, *Brain Res Rev* 47:5–17, 2004.

Triarhou LC: *Cellular structure of the cerebral cortex*, Basle, 2009, Karger.

STUDY GUIDELINES

1. The information in this chapter underpins the science of clinical electrophysiology.
2. Appreciate that neuronal membranes carry an electrical charge based on passive ion diffusion along specific ion channels and regulated by a sodium–potassium pump, and that action potentials are abrupt changes in membrane voltage caused by activation of voltage-gated ion channels.
3. Note that impulse propagation is an all-or-nothing event and of the same magnitude all the way along the nerve fiber and its branches.
4. Myelination dramatically increases the speed of impulse conduction.
5. Examples of clinical neurophysiology related to the peripheral nervous system await your attention in Chapter 12.

STRUCTURE OF THE PLASMA MEMBRANE

In common with cells elsewhere, the plasma membrane of neurons is a double layer (bilayer) of phospholipids made up of phosphate heads facing the aqueous media of the extracellular and intracellular spaces, and paired lipid tails forming a fatty membrane in between (Figure 7.1). The phosphate layer is water-soluble (*hydrophilic*, or *polar*) and the double lipid layer is water-insoluble (*hydrophobic*, or *non-polar*).

Both the extracellular and the intracellular fluids are aqueous salt solutions in which many soluble molecules dissociate into positively or negatively charged atoms or groups of atoms called *ions*. Ions and molecules in aqueous solutions are in a constant state of agitation, being subject to *diffusion*, whereby they tend to move from areas of higher concentration to areas of lower concentration. In addition to passing down their concentration gradients by diffusion, ions are influenced by electrical gradients. Positively charged ions including Na^+ and K^+ are called *cations* because, in an electrical field, they migrate to the cathode. Negatively charged ions including Cl^- are called *anions* because these migrate to the anode. Like charges (e.g. Na^+ and K^+) repel one another, unlike charges (e.g. Na^+ and Cl^-) attract one another.

The cell membrane can be regarded as an electric *capacitor*, because it comprises outer and inner layers carrying ionic charges of opposite kind, with a (fatty) insulator in between. Away from the membrane, the voltage in the tissue fluid is brought to zero (0 mV) by the neutralizing effect of chloride anions on sodium and other cations, and the voltage in the cytosol away from the membrane is brought to zero by the neutralizing effect of anionic proteins on K^+ cations.

Ion channels

Ion channels are membrane-spanning proteins having a central pore that permits passage of ions across the cell membrane. Most channels are selective for a particular ion, for example Na^+, *or* K^+ *or* Cl^-

Several channel categories are recognized, of which the first three are of immediate relevance.

- *Passive* (non-gated) channels are open at all times, permitting ions to move across the membrane.
- *Voltage-gated* channels contain a voltage-sensitive string of amino acids that cause the channel pore to open or close in response to changes in membrane voltage.
- *Channel pumps* are energy-driven ion exporters and/or importers designed to maintain steady-state ion concentrations. The Na^+–K^+ exchange pump (usually referred to as the *sodium pump*) is vital to maintenance of the resting membrane potential.
- *Transmitter-gated* channels abound in postsynaptic membranes. Some are activated directly by transmitter molecules, others indirectly (see Ch. 8).
- *Transduction* channels are activated by peripheral sensory stimulation. Sensory nerve endings exhibit different stimulus specificities in different locations, for example mechanical in muscle; tactile, thermal, or chemical in skin; acoustic in the cochlea; vestibular in the labyrinth; electromagnetic in the retina; gustatory in the tongue; olfactory in the upper part of the nasal mucous membrane.

Figure 7.2 depicts the three passive channels concerned with generating the resting potential.

The existence of distinct channels for Na^+, K^+ and Cl^- ions would result in zero voltage difference across the membrane if passive diffusion of the three ions were equally free. However, the number of sodium channels is relatively small, and movement of the Na^+ ion is relatively slow because of

Figure 7.1 Structure of the neuronal cell membrane. The only membrane proteins shown here are ion channels.

its relatively large 'hydration shell' of H_2O molecules. In effect, the membrane is many times more permeable to K^+ and Cl^- than to Na^+.

The resting membrane potential

The membrane potential of the resting (inactive) neuron is generated primarily by differences in concentration of the sodium (Na^+) and potassium (K^+) ions dissolved in the aqueous environments of extracellular fluid (ECF) and cytosol. In Table 7.1, it can be seen that potassium is 20 times more concentrated in the cytosol; sodium is 10 and chloride 3.8 times more concentrated in the ECF.

In Figure 7.3, a voltmeter is connected to electrodes inserted into the ECF surrounding an axon. One of the electrodes has been inserted into a glass pipette having a minute tip. On the left side of the figure, both electrode tips are in the ECF, and there is no voltage difference; a zero value is recorded. On the right side, the pipette has been lowered, puncturing the plasma membrane of the axon and admitting the intracellular fluid of the cytosol. The electrical charge now reveals a *potential* (voltage) difference of −70 mV. In practice, the membrane potential ranges from −60 mV to −80 mV

Table 7.1 Ionic concentrations in cytosol and extracellular fluid

Ion	Concentration (mmol/L)		Equilibrium potential (mV)
	Cytosol	Extracellular fluid	
K^+	100	5	−90
Na^+	15	150	+60
Cl^-	13	50	−70

in different neurons. These values represent the *resting* membrane potential, i.e. when impulses are not being conducted.

Resting membrane permeability

Potassium ions

From what has been mentioned, it is clear that K^+ concentrations on either side of the cell membrane would be the same were there no constraint. In fact, there are two electrical constraints at the level of the ion pore, namely the attraction exerted by the protein anions on the inside, and the repulsion

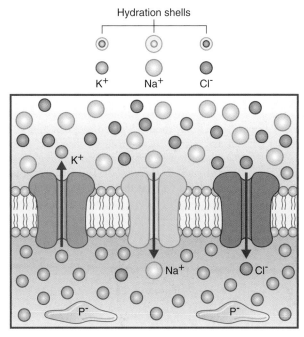

Hydration shells

K⁺   Na⁺   Cl⁻

Figure 7.2 In the resting state, Na⁺ and Cl⁻ ions are concentrated external to the membrane, because of the slow inward passage of the hydrated Na⁺ ions through their channels, combined with their attraction to Cl⁻ ions. K⁺ ions are concentrated on the inside, because of their attraction to protein anions (P⁻). The arrows are directed down the concentration gradients of the respective ions.

Figure 7.3 The resting membrane potential. **(1)** The two electrodes of a voltmeter are inserted into the extracellular fluid (ECF) surrounding an axon. The left electrode tip occupies a micropipette. There is no voltage difference registering, hence the zero value in the record below. **(2)** On the right, the pipette has been lowered (arrow), puncturing the plasma membrane to sample the intracellular fluid (ICF) immediately beneath. A voltage difference of –70 mV is recorded.

exerted by the Na⁺ cations on the outside. The equilibrium state exists when the concentration gradient is exactly balanced by the voltage gradient; the potential difference at this point is expressed as E_K, the potassium equilibrium potential. This can be expressed by means of the *Nernst equation*, which uses principles of thermodynamics to convert the concentration gradient of an ion to an equivalent voltage gradient.

$$E_K = \frac{RT}{FZ_K} \ln \frac{[K^+]_o}{[K^+]_i} \qquad \text{EQUATION 1}$$

E_K = equilibrium potential for potassium expressed as millivolts
R = universal gas constant (8.31 J/mol/°absolute)
T = temperature in degrees Kelvin (310° at 37°C)
F = Faraday (96 500 C/per mole of charge)
Z_K = valence of potassium (+1)
$\ln$ = natural logarithms
$[K^+]_o$ = potassium concentration outside the cell membrane
$[K^+]_i$ = potassium concentration inside the cell membrane

Converting the natural log to $\log_{10}$ and resolving the numeric fractions yields

$$E_K = 62 \times \log_{10}(5/100) = -90 \text{ mV}$$

Repeating the exercise for sodium and chloride yields

$$E_{Na} = +60 \text{ mV and } E_{Cl} = -70 \text{ mV}$$

The value of the resting potential can be calculated using the *Goldman* equation, from the relative distributions of the three principal ions involved (Table 7.1), and their membrane permeabilities.

$$RP = 62 \log \frac{P_{K^+}[K^+]_o + P_{Na^+}[Na^+]_o + P_{Cl^-}[Cl^-]_i}{P_{K^+}[K^+]_i + P_{Na^+}[Na^+]_i + P_{Cl^-}[Cl^-]_o} \qquad \text{EQUATION 2}$$

RP = resting potential
62 = RT/F × 2.3 (constant for converting ln to $\log_{10}$)
P = the three membrane permeabilities
o and i refer to outside and inside the cell. The concentrations of the negative chloride ions are shown inverted because –log (X/Y) = log (Y/X)
Brackets signify concentration.

The Goldman equation is nothing more than the Nernst equation for each of the three ions, with each concentration multiplied by the conductance (permeability) of that ion. The effect of the chloride ion on resting potential is insignificant, because its equilibrium potential is the same as the resting potential. The sum of the fractions for K⁺ and Na⁺ yields an outcome of –70 mV, as required by the known value.

85

Figure 7.4 The Na⁺–K⁺ pump. The diagram indicates simultaneous expulsion of three sodium ions for every two potassium ions imported.

Sodium pump

The resting potential needs to be stabilized, because of the tendency of Na^+ ions to leak inward and K^+ to leak outward along their concentration gradients. Stability is assured by the Na^+–K^+ pump making appropriate corrections for their passive flows. This channel is capable of simultaneously extruding N^+ and importing K^+. Three sodium ions are exported for every two potassium ions imported (Figure 7.4). In both cases, the movement is *against* the existing concentration gradient. The required energy for this activity is provided by the ATPase enzyme that converts ATP to ADP. The greater the amount of Na^+ in the cytosol, the greater is the activity of the enzyme.

As mentioned in Chapter 6, the axonal degeneration occurring in multiple sclerosis is attributable to failure of the sodium pump along the denuded axolemma. This leads to Na^+ overload, which in turn promotes excess Ca^{2+} release from intracellular stores.

RESPONSE TO STIMULATION: ACTION POTENTIALS

Neurons typically interact at chemical synapses, where liberation of a transmitter substance is produced by the arrival of *action potentials*, or *spikes*, at the synaptic boutons. The transmitter crosses the synaptic cleft and activates *receptors* embedded in the membranes of target neurons. The receptors activate *transmitter-gated* ion channels to alter the level of polarization of the target neuron. Receptors activated by an inhibitory transmitter cause the membrane potential to increase beyond the resting value of −70 mV, perhaps to −80 mV or more, a process known as *hyperpolarization*. Excitatory transmitters cause the membrane potential to diminish, a process of *depolarization*.

Electrotonic potentials

The initial target cell response to excitatory stimulation takes the form of local, *graded* or *electrotonic potentials* (ETPs). Positive ETPs on multipolar neurons are usually on one or more dendrites in receipt of excitatory synapses. At a low frequency of stimulation, small, decremental waves of depolarization extend for 50–100 μm along the affected dendrites, dying away after 2 or 3 ms (Figure 7.5). With increasing frequency, the waves undergo stepwise *temporal summation* to form progressively larger waves continuing on over the surface of the soma. *Spatial summation* occurs when waves traveling along two or more dendrites coalesce on the soma (Figure 7.6). About 15 mV of depolarization, to a value of −55 mV, brings the neuron to *threshold* (firing level) at its most sensitive region, or *trigger point*, in the initial segment of the axon (Figure 7.7). The initial segment is the first region to 'give way' at threshold voltage, because it is exceptionally rich in voltage-gated sodium channels. When the level of depolarization (the *generator potential*) reaches threshold, nerve impulses in the form of *action potentials* are suddenly fired off.

In sensory neurons of cranial and spinal nerves, the trigger zone generates what is known as the *receptor potential*. The trigger zone of sensory neurons is exceptionally rich in the sensation-specific transduction channels defined earlier.

In the case of myelinated nerve fibers, the trigger point is easily identified: in multipolar neurons, it is immediately proximal to the first myelin segment, and in peripheral sensory neurons it is immediately distal to the final segment.

Negative excitatory postsynaptic potentials are elicited by inhibitory transmitters. They, too, are decremental.

The shape of action potentials

A single action potential is depicted in Figure 7.8. The *spike* segment of the potential commences when the local response reaches threshold value at −55 mV. The rising phase of depolarization passes beyond zero to include an *overshoot* phase reaching about +35 mV. Overshoot phase includes the rising and falling phases above zero potential. The falling phase planes out in a brief *after-depolarization*, prior to an *undershoot* phase of *after-hyperpolarization* where the membrane potential reaches about −75 mV before returning to baseline.

It should be pointed out that standard representations such as this figure show the voltage changes plotted against a time base. When direction is substituted for time, it becomes obvious that the time-based picture matches the sequence in a peripheral sensory neuron. For all multipolar neurons, the representation should be the reverse (Figure 7.7).

When the local response to stimulation has depolarized the membrane to threshold, the sudden increase in depolarization is brought about by the opening of voltage-gated sodium channels (Figure 7.9). Sodium entry produces further depolarization, and the positive feedback causes the remaining Na^+ channels of the trigger zone to open, driving the membrane charge momentarily into a charge reversal (overshoot) of +35 mV, approaching the Nernst potential for sodium. At this point, the sodium channels commence a progressive inactivation, and the voltage-gated potassium channels are simultaneously triggered to open. Current flow switches from Na^+ inflow to K^+ outflow. The hyperpolarization phase is explained by the voltage-gated sodium channels being completely inactivated prior to closure of the potassium channels. Any remaining discrepancy is adjusted by activity of the Na^+–K^+ pump.

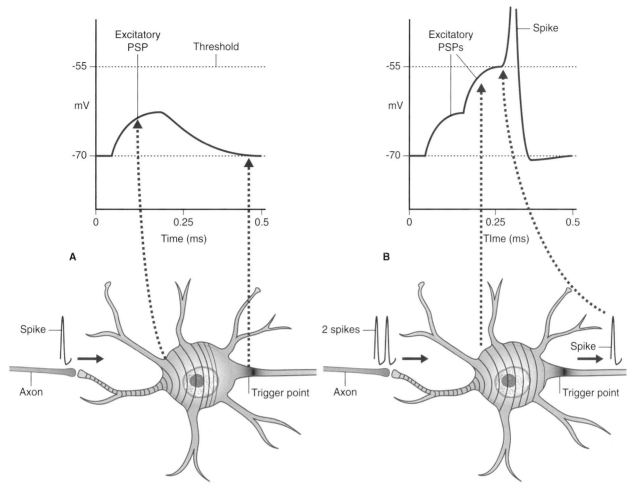

Figure 7.5 Temporal summation. **(A)** A sensory axon (blue) delivers a single spike to a motor neuron, sufficient to elicit an excitatory postsynaptic potential (PSP) that dies away. **(B)** The axon delivers two spikes that undergo temporal summation to reach firing threshold at the initial segment of the axon, which responds by generating a spike that will pass along the motor axon.

Close analyses of the sodium channels involved have revealed a dual mechanism of operation, as indicated in Figure 7.10. In the resting state, an *activation gate* in the midregion of both Na^+ and K^+ channel pores is closed. The sodium channel is the first to respond at threshold, by opening its activation gate and allowing a torrential inflow of Na^+ ions down the concentration gradient. One millisecond later, a second, *inactivation gate,* in the form of a flap of globular protein, seals the exit into the cytosol while the K^+ channel pore is opening. When the membrane potential approaches normality, the sodium gating reverts to its resting inactive state.

The action potential response to depolarization is *all or none,* a term signifying that if it occurs at all, it is total. In this respect, it is quite unlike the graded potentials that summate to initiate action potentials. Action potentials are also distinguished from graded potentials in being *non-decremental;* they are propagated at full strength along the nerve fiber all the way to the nerve endings, which in the case of lower limb neurons may be more than a meter away from the parent somas.

During the rising and early falling phases of the action potential, the neuron passes through an *absolute refractory period* where it is incapable of initiating a second impulse because too many voltage-gated channels are already open (Figure 7.11). This is followed by a *relative refractory period,* where stimuli in excess of the standard 15-mV requirement can elicit a response. It is quite common for the generator potential to reach up to 35 mV, triggering impulses at 50–100 impulses per second, expressed as 50–100 Hz (Hertz = times per second).

Propagation

Reversal of potential at the trigger zone is propagated (conducted) along the axon in accordance with the electrotonic circuit shown in Figure 7.12. The positive internal membrane charge passes in both directions within the axoplasm, while positive outside charge passes in both directions within the ECF to neutralize the negative external potential. The membrane immediately proximal is sufficiently refractory to resist depolarization, whereas that immediately distal undergoes a

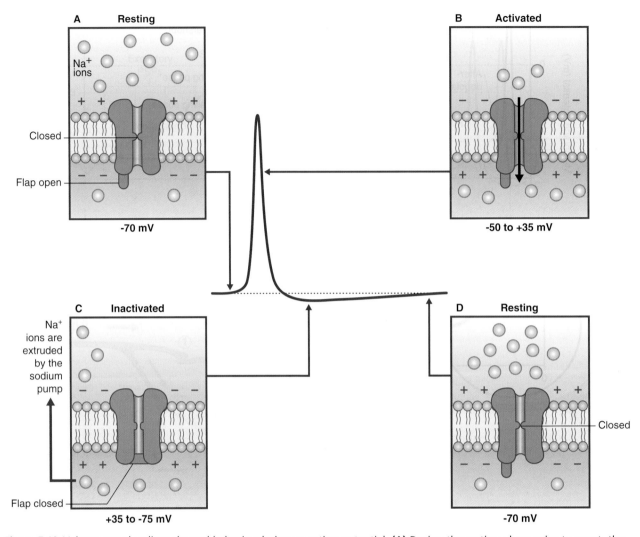

Figure 7.10 Voltage-gated sodium channel behavior during an action potential. **(A)** During the resting phase prior to onset, the midregion of the channel pore is closed and the inactivation flap is open. **(B)** When the threshold level is crossed, activation of the channel opens the pore completely, with a time limit of 1 ms. **(C)** The pore is closed by the inactivation flap. **(D)** Restoration of the resting potential causes the midregion to close and the flap to open.

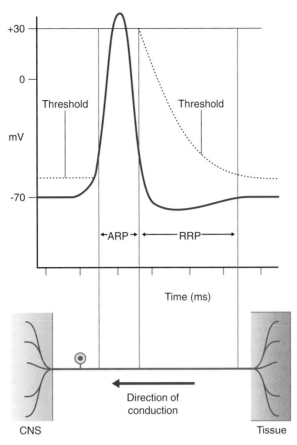

Figure 7.11 Refractory periods. ARP, absolute refractory period; CNS, central nervous system; RRP, relative refractory period.

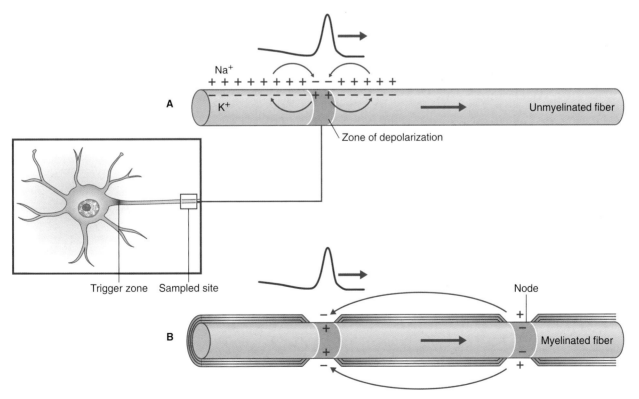

Figure 7.12 Current flow during impulse propagation, represented as movement of positive charges. (A) Continuous conduction along an unmyelinated fiber. (B) Saltatory conduction along a myelinated fiber.

Clinical Panel 7.1 Local anesthetics: how they work

Locally applied anesthetics reversibly block nerve conduction by inactivating sodium channels – especially voltage-gated sodium channels – thereby preventing depolarization. The more firmly they bind to the protein surround of the ion channels, the longer their duration of action. A high lipid solubility is required to access these proteins. When injected close to a peripheral nerve, unmyelinated and finely myelinated (Aδ) fibers are the first to be inactivated, thereby relieving both aching and stabbing pain sensation. If the nerve is mixed, some temporary motor paralysis may follow.

Most local anesthetics are either *amides* (including bupivacaine and lidocaine) or *esters* (including benzocaine and novocaine). Both groups cause local vasodilation by directly relaxing arteriolar smooth muscle. Because this accelerates their clearance, epinephrine is often included in anesthetic solutions as it causes smooth muscle contraction or vasoconstriction.

REFERENCE
Scholz A: Mechanisms of local anaesthetics on voltage-gated sodium and other ion channels, *Br J Anaesthesia* 89:52–61, 2002.

Core Information

Ions are electrically charged atoms or groups of atoms. Na^+ and K^+ are cations, Cl^- and P^- (proteins) are anions. Cell membranes are charged capacitors carrying a resting potential (voltage) of -70 mV.

Passive ion channels for Na^+, K^+, and Cl^- are open at all times, and the ions diffuse down their concentration gradient through their respective channels. However, Na^+ channels are relatively scarce, whereas K^+ and Cl^- are numerous. K^+ ions are abundant in the cytosol, being attracted by protein anions in the cytoskeleton and repelled by the Na^+ ions outside. A Na^+–K^+ channel pump maintains the resting steady state of the membrane potential.

The initial response of a multipolar neuron to an excitatory stimulus takes the form of decremental waves of positive electrotonus. Temporal and/or spatial summation of such waves produces a generator potential at the initial segment of the axon. At a threshold value of 50 mV, action potentials are fired off along the nerve fiber. On the other hand, inhibitory stimulation takes the form of negative electrotonic waves that summate to produce overall hyperpolarization.

The action potential (spike) is characterized by a rising phase from baseline up to $+35$ mV, a falling phase down to baseline followed by a hyperpolarization phase down to -75 mV with return to baseline. Triggering the rapid depolarization is activation of voltage-gated ion channels, whereby the ion channel is briefly (1 ms) opened completely, allowing massive Na^+ inflow tipping the potential to $+35$ mV, whereupon the channels are shut by inactivation gates and voltage-gated K^+ channels are opened, with a current switch from Na^+ inflow to K^+ outflow.

For about 1 ms following impulse initiation, the trigger zone initial segment is absolutely refractory to further stimulation; for the following 3 ms, it is relatively refractory.

Action potentials are propagated in an all-or-none manner and at full strength along the fiber and its branches. Propagation is continuous along unmyelinated axons, saltatory (from node to node) along myelinated axons. Saltatory conduction is much faster. The widest fibers have the longest internodal segments and the fastest conduction rates.

REFERENCE

Koester J, Siegelbaum SA: Peripheral signaling: the action potential. In: Kandel ER, Schwarz JH, Jessell TJ, editors: *Principles of neural science*, ed 4, New York, 2000, McGraw-Hill, pp 150–170.

Transmitters and receptors

STUDY GUIDELINES

1 This chapter dwells on chemical neurotransmission. The information is intended to set the stage for learning about therapeutic applications, notably in relation to the autonomic nervous system and to emotional or behavioral disorders including the psychoses.
2 The numbered flow diagrams are meant to convey a sense of motion. It may be a good idea to 'go with the flow' by following the possible paths taken by a given transmitter molecule (e.g. five for catecholamines).
3 Learn to distinguish between the nature of fast (ionotropic) and slow (metabotropic) receptors.
4 The transmitter or receptor agonists and antagonists mentioned here will come up in later chapters.

ELECTRICAL SYNAPSES

Electrical synapses are scarce in the mammalian nervous system. As seen in Figure 8.1, they consist of gap junctions (nexuses) between dendrites or somas of contiguous neurons, where there is cytoplasmic continuity through 1.5-nm channels. No transmitter is involved, and there is no synaptic delay.

The gap junctions are bridged by tightly packed ion channels, each comprising mirror image pairs of connexons, which are transmembrane protein groups (*connexins*) disposed in hexagonal format around an ion pore. Wedge-shaped connexin subunits bordering each ion pore are closely apposed when the neurons are inactive. Action potentials passing along the cell membrane cause the subunits to rotate individually, creating a pore large enough to permit free diffusion of ions and small molecules down their concentration gradients.

The overall function of these gap junctions is to ensure synchronous activity of neurons having a common action. An example is the inspiratory center in the medulla oblongata, where all the cells exhibit synchronous discharge during inspiration. A second example is among neuronal circuits controlling *saccades,* where the gaze darts from one object of interest to another.

CHEMICAL SYNAPSES

Transmitter liberation (Table 8.1 and Figure 8.2)

At resting nerve terminals, synaptic vesicles accumulate in the active zones, where they are tethered to the presynaptic densities by strands of *docking proteins* including actin. With the arrival of action potentials, myriads of voltage-gated calcium channels located in the presynaptic membrane are opened, leading to instant flooding of the active zone with Ca^{2+} ions. These ions cause contraction of actin filaments to bring the nearest vesicles into direct contact with the presynaptic membrane.

When the vesicle protein *synaptophysin* contacts the vesicle membrane, it becomes embedded in it and hollows out to create a *fusion pore* through which the vesicle discharges its contents into the synaptic cleft. The act of expulsion appears to be a function of another vesicle protein, *calmodulin,* activated by Ca^{2+} ions. These and other local protein responses to calcium entry are extremely rapid, the time elapsing between calcium entry and transmitter expulsion being less than 1 ms. In the case of small synaptic vesicles such as those containing glutamate or γ-aminobutyric acid (GABA), single spikes are sufficient to yield some transmitter release. In the case of peptidergic neurons, impulse frequencies of 10 Hz or more are required to induce typically slow (delay of 50 ms or more) transmitter release from the large, dense-cored vesicles.

Table 8.1 Some named proteins involved in transmitter transport and vesicle recycling

Named protein	Function
Actin	Brings vesicle into contact with presynaptic membrane
Synaptophysin	Creates the membrane fusion pore
Calmodulin	Expels vesicle content into synaptic cleft
Clathrin	Withdraws vesicle membrane from synaptic cleft
Dynamin	Pinches the neck of the developing vesicle to complete its separation
Ligand	Receptor protein that binds with the transmitter molecule

Figure 8.1 Structure of an electrical synapse. **(A)** Synaptic contact between two dendrites. **(B)** Enlargement from (A). **(C)** The gap junction between the cell membranes is bridged by close-packed ion channels. **(D)** Each ion channel comprises a mirror image pair of connexons. **(E)** Each connexon comprises six connexins, each having a wedge-shaped subunit bordering the ion channel. **(F)** The subunits open the ion channel by synchronous rotation.

Target cell receptor binding

Transmitter molecules bind with receptor protein molecules in the postsynaptic membrane. The two great categories of receptor are known as *ionotropic* and *metabotropic*. Each category contains some receptors whose activation leads to opening of ion pores and others whose activation leads to closure.

Ionotropic receptors

Ionotropic receptors are characterized by the presence of an ion channel within each receptor macromolecule (Figure 8.2). The transmitter binds with its specific receptor facing the synaptic cleft, causing it to change its conformation so as to open or close its ion pore. Ionotropic receptor channels are said to be transmitter-gated, or *ligand*-gated (from the Latin *ligandum*, 'binding'), signifying their capacity to bind a transmitter molecule or a drug substitute.

In Figure 8.3A, the excitatory channel has been opened by the transmitter, causing a major influx of sodium and a minor efflux of potassium; the excitatory postsynaptic potential (EPSP) has depolarized the cell membrane almost to firing point. In Figure 8.3B, the membrane can be hyperpolarized only to –70 mV, the chloride equilibrium potential. A greater level of depolarization requires a second messenger system (see below).

Ionotropic receptors are called *fast* receptors on account of their immediate and brief effects on ion channels.

Metabotropic receptors

Metabotropic receptors are so called because many are capable of generating multiple metabolic effects within the cytoplasm of the neuron. The receptor macromolecule is an intrinsic membrane protein devoid of an ion channel. Its function is initiated by one or other of two subunits (α subunit, β subunit) that detaches in response to transmitter activation and moves along the inner surface of the membrane. The subunits are called *G proteins,* because most bind with guanine nucleotides such as guanine triphosphate (GTP) or guanine diphosphate. Their action on ion channels is usually indirect, via a *second messenger system.* However, some G proteins do not bind with nucleotides; instead, they activate ion channels *directly* (see later).

A G protein having a stimulatory effect is known as a G_s protein; a G_i protein is one with an inhibitory effect.

Three second messenger systems are well recognized.

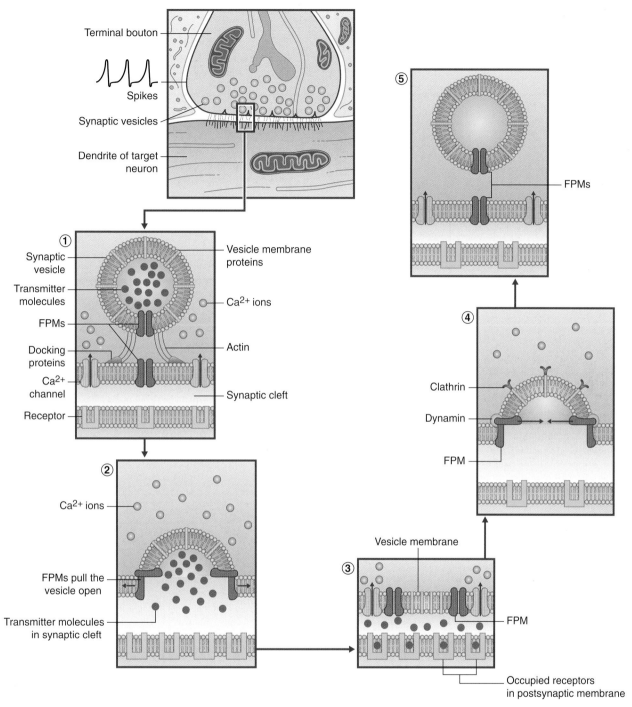

Figure 8.2 Sequence of events following depolarization of the presynaptic membrane. **(1)** Opening of calcium channels *(arrows)* causes synaptic vesicles to be pulled into contact with the presynaptic membrane by actin filaments. Matching pairs of fusion protein macromolecules (FPMs) in the vesicle and presynaptic membrane are aligned. **(2)** The FPMs separate *(outward arrows)*, permitting transmitter molecules to enter the synaptic cleft. **(3)** Vesicle membrane is incorporated into the presynaptic membrane while transmitter is activating the specific receptors. **(4)** Clathrin molecules assist inward movement of vesicle membrane. Dynamin molecules *(green)* assist approximation of FPM pairs *(inward arrows)* and pinch the neck of the emerging vesicle. **(5)** The vesicle is now free for recycling.

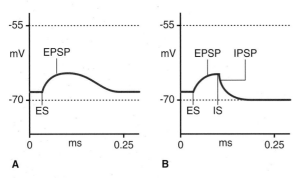

Figure 8.3 (A) A transmitter-gated excitatory ionotropic receptor. Binding of the transmitter *(red,* in this example representing glutamate) has opened the pore of a 'mixed' Na⁺–K⁺ cation channel. A large influx of sodium ions has depolarized the membrane, as shown by the excitatory postsynaptic potential (EPSP). **(B)** A transmitter-gated inhibitory ionotropic receptor. Binding of the transmitter *(blue,* representing GABA$_A$) has opened the pore of a chloride channel. Inward chloride conductance has been increased, and the inhibitory postsynaptic potential (IPSP) restores the membrane potential to its resting state.

1 The cyclic AMP system, responsible for phosphorylation of proteins.
2 The phosphoinositol system, responsible for liberating calcium from cytoplasmic stores.
3 The arachidonic acid system, responsible for production of arachidonic acid metabolites.

Cyclic AMP system

(The abbreviation cyclic AMP represents cyclic adenosine monophosphate.) In the examples shown in Figure 8.4, transmitter–receptor binding releases the alpha subunit of a G$_s$ protein, leaving it free to link with GTP, which in turn facilitates *adenosine cyclase* to convert ATP to cyclic AMP. Protein kinase A in the membrane is stimulated by cyclic AMP to transfer phosphate ions from ATP to an ion channel, causing its pore to admit sodium ions, initiating depolarization of the target neuron. When the G$_s$ protein is switched off, the membrane-attached enzyme *protein phosphatase* catalyzes extraction of the phosphate ions, resulting in pore closure.

Phosphoinositol system

In the example shown in Figure 8.5, activation of another kind of G$_s$ protein alpha subunit causes the effector enzyme *phospholipase C* to split a membrane phospholipid (PIP$_2$) into a pair of second messengers: *diacylglycerol* (DAG) and *inositol phosphate* (IP$_3$). DAG activates protein kinase C, which initiates protein phosphorylation. IP$_3$ diffuses into the cytosol, where it opens calcium-gated channels, mainly in nearby membranes of smooth endoplasmic reticulum. The Ca^{2+} ions activate certain calcium-dependent enzymes downstream, and may open calcium-gated K⁺ (outward) and Cl⁻ (inward) channels with excitatory effect.

Figure 8.4 The cyclic AMP (cAMP) system. The diagram shows the basic steps along the path from a G$_s$ protein-linked receptor via cyclic AMP to an ion channel. **(1)** Transmitter is activating the receptor macromolecule. **(2)** G$_s$ protein α subunit is freed to bind with guanosine triphosphate (GTP). **(3)** GTP links the unit to adenylate cyclase. **(4)** Adenylate cyclase catalyzes synthesis of cyclic AMP from ATP. **(5)** Cyclic AMP activates protein kinase A (PKA). **(6)** PKA transfers phosphate groups from ATP to a sodium ion channel, causing its pore to open and Na⁺ ions to rush into the cytosol, with a depolarizing effect. **(7)** Following inactivation of the G$_s$ protein, dephosphorylation of the channel by a phosphatase enzyme allows the channel pore to close.

Figure 8.5 The phosphoinositol system. The steps indicate the dual function of this system. **(1)** The transmitter activates the receptor macromolecule. **(2)** The G_s protein α subunit is freed to bind with guanosine triphosphate (GTP), which links it to phospholipase C (PLC). **(3)** PLC moves along the membrane and splits the enzyme phospholipase C (PLC) into diacylglycerol (DAG) and inositol triphosphate (IP_3). **(4)** DAG attracts enzyme protein kinase C (PKC) into the membrane, where **(5)** DAG is triggered to phosphorylate several proteins, potentially including ion channels. **(6)** IP_3 activates calcium channels in sacs of smooth endoplasmic reticulum. **(7)** Stored calcium spills out of the channel pore into the cytosol. **(8)** Ca^{2+}-dependent enzymes are activated.

Arachidonic acid system

This is described later, in connection with histamine.

Metabotropic receptors are in general *slow* receptors. Membrane channel effects may continue for hundreds of milliseconds after a single stimulus.

Gene transcription effects

It is also well established that the reflex responses to repetitive stimuli may be either progressively increased (a state of *sensitization,* usually induced by noxious stimuli) or diminished (a state of habituation induced by harmless stimuli). Animal experiments involving reflex arcs involving sets of sensory, internuncial, and motor neurons have shown that a characteristic of sensitization is the development of additional synaptic contacts between the internuncials and the motor neurons, together with additional transmitter synthesis and release. Characteristic of habituation is a reduction of transmitter synthesis and release. All these changes result from *alterations of gene transcription.* Repetitive noxious stimuli cause cyclic AMP to increase its normal rate of activation of protein kinases involved in phosphorylation of proteins that regulate gene transcription. The outcome is increased production of proteins (including enzymes) required for transmitter synthesis, and of other proteins for construction of additional channels and synaptic cytoskeletons. Repetitive harmless stimuli merely reduce the rate of transmitter synthesis and release.

Gene transcription effects are especially important in the context of forming long-term memories (Ch. 34).

TRANSMITTERS AND MODULATORS

Several criteria should be fulfilled for a substance to be accepted as a neurotransmitter.

- The substance must be present within neurons, together with the molecules, including enzymes, required to synthesize it.
- The substance must be released following depolarization of the nerve endings that contain it, and this release must be induced by entry of calcium.
- The postsynaptic membrane must contain specific receptors that will modify the membrane potential of the target neuron.
- The isolated substance must exert the same effect when applied to a target neuron via a micropipette (microiontophoresis).

- Specific antagonist molecules, whether delivered through the circulation or by iontophoresis, must block the effect of the putative ('thought to be') transmitter.
- The physiologic mode of termination of the transmitter effect must be identified, whether it be by enzymatic degradation or by active transport into the parent neuron or adjacent neuroglial cells.

Many transmitters limit their own rate of release by negative feedback activation of autoreceptors in the presynaptic membrane, having the effect of inhibiting further release. Ideally, the existence of specific inhibitory autoreceptors should be established.

The term *neuromodulator* (L. *modulare*, to regulate) has been subject to several interpretations. The most satisfactory appears to derive from the terms *amplitude modulation* and *frequency modulation* in electrical engineering, signifying superimposition of one wave or signal onto another. Figure 8.6 represents a sympathetic and a parasympathetic nerve ending, close to a pacemaker cell (modified cardiac myocyte). This neighborly arrangement of nerve endings is common in the heart, and allows the respective transmitters to modulate each other's activity. The sympathetic nerve ending liberates norepinephrine (noradrenaline), which has a stimulatory effect. The three modulators shown exert their effects via second messenger systems.

The figure caption also refers to *autoreceptors* and *heteroreceptors*. Receptors for a particular transmitter often occur in the presynaptic as well as in the postsynaptic membrane.

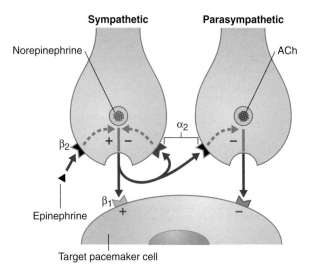

Figure 8.6 Neuromodulation occurs at nerve endings in the sinuatrial node of the heart, where sympathetic and parasympathetic nerve endings often occur in pairs. In this representation, the sympathetic system is the more active, releasing the transmitter norepinephrine, which depolarizes cardiac pacemaker cells via β_1 pacemaker membrane receptors. Circulating epinephrine exerts positive modulation on the nerve ending by increasing transmitter release via β_2 presynaptic membrane heteroreceptors. Inhibitory modulation of excess norepinephrine release is expressed via α_2 presynaptic membrane autoreceptors. At the same time, release of the inhibitory transmitter acetylcholine (ACh) from the parasympathetic bouton is inhibited via α_2 heteroreceptors.

They are called *autoreceptors*. These are activated by high transmitter concentration in the synaptic cleft, and they have a negative feedback effect, inhibiting further transmitter release from the synaptic bouton. *Heteroreceptors* occupy the plasma membrane of neurons that do not liberate the specific transmitter. In the example shown, activity at sympathetic nerve endings is accompanied by inhibition of parasympathetic activity through the medium of heteroreceptors located on parasympathetic nerve endings.

Fate of neurotransmitters

The ultimate fate of transmitters released into synaptic clefts is highly variable. Some transmitters are inactivated within the cleft, some diffuse away into the cerebrospinal fluid via the extracellular fluid, and some are recycled either by direct uptake or indirectly via glial cells.

The principal transmitters and modulators are shown in Table 8.2. Respective receptor types are in Table 8.3.

Table 8.2 Main types of transmitters and modulators, with examples of each[a] The neuropeptides are modulators

Type	Example(s)
Amino acids	Glutamate
	γ-Aminobutyric acid (GABA)
	Glycine
Biogenic amines	Acetylcholine
	Monoamines
	Catecholamines (dopamine, norepinephrine [noradrenaline], epinephrine [adrenaline])
	Serotonin
	Histamine
Neuropeptides	Vasoactive intestinal polypeptide
	Substance P
	Enkephalin
	Endorphins
	Many others
Adenosine	—
Gaseous	Nitric oxide

[a]*The five monoamines contain a single amine group. Catecholamines also contain a catechol nucleus.*

Table 8.3 Receptor types activated by different neurotransmitters

Ionotropic receptors	Metabotropic receptors
Glutamate (AMPA/K)	Glutamate (mGluR)
GABA$_A$	GABA$_A$
Acetylcholine (nicotinic)	Acetylcholine (muscarinic)
Glycine	Dopamine (D$_1$, D$_2$)
Serotonin (5-HT$_3$)	Serotonin (5-HT$_1$, 5-HT$_2$)
	Norepinephrine (noradrenaline) (α_1, α_2), epinephrine (adrenaline)
	Histamine (H$_1$, H$_2$, H$_3$)
	All neuropeptides
	Adenosine

Figure 8.7 The three amino acid transmitters. Glutamate is derived from α-ketoglutarate by the enzyme GABA transaminase (GABA-T); γ-aminobutyric acid (GABA) is derived from glutamate by glutamic acid decarboxylase (GAD). Glycine is the simplest amino acid.

Amino acid transmitters

The most prevalent excitatory transmitter in the brain and spinal cord is the amino acid L-*glutamate* (Figure 8.7). As an important example, *all* neurons projecting into the white matter from the cerebral cortex, regardless of their destinations in other areas of cortex or brainstem or spinal cord, are excitatory and use glutamate as transmitter. Glutamate is derived from α-ketoglutarate; it also provides the substrate for formation of the most common inhibitory transmitter, *GABA*.

GABA is widely distributed in the brain and spinal cord, being the transmitter in approximately one-third of all synapses. Millions of GABAergic neurons form the bulk of the caudate and lentiform nuclei, and they are also concentrated in the hypothalamus, periaqueductal gray matter, and hippocampus. Moreover, GABA is the transmitter for the large Purkinje cells, which are the *only* output cells of the cerebellar cortex, projecting to the dentate and other cerebellar nuclei.

GABA is synthesized from glutamate by the enzyme *glutamic acid decarboxylase.*

A third amino acid transmitter, *glycine*, is the same molecule that is used in the synthesis of proteins in all tissues. It is the simplest of the amino acids, being synthesized from glucose via serine. It is an inhibitory transmitter largely confined to internuncial neurons of the brainstem and spinal cord.

Glutamate

Glutamate acts on specific receptors of both ionotropic and metabotropic kinds. The three ionotropic ones, named after synthetic agonists that activate them, are known as *AMPA, kainate,* and *NMDA* (referring to amino-methylisoxazole propionic acid, kainate, and *N*-methyl-D-aspartate, respectively). Kainate receptors are scarce; they occur in company with AMPA, hence the common use of either AMPA–K or non-NMDA to include both.

Ionotropic glutamate receptors

Activation of AMPA–K receptor channels in the postsynaptic membrane allows an immediate inrush of Na^+ together with a small outward movement of K^+ ions (Figure 8.8), generating the early component of the EPSP in the target neuron. Should this component depolarize the target cell membrane from −65 mV to −50 mV, this will suffice to generate electrostatic repulsion of Mg^{2+} cations that plug the NMDA receptor ion pore at rest. Na^+ ions enter via the pore and generate action potentials. Significantly, Ca^{2+} ions also enter, and the extended period of depolarization (up to 500 ms from a single action potential) allows activation of calcium-dependent enzymes with knock-on capacity to modify the structure and even the number of synaptic contacts in the target cell. The phenomenon of *activity-dependent synaptic modification* is especially detectable in experimental studies of cultured slices of rat hippocampus, and is likely to be important in the generation of short-term memory traces. (For example, the anesthetic drug *ketamine*, which blocks the NMDA channel, also blocks memory formation.) A characteristic effect of repetitive activation of the NMDA receptor is *long-term potentiation*, represented by above-normal EPSP responses even some days after 'training'. (See *long-term depression*, later.)

The role of NMDA receptors in the phenomenon called *glutamate excitotoxicity* has been demonstrated in vascular strokes produced in experimental animals. The mass death of neurons in this kind of experiment is thought to be the result of degradation caused by excess calcium influx in accordance with the following sequence: ischemia > excess calcium influx > activation of calcium-dependent proteases and lipases > degradation of proteins and lipids > cell death. Ischemic damage may be less severe if an NMDA antagonist drug is administered soon after the initial insult.

Metabotropic glutamate receptors

More than 100 different metabotropic glutamate receptors have been identified, all of them being intrinsic membrane proteins, most occupying postsynaptic membranes and having an excitatory function, others occupying presynaptic membranes where they act as inhibitory autoreceptors.

GABA

Two major classes of GABA receptor are recognized, one being ionotropic and the other metabotropic.

Ionotropic GABA receptors

Termed $GABA_A$, these are especially abundant in the limbic lobe of the brain. Each is directly linked to a chloride ion channel (Figure 8.9). Following activation of $GABA_A$ receptors, channel pores are opened and Cl^- ions diffuse down their concentration gradient from synaptic cleft to cytosol. Hyperpolarization up to −80 mV or more is brought about by summation of successive inhibitory postsynaptic potentials (IPSPs) (Figure 8.10).

The *sedative, hypnotic* barbiturates and benzodiazepines, for example diazepam (Valium), exert their effects by activating the natural receptor. So, too, does ethanol. (Loss of

Figure 8.8 Ionotropic glutamate receptors. **(1)** On arrival of action potentials at the nerve terminal, **(2)** calcium channels open, and **(3)** Ca^{2+} ions cause synaptic vesicles to be pulled against the cell membrane. **(4)** Glutamate molecules undergo exocytosis into the synaptic cleft. **(5)** Transmitter binding to the AMPA–K receptor opens the ion channel, permitting large influx of sodium and a small efflux of potassium. **(6)** The resulting excitatory postsynaptic potential (EPSP) produces some 20 mV of depolarization, which **(7)** permits the glutamate ligand to activate the NMDA receptor by expulsion of its Mg^{2+} 'plug'. Both sodium and calcium ions are admitted. **(8)** The NMDA-induced EPSP is sufficient to **(9)** trigger action potentials having an extended repolarization period.

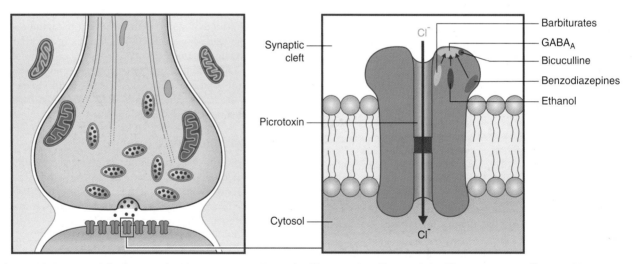

Figure 8.9 Drugs and the ionotropic GABA$_A$ receptor, *Green* signifies agonist effect, *red* signifies antagonist effect. Barbiturates, benzodiazepines, and ethanol exert their hyperpolarizing effect via the natural receptor. Bicuculline antagonizes the receptor, whereas picrotoxin closes the ion pore by direct action locally.

social control under the influence of ethanol may follow the release of target excitatory neurons normally held in check by tonic GABAergic activity.) Some volatile anesthetics also bind with the natural receptor, prolonging the open state of the ion channel.

The chief antagonist at the receptor site is the convulsant drug bicuculline. Another convulsant is picrotoxin, which binds with protein subunits that choke the ion pore when activated.

Metabotropic GABA receptors

Termed *GABA$_B$*, these are relatively uniformly distributed throughout the brain. They are also found within peripheral autonomic nerve plexuses. Although most of their G proteins operate via second messengers, a significant number act *directly*, on a special class of postsynaptic K$^+$ channels known as *GIRK* channels (G protein inwardly rectifying K$^+$ channels). As shown in Figure 8.11, transmitter-binding releases

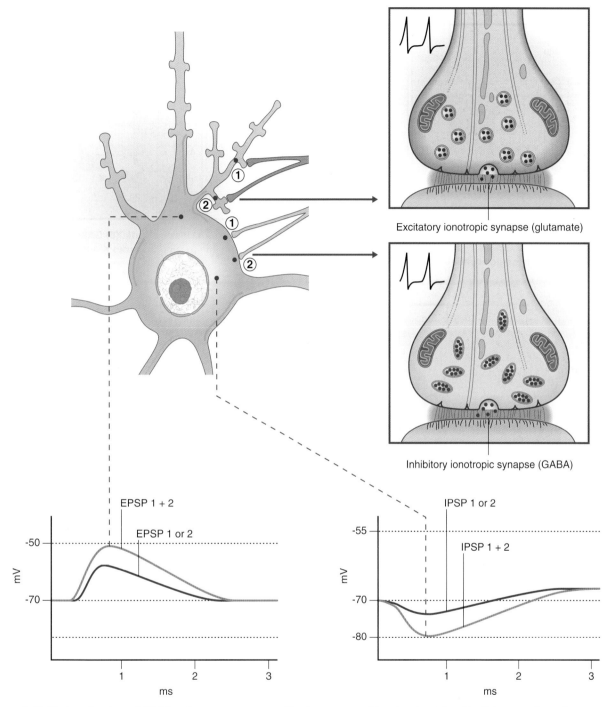

Figure 8.10 Glutamatergic and GABAergic synapses on a multipolar neuron with spiny dendrites. Spatial summation of postsynaptic potentials is illustrated for each pair of synapses.

the βγ subunit, which *expels* K⁺ ions through the GIRK channel, thereby producing an IPSP.

The response properties of the target neuronal receptors are slower and weaker than those of GABA$_A$ ionophores, requiring higher-frequency stimulation to be activated. This has led to the belief that they may be extrasynaptic in position rather than facing the synaptic cleft. This is indicated in Figure 8.12, where the belief is supported by the existence of another type of G-direct channel in extrasynaptic locations. This is a calcium channel that is also voltage-gated, and therefore participates in provision of the calcium ions needed to draw synaptic vesicles against the presynaptic membrane.

Activation of a G–Ca²⁺ ligand site closes Ca²⁺ channels, thereby reducing the effectiveness of action potentials, with inhibitory effect on the parent neuron and on any nearby glutamatergic neurons.

In clinical disorders that involve excessive tonic muscle reflex responses (the state of *spasticity*, Ch. 16), the muscle relaxant *baclofen* is sometimes injected into the subarachnoid space surrounding the spinal cord. The drug seeps into the cord and inhibits release of glutamate from the terminals of muscle afferents, mainly by diminishing the massive calcium entry associated with excessively frequent action potentials.

Figure 8.17 Synthetic pathway of the catecholamine transmitters.

Dopamine Dopamine is of particular interest in the clinical contexts of Parkinson disease, drug addiction, and schizophrenia. It is synthesized from tyrosine in two steps (Figure 8.17), being converted to DOPA (dihydroxyphenylalanine) by *amino acid hydroxylase*, and from DOPA to dopamine by *dopa decarboxylase*, an enzyme restricted to catecholaminergic neurons. The two main sets of dopaminergic neurons are located in the midbrain. They are the substantia nigra and the ventral part of the tegmentum called the ventral tegmental area (VTA).

The substantia nigra belongs functionally to the basal ganglia (Ch. 28). A dopaminergic *nigrostrial pathway* projects from substantia nigra to striatum (caudate nucleus and putamen). This pathway controls a motor loop of neurons feeding forward to the motor cortex. Degeneration of neurons in the substantia nigra is a classic feature of *Parkinson disease*, in which normal movements are disrupted by rigidity of the musculature and/or tremor.

The VTA projects groups of dopaminergic neurons into the forebrain. One group, called *mesocortical,* projects to the prefrontal cortex; overactivity of this system has been invoked to explain some clinical features of schizophrenia (Ch. 29). The other, called *mesolimbic*, projects to several limbic nuclei including the nucleus accumbens (bedded in the ventral striatum); dopamine liberation within the nucleus accumbens appears to be the basis of the *dopamine rush*, or *dopamine high*, associated with several kinds of drug addiction (Ch. 34).

Receptors Dopamine receptors are all G protein-coupled. D_1 and D_2 receptors are recognized, each having more than one subtype. D_1 receptors activate G_s proteins and are excitatory, activating adenylate cyclase with consequent receptor phosphorylation. D_2 receptors activate G_i proteins and are inhibitory; they may inactivate adenylate cyclase, and may also promote hyperpolarization by opening GIRK ion channels and/or inhibiting voltage-gated Ca^{2+} channels. Both kinds are numerous in the striatum, where they are required for the proper execution of learned motor programs including locomotion (Ch. 28).

Norepinephrine In the CNS, noradrenergic neurons are concentrated in the cerulean nucleus (locus ceruleus) in the floor of the fourth ventricle. From here, they project to all parts of the gray matter of the brain and spinal cord (see Figure 24.4). These neurons are important for regulation of the sleep–wake cycle and the control of mood.

In the PNS, norepinephrine is liberated by sympathetic nerve endings, notably throughout the cardiovascular system, where it maintains the blood pressure. It is an integral component of the 'fight or flight' response to danger. Formation of norepinephrine takes place in neurons containing *dopamine β-hydroxylase*. This enzyme is remarkable in being restricted to the inner surface of the membrane of synaptic vesicles.

Receptors All are G protein-gated. They are broadly grouped into alpha and beta sets, with two principal subtypes within each. Some details are provided in Table 8.4.

Catecholamine recycling Recycling of dopamine and norepinephrine occurs via specific reuptake transporters, as indicated in Figure 8.18. The figure indicates that not all the molecules are recycled into synaptic vesicles within the parent neuron. Any of three other fates are possible: some are metabolized in or near the synaptic cleft by the enzyme *COMT;* others are carried for up to 100 μm by the extracellular fluid, perhaps bonding to isolated specific membrane heteroreceptors on other neurons as depicted in Figure 6.6 ('volume transmission'); and others achieve reuptake only to be metabolized by the enzyme *MAO* liberated by nearby mitochondria.

Epinephrine Neuronal production of epinephrine in the CNS appears to be confined to a group of cells in the upper lateral part of the medulla oblongata. Only these contain the enzyme *(phentolamine N-methyltransferase)* that provides the final link in the catecholamine chain (Figure 8.17). Some of these neurons project upward to the hypothalamus, others to the lateral gray horn of the spinal cord. Their functions are not yet clear.

In the PNS, the *chromaffin cells* of the adrenal medulla liberate epinephrine as a hormone into the capillary bed. The

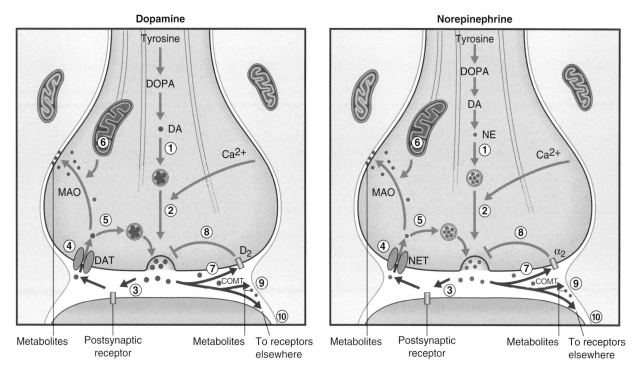

Figure 8.18 History of the main catecholamine transmitter molecules. **(1)** Transmitter dopamine (DA) or norepinephrine (NE) molecules are transported into synaptic vesicles. **(2)** Following depolarization-induced calcium entry to the cytosol, synaptic vesicles are pulled into contact with the presynaptic membrane of the terminal bouton. **(3)** Liberated transmitter molecules have three possible fates. Most bind with G protein-coupled receptors in the postsynaptic membrane, initiating second messenger events. **(4)** Specific transmitter reuptake transporters (DAT, NET) return transmitter molecules to the cytosol. **(5)** Some of these molecules are repackaged for further use. **(6)** Surplus molecules in the cytosol are degraded by mitochondria-derived monoamine oxidase (MAO) enzyme. The metabolites float away in extracellular fluid destined to weep through ventricular walls into the cerebrospinal fluid, where some metabolites may be detected. **(7)** A second group of transmitter molecules within the synaptic cleft are broken down by catechol-O-methyl transferase (COMT). **(8)** A third group function as D_2 or α_2 autoreceptors, inhibiting further transmitter release. **(9)** A second set of metabolites drifting away in the extracellular fluid. **(10)** Some intact transmitter molecules drifting away to activate receptors elsewhere.

Table 8.4 Main features of noradrenergic receptors

Receptor type	Location on neuron	Regions found	Second messenger	Effects
α_1	Postsynaptic	Smooth muscle, brain	Phosphoinositol	Excitatory. Opens calcium channels
α_2	Mainly presynaptic	—	G protein direct	Inhibitory. Opens GIRK channels
β_1	Postsynaptic	Heart, brain	Adenylate cyclase +	Excitatory. Opens calcium channels
β_2	Postsynaptic	Smooth muscle, liver, brain	Adenylate cyclase ±	Inhibitory to smooth muscle. Glycogen breakdown + in liver. Excitatory in brain

epinephrine augments sympathetic effects on the circulatory and other systems during the alarm response to danger. As shown in Figure 13.6, the chromaffin cells are modified sympathetic ganglion cells receiving synaptic contacts from preganglionic cholinergic neurons. One function of circulating epinephrine, illustrated in Figure 13.5, is to boost norepinephrine output at sympathetic nerve terminals by activating β_2 heteroreceptors there.

Serotonin

In the medical literature, more has been written about serotonin than about any other neurotransmitter. Depletion of serotonin has a well-established connection with depression. Abnormalities of serotonin metabolism have been implicated in other behavioral disorders, including anxiety states, obsessive-compulsive disorders, and bulimia.

As indicated in Figures 21.2 and 21.5, serotonergic cell bodies occupy the midregion or raphe (seam) of the brainstem. Their axonal ramifications are quite prodigious, penetrating to every region of the gray matter of brain and spinal cord.

Serotonin, commonly referred to as *5-HT* because it is 5-hydroxytryptamine, is derived from the dietary amino acid tryptophan, present in the circulation. It is actively transported across the blood–brain barrier into the brain extracellular fluid, then transported into serotonergic neurons. Formation of serotonin from tryptophan is a two-step process (Figure 8.19). Tryptophan is converted to 5-hydroxytryptophan by the enzyme *tryptophan hydroxylase*, and this is converted to serotonin by *5-hydroxytrytophan decarboxylase.*

Receptors Seven groups of receptors have been identified. Ongoing research seeks to refine drug therapy so as to target individual receptors thought to be responsible, by either over- or underactivity, for specific disorders, notably in the psychiatric domain.

Table 8.5 provides some details for a selected shortlist of serotonin receptors. The table includes a reference to receptors on the somas and dendrites of the parent cell. These are targets of recurrent axon collaterals, as indicated in Figure 8.20.

Recycling Recycling follows the same general pattern as for the catecholamines. Here again, the final step of transmitter synthesis takes place within the terminal bouton, and the released molecules may activate either presynaptic autoreceptors on the parent neuron or isolated heteroreceptors on other neurons nearby. There appears to be no degradatory enzyme in or near the synaptic cleft comparable with COMT, but MAO is present within the parent bouton (as shown in Figure 8.21).

Monoamines and abnormal emotional or behavioral states

Abnormal monoamine function has been implicated in a great variety of abnormal emotional or behavioral states,

Figure 8.19 Synthesis of serotonin from tryptophan.

Figure 8.20 Serotonergic autoreceptors. 5-HT$_{1A}$ reduce both excitability and serotonin synthesis. 5-HT$_{1D}$ reduce serotonin release. (After Nestler et al. 2001, with permission of McGraw-Hill)

Table 8.5 Some serotonin receptors of clinical interest

Receptor type	Neuronal location	Second messenger	Effect	Activity contributes to
5-HT$_{1A}$	Parent cell somas and dendrites	Inhibits cyclic AMP	Inhibitory	Anxiety, depression, pain
5-HT$_{1D}$	Presynaptic autoreceptors	Inhibits cyclic AMP, opens GIRK channels	Inhibitory	Vasoconstriction. Activation relieves migraine
5-HT$_{2A}$	Target cell somas and dendrites	Stimulates phosphoinositol	Excitatory	Overactivity causes hallucinations
5-HT$_{2C}$	Target cell somas and dendrites	Stimulates phosphoinositol	Excitatory	Overactivity causes increased appetite
5-HT$_3$	Target cell somas and dendrites in area postrema	No: it is ionotropic	Excitatory	Stimulation causes emesis (vomiting)

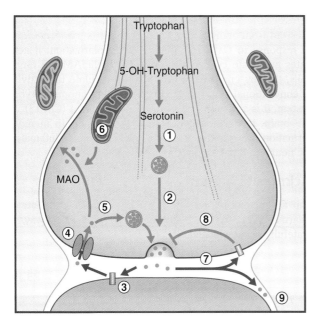

Figure 8.21 History of serotonin transmitter molecules in the central nervous system. **(1)** Serotonin is transported into synaptic vesicles. **(2)** Transmitter molecules undergo exocytosis into the synaptic cleft. **(3)** A postsynaptic serotonin receptor is being targeted. **(4)** The (therapeutically important) serotonin reuptake transporter returns transmitter to the terminal cytosol. **(5)** Some transmitter is repackaged into synaptic vesicles. **(6)** Some is degraded instead by (therapeutically important) monoamine oxidase (MAO). **(7)** Some activates presynaptic autoreceptors. **(8)** A 5-HT$_{1D}$ presynaptic autoreceptor is retarding further transmitter release. **(9)** Some diffuses through the extracellular space, using 'volume transmission' to activate receptors on other neurons.

Figure 8.22 Synthesis of histamine from histidine.

including depression, insomnia, anxiety disorders, panic attacks, and specific phobias. Brain areas involved are discussed in Chapters 23 and 29.

Histamine

Histamine is synthesized from histidine by *histidine decaboxylase,* as shown in Figure 8.22. The somas of histaminergic neurons appear to be confined to the posterior part of the hypothalamus, where they occupy the small *tuberomammillary nucleus* shown in Figure 26.1. However, their axons extend widely, mainly to all parts of the cerebral cortex. The main function of histaminergic neurons is to participate with cholinergic and serotonergic neurons in maintaining the awake state. These neurons are active in the awake state and silent during sleep (see Ch. 24). Activation is a function of the peptide orexin locally produced by lateral hypothalamic neurons. The compulsive daytime sleep disorder known as narcolepsy (Ch. 30) appears to result from failure of orexin production.

Receptors H$_1$, H$_2$ and H$_3$ receptors on target neurons are known. All three activate G proteins. H$_1$ and H$_2$ receptors activate G$_s$ proteins, acting via arachidonic acid production. The acid is processed further to yield prostaglandins and other endoperoxides, some of which modify cyclic AMP activity and others that bind directly to ion channels. The H$_3$ group are inhibitory autoreceptors.

In clinical practice, *antihistamines* are widely prescribed for the purpose of blocking H$_2$ receptors involved in gastric acid secretion and various allergic responses. Drowsiness has been a common side effect of such drugs prior to production of cimetidine and others that are not able to cross the blood–brain barrier.

Neuropeptides

More than 50 neuropeptides have been isolated. All of them are linear chains of amino acids linked by peptide bonds. Peptide precursor chains (called propeptides) are passed through the Golgi complex and budded off in large, dense-cored vesicles that are rapidly transported to the nerve endings, where peptide formation is completed. As previously illustrated in Figure 6.5, peptides undergo non-synaptic release and may travel some distance to reach their receptors.

Receptors

These are all G protein-coupled. In general, they are cotransmitters, and their function is to modulate the effect of principal, small-molecule transmitters such as glutamate or ACh. Calcium channels are relatively scarce outside the synaptic cleft, and peptide liberation characteristically requires relatively high-frequency action potentials. An example is mentioned in Chapter 13: sweat glands are supplied by cholinergic neurons having vasoactive intestinal polypeptide (VIP) as cotransmitter. At low-frequency stimulation, ACh alone is sufficient to provide routine 'insensible perspiration', which is also invisible. *Sweating* for any length of time requires local vasodilatation in addition to an abundance of ACh, and this is provided by VIP, a potent dilator of arterioles.

Within the CNS, naturally occurring *opioid* (opium-like) peptides, called *endorphins,* are highly significant in relation to the control of pain perception, as discussed in Chapter 24.

Adenosine

Adenosine, derived from ATP, is a well-established excitatory cotransmitter with ACh in parasympathetic neurons

9 Peripheral nerves

STUDY GUIDELINES

1. Understand where the limb plexuses fit into the general scheme of the spinal nerves.
2. Be able to name the connective tissue sheath surrounding a nerve trunk, a nerve fascicle, a nerve fiber.
3. Understand how myelin sheaths are composed of cell membranes.
4. Appreciate the functional significance of the nodes of Ranvier, and why thicker nerve fibers conduct faster.
5. Understand why nerves regenerate better following a crush injury than a cut.
6. Recognize the two kinds of transneuronal atrophy.
7. To appreciate the clinical importance of peripheral nerves, we suggest you pay a preliminary visit to the Clinical Panels in Chapter 12.

GENERAL FEATURES

The peripheral nerves comprise the cranial and spinal nerves linking the brain and spinal cord to the peripheral tissues. The spinal nerves are formed by the union of **anterior** and **posterior nerve roots** at their points of exit from the vertebral canal (Figure 9.1). The swelling on each posterior root is a **spinal** or **posterior root ganglion**. The **spinal nerve** is only 1 cm long and occupies an intervertebral foramen. On emerging from the foramen, it divides into **anterior** and **posterior rami**.

The posterior rami supply the erector spinae muscles and the overlying skin of the trunk. The anterior rami supply the muscles and skin of the side and front of the trunk, including the muscles and skin of the limbs; they also supply sensory fibers to the parietal pleura and parietal peritoneum.

The cervical, brachial, and lumbosacral plexuses are derived from anterior rami, which form the *roots* of the plexuses. The term *root* therefore has two different meanings

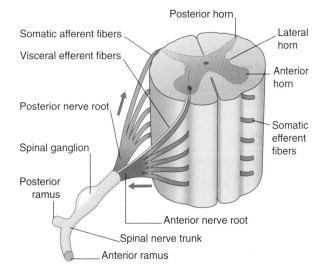

Figure 9.1 Segment of thoracic spinal cord with attached nerve roots. *Arrows* indicate directions of impulse conduction. Green indicates sympathetic outflow.

depending on the context. (Details of the plexuses are in standard anatomy texts.)

The neurons contributing to peripheral nerves are partly contained within the central nervous system (CNS) (Figure 9.2). The cells giving rise to the motor (*efferent*) nerves to skeletal muscles are **multipolar** *alpha* and *gamma* **neurons** of similar configuration to the one depicted in Figure 6.4; in the spinal cord, they occupy the anterior horn of gray matter. Further details are in Chapter 10. Those giving rise to posterior nerve roots are **unipolar neurons** whose cell bodies lie in posterior root ganglia and whose sensory (afferent) central processes enter the posterior horn of gray matter.

The spinal nerves supply *somatic efferent fibers* to the skeletal muscles of the trunk and limbs, and *somatic afferent fibers* to the skin, muscles, and joints. They all carry *visceral efferent,* autonomic fibers, and some spinal nerves contain visceral afferent fibers too.

MICROSCOPIC STRUCTURE OF PERIPHERAL NERVES

Figure 9.3 illustrates the structure of a typical peripheral nerve. It is not possible to designate individual nerve fibers as motor or sensory on the basis of structural features alone.

Peripheral nerves are invested with **epineurium**, a loose, vascular connective tissue sheath surrounding the fascicles (bundles of fibers) that make up the nerve. Nerve fibers are exchanged between fascicles along the course of the nerve.

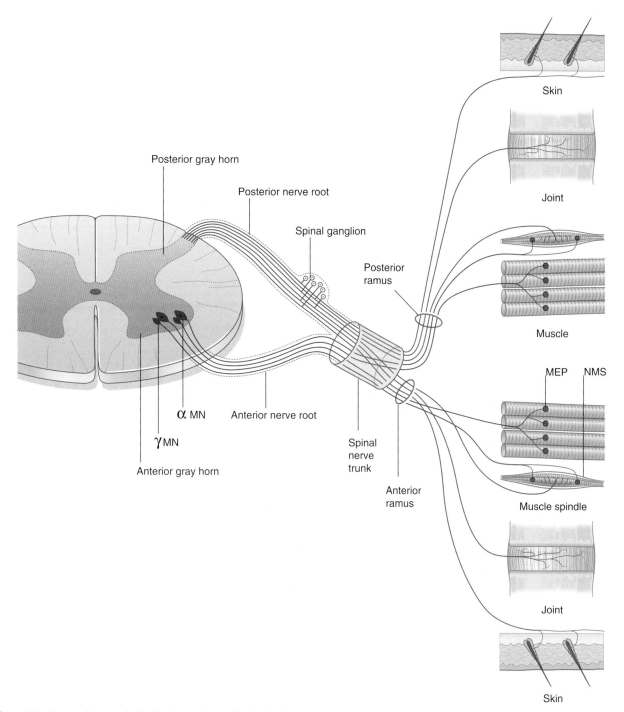

Figure 9.2 Composition and distribution of a cervical spinal nerve. *Note*: The sympathetic component is not shown. MEP, motor end plate; MN, multipolar neurons; NMS, neuromuscular spindle.

Each fascicle is covered by **perineurium**, composed of several layers of pavement epithelium bonded by tight junctions. Surrounding the individual Schwann cells is a network of reticular collagenous fibers, the **endoneurium**.

Less than half of the nerve fibers are enclosed in myelin sheaths. The remaining, unmyelinated fibers travel in deep gutters along the surface of Schwann cells.

The term *nerve fiber* is usually used in the context of nerve impulse conduction, where it is equivalent to *axon.* An anatomic definition is possible for a myelinated fiber: it comprises axon, myelin, and neurolemmal sheaths, and endoneurium. It is not possible for unmyelinated axons because they share *neurolemmal* (Schwann cell) and endoneurial sheaths.

Myelin formation

The **Schwann cell** is the representative neuroglial cell of the peripheral nervous system (PNS). It forms chains of neurolemmal cells along the nerves. Modified Schwann cells form

Figure 9.3 Transverse section of a nerve trunk. **(A)** Light microscopy. **(B)** Electron microscopy.

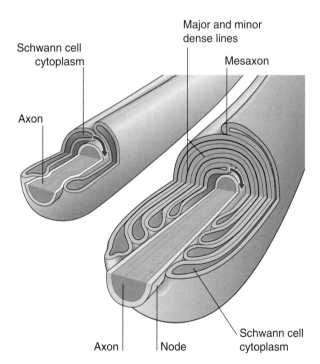

Figure 9.4 Myelination in peripheral nervous system. *Arrows* indicate movement of flange of Schwann cell cytoplasm.

satellite cells in posterior root ganglia and in autonomic ganglia, and **teloglia** at encapsulated sensory nerve endings (Ch. 11).

If an axon is to be myelinated, it receives the simultaneous attention of a sequence of Schwann cells along its length. Each one encloses the axon completely, creating a 'mesentery' of plasma membrane, the **mesaxon** (Figure 9.4). The mesaxon is displaced progressively, being rotated around

the axon. Successive layers of plasma membrane come into apposition to form the **major** and **minor dense lines** (Figure 9.4).

Paranodal pockets of cytoplasm persist at the ends of the myelin segments, on each side of the nodes of Ranvier.

Myelin expedites conduction

Along unmyelinated fibers, impulse conduction is *continuous* (uninterrupted). Its maximum speed is 15 m/s. Along myelinated fibers, excitable membrane is confined to the nodes of Ranvier, because myelin is an electrical insulator. Impulse conduction is called *saltatory* ('jumping'), because it leaps from node to node. Speed of conduction is much greater along myelinated fibers, with a maximum of 120 m/s. The number of impulses that can be conducted by myelinated fibers is also much greater than by unmyelinated ones.

The larger the myelinated fiber, the more rapid the conduction, because larger fibers have longer internodal segments and the nerve impulses take longer 'strides' between nodes. A 'rule of six' can be used to express the ratio between size and speed: a fiber of 10 μm external diameter (i.e. including myelin) will conduct at 60 m/s, one of 15 μm at 90 m/s, and so on.

In physiologic recordings, peripheral nerve fibers are classified in accordance with conduction velocities and other criteria. Motor fibers are classified into groups A, B, and C in descending order. Sensory fibers are classified into types I–IV. In practice, there is some interchange of usage: for example, unmyelinated sensory fibers are usually called C fibers rather than type IV.

Details of diameters and sources are given in Tables 9.1 and 9.2.

The electron micrograph in Figure 9.5 illustrates a myelinated peripheral nerve fiber with attendant Schwann cell, that in Figure 9.6 a group of unmyelinated fibers bedded in the cytoplasm of a Schwann cell, and Figure 9.7 a nodal region within the CNS.

Table 9.1 Classification of peripheral nerve fibers

Nerve type	Number	Letter	Diameter (µm)	Conduction velocity (m/s)
Myelinated				
Large	I	Aα	12–20	70–120
Medium	II	Aβ	6–12	35–70
Small	III	Aγ	3–6	10–40
Small	–	Aδ	2–5	5–35
Unmyelinated	IV	C	0.2–1.5	0.5–2

Table 9.2 Locations of peripheral nerve fiber types

Fiber type	Origin
Sensory	
Ia	Muscle spindle annulospiral endings
Ib	Golgi tendon organs
II (Aβ)	Muscle spindle flower spray endings; touch or pressure receptors in skin and elsewhere
III (Aδ)	Follicular endings; fast pain and thermal receptors
IV (C)	Slow pain, itch, touch receptors
Motor	
Aα	Alpha motor neurons supplying extrafusal muscle fibers
Aγ	Gamma motor neurons supplying intrafusal muscle fibers

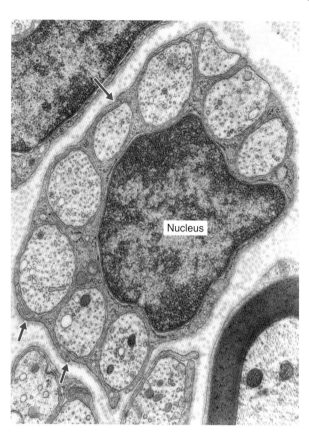

Figure 9.6 Unmyelinated nerve fibers. Nine unmyelinated fibers are lodged in the cytoplasm of this Schwann cell. Mesaxons (*arrows* indicate examples) are detectable where the axons are fully embedded. Two incompletely embedded axons at top right are covered by the basal lamina of the Schwann cell. (From Pannese 1994, with permission of Thieme.)

Central nervous system–peripheral nervous system transitional region

Close to the brainstem and spinal cord, peripheral nerves enter the *CNS–PNS transitional zone* (Figure 9.8). Astrocyte processes reach out of the CNS into the endoneurial compartments of peripheral nerve rootlets and interdigitate with the Schwann cells. In unmyelinated fibers, the astrocytes burrow into the space between axons and Schwann cells. In myelinated fibers, nodes are bounded by Schwann cell myelin (showing some transitional features) on the peripheral side, and by oligodendrocytic myelin centrally.

DEGENERATION AND REGENERATION

When nerves are cut or crushed, their axons degenerate distal to the lesion, because axons are pseudopodial outgrowths and depend on their parent cells for survival. In the PNS, regeneration is vigorous and it is often complete. In the CNS, on the other hand, it is neither vigorous nor complete.

Figure 9.5 Myelinated nerve fiber. Ten lamellae of myelin form a continuous spiral from the outer to the inner mesaxon of the Schwann cell (*arrows*). A basal lamina surrounds the Schwann cell. (From Pannese 1994, with permission of Thieme.)

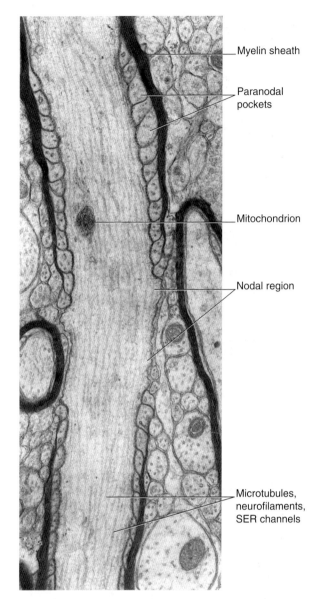

Figure 9.7 Central nervous system nodal region. The myelin sheaths taper as they approach the nodal region, successive wrappings terminating in paranodal pockets of oligodendrocyte cytoplasm. The nodal region is about 10 μm long and lacks any basal lamina. The longitudinal streaks are created by microtubules, neurofilaments, and elongated sacs of smooth endoplasmic reticulum (SER). (From Pannese 1994, with permission of Thieme.)

Wallerian degeneration of peripheral nerves

The principal events in peripheral nerve degeneration are represented in Figure 9.9 and described in the caption. Following a crush or cut injury to a nerve, the axons and myelin sheaths distal to the cut break up into 'elipsoids within the first 48 h – mainly because of Ca^{2+}-activated release of proteases by Schwann cells. The debris is cleared by monocytes that enter the damaged endoneurial sheaths from the blood and become macrophages. In addition to their phagocytic function, the macrophages are mitogenic to Schwann

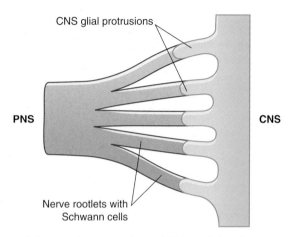

Figure 9.8 Central nervous system (CNS)–peripheral nervous system (PNS) transitional zone.

cells and participate with Schwann cells in provision of trophic (feeding) and tropic (guidance) factors for regenerating axons.

The end result of degeneration is a shrunken nerve skeleton with intact connective tissue and perineurial sheaths, and a core of intact, multiplying Schwann cells.

Regeneration of peripheral nerves

The principal events in regeneration of a peripheral nerve are summarized in Figure 9.9B. Following a clean cut, axons begin to sprout from the face of the proximal stump within a few hours, but in the more common crush or tear injuries seen clinically, the axons die back for 1 cm or more and sprouting may be delayed for a week. Successful regeneration requires that the axons make contact with Schwann cells of the distal stump. Failure to make contact leads to production of a *pseudoneuroma* consisting of whorls of regenerating axons trapped in scar tissue at the site of the initial injury. Following amputation of a limb, an *amputation pseudoneuroma* can be a source of severe pain.

Two reparative events are in simultaneous progress within hours of the injury. In the proximal stump, multiple branchlets begin to extend distally, their tips exhibiting swellings called **growth cones**; in the distal stump, Schwann cells send processes in the direction of the growth cones. The cones are surmounted by antenna-like **filopodia**, and these develop surface receptors that become anchored temporarily to complementary *cell surface adhesion molecules* in Schwann cell basement membranes. Filaments of actin within the filopodia become attached to the surface receptors; from these points of anchorage, they are able to exert onward traction on the growth cones.

Growth cones are mitogenic to Schwann cells, which divide further before wrapping the larger axons with myelin lamellae.

Regeneration proceeds at about 5 mm/day in the larger nerve trunks, slowing down to 2 mm/day in the finer branches. Not surprisingly, the functional outlook is better after a crush injury (endoneurium preserved) than after complete severance. At the same time, filopodia of motor and sensory axons 'recognize' Schwann cell basement membranes previously occupied by axons of similar kind.

Figure 9.9 Events in degeneration of a single myelinated nerve fiber. **(A)** Intact fiber, showing its four components. The fiber is being pinched at its upper end. **(B)** The myelin and axon have broken up into 'ellipsoids' and droplets. Monocytes are entering the endoneurial tube from the blood. **(C)** The droplets are being engulfed by monocytes. **(D)** Clearance of debris is almost complete. Schwann cells and endoneurium remain intact. Events in regeneration. **(E)** An axonal sprout has entered the distal stump. The sprout is mitogenic to each Schwann cell it encounters. **(F)** The growth cone is extending distally along the surface of Schwann cells. **(G)** Myelination is commencing along the proximal part of the regenerating axon. **(H)** When regeneration is complete, the fiber has a normal appearance, but the myelin segments are shorter than the originals.

STUDY GUIDELINES

1 Try to appreciate the vast significance of motor units with respect to movements of all kinds, and to appreciate the functional significance of their sizes and muscle chemistries.
2 Learn to sketch a motor end plate, indicating locations of transmitter, receptor, and hydrolytic enzyme.
3 Sketch an intrafusal muscle fiber, indicating locations of two motor and three sensory nerve endings.
4 Appreciate the functional significance of coactivation of alpha and gamma motor neurons during voluntary movements.
5 With the essentials of this chapter still in mind, consider a first read through the Electromyography section of Chapter 12.

In gross anatomy, the nerves to skeletal muscles are branches of mixed peripheral nerves. The branches enter the muscles about one-third of the way along their length, at *motor points* (Figure 10.1). Motor points have been identified for all major muscle groups for the purpose of *functional electrical stimulation* by physical therapists, in order to increase muscle power.

Only 60% of the axons in the nerve to a given muscle are motor to the muscle fibers that make up the bulk of the muscle. The rest are sensory in nature, although the largest sensory receptors—the neuromuscular spindles—have a motor supply of their own.

MOTOR INNERVATION OF SKELETAL MUSCLE

The nerve of supply branches within the muscle belly, forming a plexus from which groups of axons emerge to

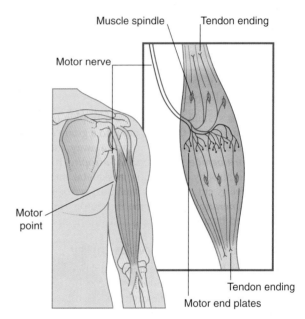

Figure 10.1 Pattern of innervation of skeletal muscle.

supply the muscle fibers (Box 10.1 and Figure 10.1). The axons supply single motor end plates placed about halfway along the muscle fibers (Figure 10.2A).

A *motor unit* comprises a motor neuron in the spinal cord or brainstem together with the *squad* of muscle fibers it innervates. In large muscles (e.g. the flexors of the hip or knee), each motor unit contains 1200 muscle fibers or more. In small muscles (e.g. the intrinsic muscles of the hand), each unit contains 12 muscle fibers or less. Small units contribute to the finely graded contractions used for delicate manipulations.

There are three different types of skeletal muscle fiber.

1 *Slow-twitch, oxidative fibers* are small, rich in mitochondria and blood capillaries (hence, red). They exert small forces and are fatigue-resistant. They are deeply placed and suited to sustained postural activities, including standing.
2 *Fast, glycolytic (FG) fibers* are large, mitochondria-poor, and capillary-poor (hence, white). They produce brief, powerful contractions. They predominate in superficial muscles.
3 *Intermediate (fast, oxidative–glycolytic, FOG)* fibers have properties intermediate between the other two. Every muscle contains all three kinds of fiber, but a given motor unit contains only one kind. The fibers of each unit interdigitate with those of other units.

Box 10.1 Muscle fiber: internal details

A Structures

Six myofibrils

Waves of depolarization

T tubule openings in plasma membrane

Motor end plate

Filaments in a sarcomere

The contractile apparatus consists of myofibrils containing interleaved thick and thin filaments.

Ca^{2+} ions are stored in sacs of sarcoplasmic reticulum

Thick (myosin) filaments float in the sarcoplasm

T tubule

Synaptic vesicles in motor end plate

Thin (actin) filaments are bonded to Z disks

B Sarcomere at rest

ACh receptors on junctional folds initiate action potentials, which enter the tubules and release calcium from the sacs

Released Ca^{2+} ions initiate filament sliding

C Contraction Actin filaments slide along myosin filaments, thus bringing the Z disks closer together and shortening the muscle fiber as a whole

Synaptic vesicles are retrieved

Ca^{2+} ions are retrieved by the sacs

D Relaxation Actin filaments return to starting position

Actin–myosin cross bridges

Myosin filaments

Actin filaments

Troponin

Myosin heads

A Sarcomere at rest

The myosin filaments have globular heads projecting from the sides. Molecules of troponin are studded along the surface of the actin molecules. In the resting state, these two sets of molecules should not be in contact.

B

Actin

Active myosin head

C

D

E

B–E Contraction

Because the sarcomeres are cylindric, the myosin heads project like spokes of a wheel rather than oars of a boat. But their action resembles that of pairs of oars: successive groups grab the troponin studs and flick the actin filaments along at great speed. Maximal muscle contraction results in a 'crumple' of actin filaments arriving in the middle of the sarcomeres from opposite halves.

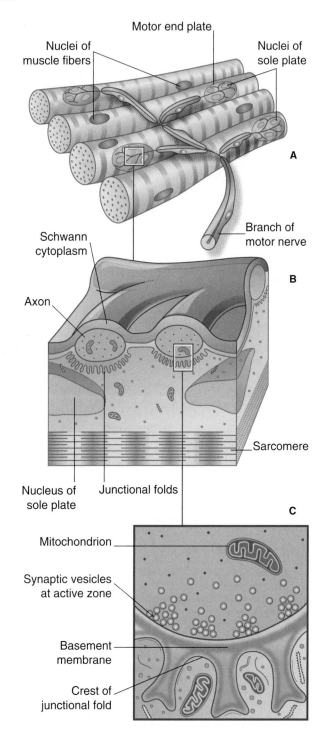

Figure 10.2 Motor nerve supply to skeletal muscle. **(A)** Four motor end plates supplied from a single axon. **(B)** Enlargement from (A). **(C)** Enlargement from (B), showing active zones.

Motor end plates

At the **myoneural junction**, the axon divides into a handful of branchlets that groove the surface of the muscle fiber (Figure 10.2B). The underlying sarcolemma is thrown into **junctional folds**. The basement membrane of the muscle fiber traverses the synaptic cleft and lines the folds. The underlying sarcoplasm shows an accumulation of nuclei, mitochondria, and ribosomes known as a **sole plate**.

Each axonal branchlet forms an elongated terminal bouton containing thousands of synaptic vesicles loaded with acetylcholine (ACh). Synaptic transmission takes place at **active zones** facing the crests of the junctional folds (Figure 10.2C). Vesicular ACh is extruded at great speed by exocytosis into the synaptic cleft. The ACh diffuses through the basement membrane to bind with ACh receptors in the sarcolemma.

Activation of the receptors leads to depolarization of the sarcolemma. The depolarization is led into the interior of the muscle fiber by **T tubules**. The sarcoplasmic reticulum liberates Ca^{2+} ions that initiate contraction of the sarcomeres.

Acetylcholinesterase enzyme is concentrated in the basement membrane, and about 30% of released ACh is hydrolyzed without reaching the postsynaptic membrane. Following hydrolysis, the choline moiety is returned to the axoplasm.

Also in terminal boutons are some dense-cored vesicles containing one or more peptides (Figure 12.2C). Best known is *calcitonin gene-related peptide*, a potent vasodilator.

Details of the muscle fiber contraction process are in Box 10.2.

Motor units in the elderly

Progressive wasting of muscles seen in the elderly is mainly due to loss of motor neurons from the spinal cord and brainstem, often due in part to low-grade peripheral neuropathy arising from vascular disease and/or nutritional deficiency. Electromyographic records taken from contracting muscles show *giant motor unit potentials* during the seventh and eighth decades. The extra-large potentials result from takeover of vacated motor end plates of lost motor neurons by collateral sprouts from the axons of adjacent healthy motor units. Details of electromyography, and of clinical neuromuscular disorders, are in Chapter 12.

SENSORY INNERVATION OF SKELETAL MUSCLE

Neuromuscular spindles

Muscle spindles are up to 1 cm in length and vary in number from a dozen to several hundred in different muscles. They are abundant (a) in the antigravity muscles along the vertebral column, femur, and tibia; (b) in the muscles of the neck; and (c) in the intrinsic muscles of the hand. All these muscles are rich in slow, oxidative muscle fibers. Spindles are scarce where FG or FOG fibers predominate.

Muscle spindles contain up to a dozen **intrafusal muscle fibers** (Figure 10.3). (Ordinary muscle fibers are extrafusal in this context.) The larger intrafusal fibers emerge from the **poles** (ends) of the spindles and are anchored to connective tissue (perimysium). Smaller ones are anchored to the collagenous spindle capsule. At the spindle **equator** (middle), the sarcomeres are replaced almost entirely by nuclei, in the form of 'bags' (in wide fibers) or 'chains' (in slender fibers).

Innervation

Muscle spindles have both a motor and a sensory nerve supply. The motor fibers, called *fusimotor*, are in the Aγ size range, in contrast to the Aα fibers supplying extrafusal

Box 10.2 Muscle fiber contraction

This flow diagram shows the sequential events taking place during the contraction of a single striated muscle fiber.

Muscle fiber diagram revealing internal details. T tubules join up to form rings, completing 'triads' of rings around the sarcomeres along with neighboring pairs of sarcoplasmic sacs, having the function of releasing calcium ions from the sacs when the tubules are depolarized.

Muscle fiber actin comprises a twisted pair of polymerized actin monomers, a double strand of tropomyosin, and a troponin molecular complex at regular intervals.

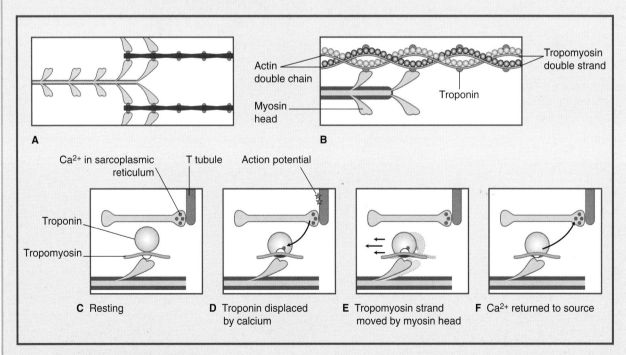

Excitation–contraction coupling:
Calcium liberated by tubule depolarization causes displacement of troponin, with exposure of actin binding sites to which myosin heads attach and pull the thin fiber toward the center of the sarcomere. The required energy is provided by ATPase enzyme contained in the myosin heads. Calcium is returned to source and the muscle actively relaxes by using ATPase to detach the myosin heads from the binding sites.

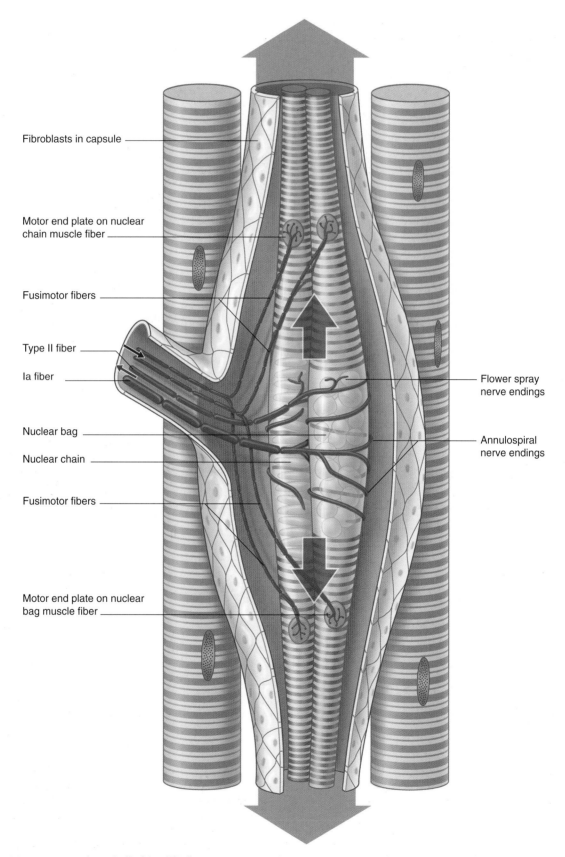

Fibroblasts in capsule

Motor end plate on nuclear chain muscle fiber

Fusimotor fibers

Type II fiber

Ia fiber

Nuclear bag

Nuclear chain

Fusimotor fibers

Motor end plate on nuclear bag muscle fiber

Flower spray nerve endings

Annulospiral nerve endings

Figure 10.3 Neuromuscular spindle (simplified). *Large arrows* indicate passive stretch of the annulospiral endings produced by lengthening of the relaxed muscle as a whole. *Medium arrows* indicate active stretch of annulospiral endings produced by activity of fusimotor nerve fibers. Active stretch more than compensates for the unloading effect of simultaneous extrafusal muscle fiber contraction. *Small arrows* indicate directions of impulse conduction to and from the spindle when the parent muscle is in use.

muscle. The fusimotor axons divide to supply the striated segments at both ends of the intrafusal muscles (Figure 10.3). A single *primary* sensory fiber of type Ia caliber applies *annulospiral* wrappings around the bag or chain segments of the intrafusal muscle fibers. *Secondary*, 'flower spray' sensory endings on one or both sides of the primary are supplied by type II fibers.

Activation

Muscle spindles are *stretch receptors*. Ion channels in the surface membrane of the sensory terminals are opened by stretch, creating positive electronic waves that summate close to the final heminode of the parent sensory fiber. Summation produces a *receptor potential* that will fire off nerve impulses when it reaches threshold.

Muscle spindles may be stretched either *passively* or *actively*.

Passive stretch

Passive stretch of muscle spindles occurs when an entire muscle belly is passively lengthened. For example, in eliciting a tendon reflex such as the *knee jerk*, the spindles in the belly of the quadriceps muscle are passively stretched when the tendon is struck. The type Ia and type II fibers discharge to the spinal cord, where they synapse on the dendrites of α motor neurons (Figure 10.4). (α Motor neurons are so called because they give rise to axons of Aα diameter.) The response to the *positive feedback* from spindles is a twitch of contraction in the extrafusal muscle fibers of quadriceps. The spindles, because they lie in parallel with the extrafusal muscle, are passively shortened; they are described as being *unloaded*.

Tendon reflexes are monosynaptic reflexes. They have a *latency* (stimulus–response interval) of about 15–25 ms.

In addition to exciting homonymous motor neurons (i.e. motor neurons supplying the same muscles), the spindle afferents *inhibit* the α motor neurons supplying the antagonist muscles, through the medium of inhibitory internuncial (interposed) neurons (Figure 10.4). This effect is called *reciprocal inhibition*. The inhibitory neurons involved are called *Ia internuncials*.

Information coding

Spindle primary afferents are most active *during* the stretching process. The more rapid the stretch, the more impulses they fire off. They therefore encode the *rate* of muscle stretch.

Spindle secondary afferents are more active than the primaries when a given position is held. The greater the degree of *maintained* stretch, the more impulses they fire off. They therefore encode the *degree* of muscle stretch.

Active stretch

Active stretch is produced by the fusimotor neurons, which elicit contraction of the striated segments of the intrafusal muscle fibers. Because the connective tissue attachments are relatively fixed, the intrafusal fibers stretch the spindle equators by pulling them in the direction of the spindle poles (Figure 10.5). (This could be called a 'Christmas cracker' effect.)

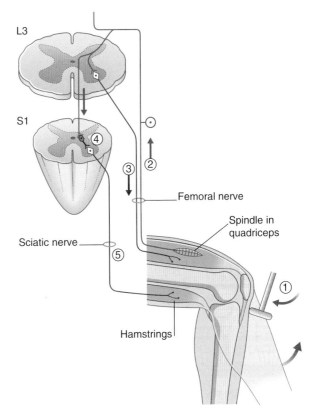

Figure 10.4 Patellar reflex, including reciprocal inhibition. *Arrows* indicate nerve impulses. **(1)** A tap to the patellar ligament stretches the spindles in quadriceps femoris. **(2)** Spindles discharge excitatory impulses to the spinal cord. **(3)** Alpha motor neurons respond by eliciting a twitch in quadriceps, with extension of the knee. **(4 and 5)** Ia inhibitory internuncials respond by suppressing any activity in the hamstrings.

During all voluntary movements, *Aα and Aγ motor neurons are coactivated by the corticospinal (pyramidal) tract.* As a result, the spindles are *not* unloaded by extrafusal muscle contraction. Through ascending connections, the spindle afferents on both sides of the relevant joints are able to keep the brain informed about contractions and relaxations during any given movement.

Tendon endings

Golgi tendon organs are found at muscle–tendon junctions (Figure 10.6). A single Ib caliber nerve fiber forms elaborate sprays that intertwine with tendon fiber bundles enclosed within a connective tissue capsule.

A dozen or more muscle fibers insert into the intracapsular tendon fibers, which are *in series* with the muscle fibers. The bulbous nerve endings are activated by the tension that develops during muscle contraction. Because the rate of impulse discharge along the parent fiber is related to the applied tension, tendon endings signal the *force* of muscle contraction.

The Ib afferents exert *negative feedback* on to the homonymous motor neurons, in contrast to the positive feedback exerted by muscle spindle afferents. The effect is called *autogenetic inhibition*, and the reflex arc is disynaptic

COMPONENTS OF THE AUTONOMIC NERVOUS SYSTEM

The autonomic ('self-regulating') nervous system is distributed to the peripheral tissues and organs by way of outlying autonomic ganglia. Controlling centers in the hypothalamus and brainstem send central autonomic fibers to synapse upon preganglionic neurons located in the gray matter of the brainstem and spinal cord. From these neurons, *preganglionic fibers* (mostly myelinated) project out of the CNS to synapse upon multipolar neurons in the autonomic ganglia. Unmyelinated *postganglionic fibers* emerge and form terminal networks in the target tissues.

Both anatomically and functionally, the autonomic system is composed of sympathetic and parasympathetic divisions.

SYMPATHETIC NERVOUS SYSTEM

The sympathetic system is so called because it acts in sympathy with the emotions. In association with rage or fear, the sympathetic system prepares the body for 'fight or flight': the heart rate is increased, the pupils dilate, and the skin sweats. Blood is diverted from the skin and intestinal tract to the skeletal muscles, and the sphincters of the alimentary and urinary tracts are closed.

The sympathetic outflow from the nervous system is *thoracolumbar*, the preganglionic neurons being located in the lateral gray horn of the spinal cord at thoracic and upper two (or three) lumbar segmental levels. From these neurons, preganglionic fibers emerge in the corresponding anterior nerve roots and enter the paravertebral sympathetic chain. The fibers do one of four things (Figure 13.1):

1 Some fibers synapse in the nearest ganglion. Postganglionic fibers enter spinal nerves T1–L2 and supply blood vessels, sweat glands and erector pili (hair-raising) muscles in the territory of these nerves.
2 Some fibers *ascend* the sympathetic chain and synapse in the superior or middle cervical ganglion, or in the stellate ganglion. (The stellate consists of the fused inferior

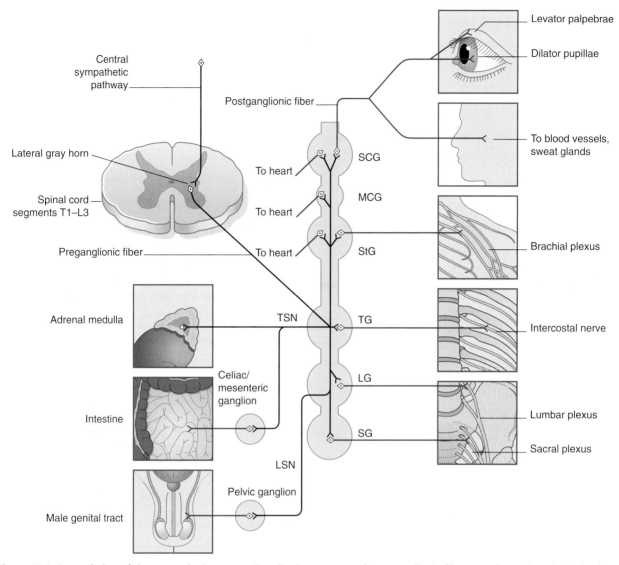

Figure 13.1 General plan of the sympathetic system. Ganglionic neurons and postganglionic fibers are shown in *red*. LG, lumbar ganglia; LSN, lumbar splanchnic nerve; MCG, middle cervical ganglion; SCG, superior cervical ganglion; SG, sacral ganglia; StG, stellate ganglion; TG, thoracic ganglia; TSN, thoracic splanchnic nerve.

cervical and first thoracic ganglia; it lies in front of the neck of the first rib.) Postganglionic fibers supply the head, neck, and upper limbs; also the heart. Of particular importance is the supply to the dilator muscle of the pupil (Clinical Panel 13.1).

3 Some fibers *descend* to synapse in lumbar or sacral ganglia of the sympathetic chain. Postganglionic fibers enter the lumbosacral plexus for distribution to the blood vessels and skin of the lower limbs.

4 Some fibers *traverse* the chain and emerge as the (preganglionic) thoracic and lumbar splanchnic nerves. The thoracic splanchnic nerves (usually called, simply, the splanchnic nerves) pass through the lower eight thoracic ganglia, pierce the diaphragm, and synapse within the abdomen in the celiac and mesenteric prevertebral ganglia, and in renal ganglia. Postganglionic fibers accompany branches of the aorta to reach the gastrointestinal tract, liver, pancreas, and kidneys. Lumbar splanchnic nerves pass through the upper three lumbar ganglia and meet in front of the bifurcation of the abdominal aorta. They enter

the pelvis as the hypogastric nerves before ending in pelvic ganglia, from which the genitourinary tract is supplied.

The medulla of the adrenal gland is the homolog of a sympathetic ganglion, being derived from the neural crest. It receives a direct input from fibers of the thoracic splanchnic nerve of its own side (see later).

The sympathetic system exerts tonic (continuous) constrictor activity on blood vessels in the limbs. In order to improve the blood flow to the hands or feet, impulse traffic along the sympathetic system can be interrupted surgically (Clinical Panel 13.1).

PARASYMPATHETIC NERVOUS SYSTEM

The parasympathetic system generally has the effect of counterbalancing the sympathetic system. It adapts the eyes for

Clinical Panel 13.1 Sympathetic interruption

Stellate block

Injection of local anesthetic around the stellate ganglion – *stellate block* – is a procedure used in order to test the effects of sympathetic interruption on blood flow to the hand. Both pre- and postganglionic fibers are inactivated, producing sympathetic paralysis in the head and neck on that side, as well as in the upper limb. A successful stellate block is demonstrated by (a) a warm, dry hand, (b) *Horner's syndrome*, which consists of a constricted pupil owing to unopposed action of the pupillary constrictor, and (c) *ptosis* (drooping) of the upper eyelid owing to paralysis of smooth muscle fibers contained in the levator muscle of the upper eyelid (Figure CP 13.1.1).

Dominance of the right stellate ganglion in control of the heart rate is shown by the marked slowing of

the pulse following a right, but not a left, stellate block. (See also Box 13.1.)

Functional sympathectomy of the upper limb may be carried out by cutting the sympathetic chain below the stellate ganglion. This is not an anatomical sympathectomy because the ganglionic supply to the limb from the middle cervical and stellate ganglia remains intact. It is a functional one because the ganglionic neurons for the limb are deprived of tonic sympathetic drive. Horner's syndrome is avoided by making the cut at the level of the second rib: the preganglionic fibers for the head and neck enter the stellate direct from the first thoracic spinal nerve.

Two indications for interruption of the sympathetic supply to one or both upper limbs are painful blanching of the fingers in cold weather (*Raynaud phenomenon*), and *hyperhidrosis* (excessive sweating) of the hands – usually an embarrassing affliction of teenage girls.

The sympathetic supply to the eye is considered further in Chapter 23.

Lumbar sympathectomy

In order to improve blood flow in the lower limb, the preganglionic nerve supply may be interrupted by cutting the upper end of the lumbar sympathetic chain. The usual procedure is to remove the second and third lumbar sympathetic ganglia. In males, bilateral lumbar sympathectomy may result in persistent, painful erections (*priapism*) because of interruption of a pathway that maintains the resting, flaccid state of the penis.

Figure CP 13.1.1 Horner's syndrome, patient's right side. Note the moderate ptosis of the eyelid, and the moderate miosis (pupillary constriction). The affected pupil reacts to light but recovers very slowly.

---

close-up viewing, slows the heart, promotes secretion of salivary and intestinal juices, and accelerates intestinal peristalsis. A notable instance of *concerted* sympathetic and parasympathetic activity occurs during sexual intercourse (Box 13.4).

The parasympathetic outflow from the CNS is *craniosacral* (Figure 13.2). Preganglionic fibers emerge from the brainstem in four cranial nerves – the oculomotor, facial, glossopharyngeal, and vagus – and from sacral segments of the spinal cord.

Cranial parasympathetic system

Preganglionic parasympathetic fibers emerge in four cranial nerves (Figure 13.3):

1 In the oculomotor nerve, to synapse in the **ciliary ganglion**. Postganglionic fibers innervate the sphincter of the pupil and the ciliary muscle. Both muscles act to produce the *accommodation reflex*.
2 In the facial nerve, to synapse in the **pterygopalatine ganglion**, which innervates the lacrimal and nasal glands; and in the **submandibular ganglion**, which innervates the submandibular and sublingual glands.

3 In the glossopharyngeal nerve, to synapse in the **otic ganglion**, which innervates the parotid gland.
4 In the vagus nerve, to synapse in **mural** ('on the wall') or **intramural** ('in the wall') ganglia of heart, lungs, lower esophagus, stomach, pancreas, gall bladder, small intestine, and ascending and transverse parts of the colon.

Sacral parasympathetic system

The sacral segments of the spinal cord occupy the conus medullaris (conus terminalis) at the lower extremity of the spinal cord, behind the body of the first lumbar vertebra. From the lateral gray matter of segments S2, S3 and S4, preganglionic fibers descend in the cauda equina within ventral nerve roots. Upon emerging from the pelvic sacral foramina, the fibers separate out as the pelvic splanchnic nerves. Some fibers of the left and right pelvic splanchnic nerves synapse on ganglion cells in the wall of the distal colon and rectum. The rest synapse in **pelvic ganglia**, close to the pelvic sympathetic ganglia already mentioned. Postganglionic parasympathetic fibers supply the detrusor muscle of the bladder; also the tunica media of the internal pudendal

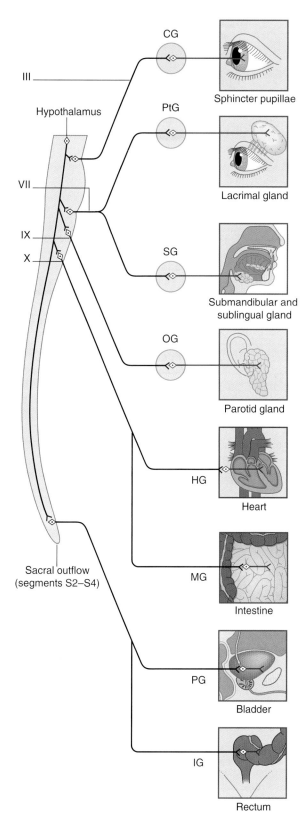

Figure 13.2 General plan of the parasympathetic system. Ganglionic neurons and postganglionic fibers are shown in *red*. CG, ciliary ganglion; HG, heart ganglia; IG, intramural ganglia; MG, myenteric ganglia; OG, otic ganglion; PtG, pterygopalatine ganglion; SG, submandibular ganglion.

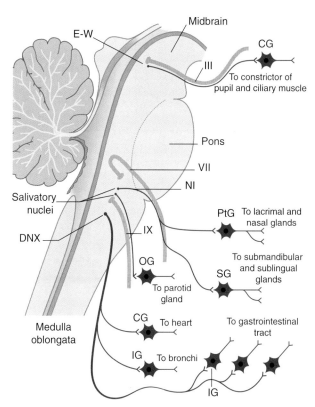

Figure 13.3 Cranial parasympathetic system. E–W, Edinger–Westphal nucleus; DNX, dorsal nucleus of vagus. Other abbreviations as in Figure 13.2.

artery and of its branches to the cavernous tissue of the penis/clitoris (see later).

NEUROTRANSMISSION IN THE AUTONOMIC SYSTEM

Ganglionic transmission

The preganglionic neurons of the sympathetic and parasympathetic systems are *cholinergic*: the neurons liberate acetylcholine (ACh) on to the ganglion cells at axodendritic synapses (Figure 13.4). The receptors on the ganglion cells are nicotinic, so named because the excitatory effect can be imitated by locally applied nicotine.

Junctional transmission

Postganglionic fibers of the sympathetic and parasympathetic systems form *neuroeffector junctions* with target tissues (Figure 13.4). Transmitter substances are liberated from innumerable varicosities strung along the course of the nerve fibers.

The chief transmitter at sympathetic neuroeffector junctions is *norepinephrine (noradrenaline)*, which is liberated from dense-cored vesicles. The postganglionic sympathetic system in general is described as *adrenergic*. An exception to the adrenergic rule is the *cholinergic* sympathetic supply to the eccrine sweat glands over the body surface.

Box 13.3 *Continued*

5 The detrusor responds to postganglionic stimulation by contracting uniformly to expel the urine.
6 The rhabdosphincter, slave to Onuf, contracts to expel urine from the urethral canal.
7 Levator ani contracts to resume its supportive role.
8 Bladder filling recommences, while the bladder wall is rendered *compliant* by tonic inhibitory α_2 action of the sympathetic system on the detrusor muscle and by β_2 receptors on parasympathetic terminals.
9 When the bladder is half-full, the stretch receptor afferents from the detrusor inform higher level neurons in the brainstem, as described in Box 21.2.

Notes on urinary incontinence
Urinary incontinence afflicts about 30% of the female population at one or more periods of their lives. Two types are described.

Stress incontinence is characterized by loss of small amounts of urine caused by a sudden brief rise in intra-abdominal pressure caused, e.g., by sneezing or coughing. Its origin is attributed to weakness of the pelvic floor following pregnancy, childbirth and/or menopause. In males it may be a problem following prostatectomy.

Urge incontinence is caused by *detrusor overactivity* and characterized by spontaneous expulsion of urine during the filling phase of the micturition cycle despite conscious attempts to inhibit it. (See Clinical Panel 24.1.)

REFERENCES
De Groat WC: Integrative control of the lower urinary tract: preclinical perspective, *Br J Pharmacol* 147:S25–S40, 2006.
FitzGerald MJT, Mueller E: Physiology of the lower urinary tract, *Clin Obstet Gynecol* 47:18–27, 2004.

---

stimulation of the anterior hypothalamus; and/or through a spinal reflex arc in response to direct genital stimulation. Activation produces smooth muscle relaxation, with flooding of the cavernous spaces. In females, a transmural exudate into the vagina acts as a lubricant for the penis. In the male, the single bulbourethral gland lubricates the urethra to facilitate passage of semen.

INTERACTION OF THE AUTONOMIC AND IMMUNE SYSTEMS

The lymphatic tissues of the thymus, lymph nodes, and spleen are richly supplied with adrenergic nerve fibers. So, too, is the bone marrow. Adrenoceptors have been found on T cells, B cells, and macrophages.

During acute psychological stress, raised levels of circulating norepinephrine may induce lymphatic tissue to respond by increasing the number of natural killer cells and cytotoxic lymphocytes. The consequent reduction of immune response to pathogens results in increased susceptibility to infections.

VISCERAL AFFERENTS

Afferents from thoracic and abdominal viscera utilize autonomic pathways to reach the CNS. They participate in important reflexes involved in the control of circulation, respiration, digestion, micturition, and coition.

Visceral activities are not normally perceived, but they do reach conscious levels in a variety of disease states. *Visceral pain is of immense importance in the context of clinical diagnosis.*

Visceral pain

There are three fundamental types of visceral pain:

1 *Pure visceral pain*, felt in the region of the affected organ.
2 *Visceral referred pain*, projected subjectively into the territory of the corresponding somatic nerves.
3 *Viscerosomatic pain*, caused by spread of disease to somatic structures.

Pure visceral pain

Pure visceral pain is characteristically vague and deep-seated. It is often accompanied by sweating or nausea. It is experienced as the initial pain in association with inflammation and/or ulceration in the alimentary tract; with obstruction of the intestine, bile duct, or ureter; or when the capsule of a solid organ (liver, kidney, pancreas) is stretched by underlying disease. In marked contrast, the viscera are completely insensitive to cutting or burning.

Visceral referred pain

As its severity increases, visceral pain is 'referred' to somatic structures innervated from the same segmental levels of the spinal cord. For example, the pain of myocardial ischemia is referred to the chest wall ('angina pectoris'), pains of biliary or intestinal origin are referred to the anterior abdominal wall, and labor pains are referred to the sacral area of the back.

According to the generally accepted 'convergence–projection' theory of referred pain, the brain falsely interprets the source of noxious stimulation because visceral and

Box 13.4 Functional innervation of male genital tract (Figure Box 13.4.1)

1 *Erection*. Psychic stimulation of the central *parasympathetic* pathway activates selected preganglionic neurons (P) to pelvic ganglia supplying parasympathetic fibers to the internal pudendal artery, where muscarinic and VIP receptors cause the artery to relax, allowing blood to distend the penile cavernous tissue spaces. Cholinergic fibers also cause the relaxant transmitter nitric oxide to be released from the lining epithelium of the cavernous spaces.

2 *Secretion*. Parasympathetic ganglia in the walls of the prostate and seminal vesicles are stimulated to cause glandular secretion (via muscarinic receptors on the acini). These secretions contribute 80% of total semen volume.

Figure Box 13.4.1 Functional innervation of male genital tract.

Box 13.4 *Continued*

3 *Emission.* Psychic stimulation of the central *sympathetic* pathway activates preganglionic neurons to pelvic ganglia supplying fibers to α_1 receptors on the smooth muscle of vas deferens, seminal vesicles, prostate and internal urethral (*preprostatic*) sphincter. Sperm and glandular contents are expelled into the urethra while the sphincter prevents backfire into the bladder. Simultaneous activation of bladder β_2 receptors prevents detrusor contraction.

4 *Ejaculation.* Entry of semen into the urethra activates somatic afferent nerve endings provided by the pudendal nerve. Through a reflex arc at S2–S4 segmental levels, somatic motor fibers in the pudendal nerve cause rhythmic contractions of the bulbospongiosus muscles to ejaculate ('throw out') the semen into the vagina.

5 *Detumescence.* Selected central sympathetic fibers activate preganglionic neurons to pelvic sympathetic ganglia supplying fibers to α_1 receptors on pudendal arterioles at points of entry into the cavernous spaces. Arteriolar constriction results in detumescence.

The sympathetic system and psychogenic impotence

In addition to the prevertebral supply of the vas deferens mentioned above (3), a second, 'paravertebral' sympathetic pathway relays in the sacral sympathetic chain to supply the trabecular tissue, rich in β_2 adrenoreceptors. The resting, flaccid state of the penis depends upon tonic activity in this pathway. In this context, the corpus cavernosum resembles a well-muscled artery. For erection to take place, the sympathetic supply must be switched off while the parasympathetic, relaxant supply is switched on. Both events may be coordinated at the level of the hypothalamus. Failure to switch off tonic sympathetic activity is regarded as the commonest immediate cause of *psychogenic impotence*, defined as impotence in the presence of intact anatomical pathways. Damage to reflex arcs, e.g. by spinal cord injury (Ch. 16), may cause *reflexive impotence*.

REFERENCE

Karadeniz T, Topsakal M, Aydogmus A, Basak D: Erectile dysfunction under age 40: etiology and role of contributing factors, *Scientific World Journal* (Suppl 1):171–174, 2004.

somatic nociceptors have some spinothalamic neurons in common; in previous experience, these neurons habitually signaled somatic pain.

Viscerosomatic pain

The parietal serous membranes (pleura and peritoneum) receive a rich sensory supply from the overlying intercostal nerves, and they are exquisitely sensitive to acute inflammatory exudates. The extension of an inflammatory process to the surface of stomach, intestine, appendix, or gallbladder gives rise to a severe, steady pain in the abdominal wall directly overlying the inflamed organ. With the onset of acute peritonitis, the abdominal wall is 'splinted' by the muscles in a protective reflex.

Tenderness

Tenderness is *pain elicited by palpation*. In the abdomen, it is sought by pressing the hand and fingers against the abdominal wall. The clinician is, in effect, clothing the finger pads with the patient's parietal peritoneum and using this to seek out an inflamed organ. If the organ is mobile, like the appendix, 'shifting tenderness' may be elicited if the patient is willing to roll from one side to the other.

Pain and the mind

Although visceral pain has well-established causative mechanisms (inflammation, spasm of smooth muscle, ischemia, distension), thoracic or abdominal pain may be experienced in the complete absence of visceral disease. Pain that recurs or persists over a long period (months), and is not accounted for by standard investigational procedures, is more likely to have a *psychological* rather than a physical explanation. This is not to deny that the pain is real, but to imply that it originates within the brain itself. An example is the abused child whose abdominal pains represent a cry for help. In adults, recurrent and rather ill-defined pains are a common manifestation of *major depression* (see Ch. 26).

Irritable bowel syndrome is a very common disorder usually arising in the third or fourth decade. In this syndrome there *is* evidence of abnormality at intestinal cellular level, but alterations of bowel behavior appear to be heightened by a *disorder of the brain–gut axis* (Clinical Panel 13.4).

Note on vascular afferents

Two *vascular* sets of unipolar neurons are customarily included in descriptions of the visceral afferent system. One supplies the carotid sinus and aortic arch with stretch receptors involved in the maintenance of the systemic blood pressure (Ch. 24); the other supplies the carotid body with chemoreceptors and is involved in respiratory control (Ch. 24). There is a progressive tendency to acknowledge *all* vascular afferents as being visceral, because those on peripheral blood vessels are morphologically and functionally the same as those serving the heart. They all contain substance P, are 'silent' in health, and subserve pain in the presence of disease or injury – as witness, the 'dragging' leg pains accompanying varicose veins, or the stab of pain when a clumsily

Clinical Panel 13.4 Irritable bowel syndrome

IBS (irritable bowel syndrome) is considered to be the the most prevalent of all GI tract disorders, affecting as much as 20% of the population in most countries. The exact incidence is uncertain because of the absence of a specific test; diagnosis is based upon a constellation of symptoms associated with a suggestive psychosocial history. The disorder is three times more common in women and onset is most frequent during the third and fourth decades.

The typical clinical picture is one of recurrent abdominal pain relieved by defecation. Some patients may have less than three bowel movements per week, others more than three per day. Both groups experience bloating (feeling of abdominal distension). Sensitivity to visceral sensations may have been triggered by a previous infectious or food-allergy gastroenteritis. The typical pyschological profile is one of introspection and hypochondriasis accompanied by feelings of mental stress and anxiety. Sometimes a history of childhood physical or sexual abuse may be elicited.

The overall situation is generally accepted as one of *dysfunction of the brain–gut axis.*

Figure 34.10 shows the position of the *emotional nociceptive area* within the cingulate gyrus. This area is activated by aversive (unpleasant) painful stimulation of any body part, as revealed by PET (positron emission tomography). In IBS patient volunteers it is activated by baloon distension of the distal colon at a lower balloon volume than in healthy controls. Heightened sensitivity to intestinal events seems to some extent *centrally* rather than peripherally generated. It is now believed that the preganglionic neurons of the parasympathetic system synapse mainly on *internuncial* neurons in the intestinal wall, rather than on the 'traditional' postganglionic motor neurons shown in Figure Box 13.2.1. The central drive of the parasympathetic may be an expression of stress, and because internuncial neurons may activate nociceptive afferents as well as motor neurons, heightened sensitivity may be maintained or even increased through this feedback loop.

At peripheral level, biopsies taken from ileum and colon indicate that heightened sensitivity may be the outcome of an immune response generated by earlier gastrointestinal infection or food allergy, as evidenced by proliferation of enterochromaffin cells in the wall of intestinal crypts, and/or mast cells in the lamina propria

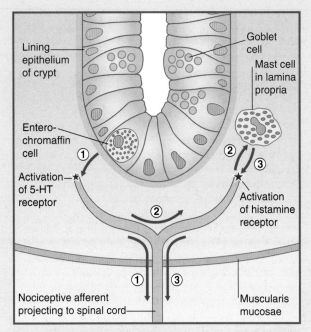

Figure CP 13.4.1 Activation of a nociceptive neuron in the wall of the colon.
1 Serotonin liberated by enterochromaffin cells has activated a nociceptive neuron projecting to posterior horn of spinal cord.
2 Antidromic impulses liberate substance P, which in turn releases histamine from mast cells.
3 Histamine reinforces the effect of serotonin.

(Figure CP 13.4.1). The peptide granules of enterochromaffin (chromate-staining) cells collectively contain more serotonin (5-HT) than does the entire brain. Serotonin liberated in response to intestinal distension has a double effect: it activates 5-HT$_3$ receptors on smooth muscle cells, thereby promoting peristaltic contractions; and it activates nociceptors on nearby visceral afferents, thereby causing mast cells to liberate histamine, which in turn may potentiate the local effect of serotonin.

Following investigations to rule out organic disease, reassurance alone may be sufficient to restore equilibrium, although many patients benefit from psychotherapy. Drug treatments are essentially symptomatic, e.g. 5-HT$_3$-receptor antagonists or M$_3$-receptor anticholinergics for diarrhea, 5-HT$_3$-receptor agonists or cholinergics for constipation.

inserted antecubital venipuncture needle strikes the brachial artery. The pathway to the posterior nerve roots is still uncertain, but it appears that (to an approximation) perivascular fibers above elbow and knee send impulses by the sympathetic route (but in the reverse direction), and that more peripheral perivascular fibers send messages in company with cutaneous nerves (and in the same direction). The notion of visceral afferents running in cutaneous nerves is reminiscent of their same service with respect to nerve fibers terminating in Golgi tendon organs at wrist and ankle.

Core Information

The autonomic nervous system contains three neuron chains of effector neurons: central neurons project from hypothalamus/brainstem to brainstem/spinal cord preganglionic neurons. These send preganglionic fibers to autonomic ganglion cells, which in turn send postganglionic fibers to target tissues.

Sympathetic preganglionic outflow to the sympathetic chain of ganglia is thoracolumbar. Some fibers synapse in nearest ganglia. Some ascend to the superior cervical, middle cervical, or stellate ganglion, whence postganglionic fibers innervate head, neck, upper limbs, and heart. Some descend to synapse in lumbar or sacral ganglia, whence postganglionic fibers enter the lumbosacral plexus to supply lower limb vessels. Some pass through the chain and synapse instead in central abdominal ganglia (for the supply of gastrointestinal and genitourinary tracts) or in the adrenal medulla.

Parasympathetic preganglionic outflow is craniosacral. Cranial nerve distributions are oculomotor nerve via ciliary ganglion to sphincter pupillae and ciliaris; facial nerve via pterygopalatine ganglion to lacrimal and nasal glands; facial nerve via submandibular ganglion to submandibular and sublingual glands; glossopharyngeal nerve via otic ganglion to parotid gland; vagus nerve via ganglia on or in walls of heart, bronchi, and alimentary tract to muscle tissue and glands. Sacral nerves 2–4 deliver preganglionic fibers to intramural ganglia of distal colon and rectum, and to pelvic ganglia for supply of bladder and internal pudendal artery.

All preganglionic neurons are cholinergic. They activate nicotinic receptors in the ganglia. All postganglionic fibers end at neuroeffector junctions. In the sympathetic system, these are generally adrenergic, liberating norepinephrine, which may activate postjunctional α_1 adrenoceptors on smooth muscle, prejunctional α_2 adrenoceptors on local nerve endings, postjunctional β_1 on cardiac muscle, or postjunctional β_2, which are more responsive to epinephrine. Epinephrine is liberated by adrenomedullary chromaffin cells and resultant activation of β_2 receptors on smooth muscle causes relaxation.

Parasympathetic postganglionic fibers are cholinergic. The cholinoceptive receptors on cardiac and smooth muscle and glands are muscarinic.

Visceral afferents
Nociceptive afferents from thoracic and abdominal viscera and from blood vessels use autonomic pathways to reach the CNS. Pure visceral pain is vague and deep-seated. Visceral referred pain is experienced in somatic structures innervated from the same segmental levels. Viscerosomatic pain arises from chemical/thermal irritation of one of the serous membranes: the pain is severe and steady, and accompanied by protective contraction of body wall muscles.

REFERENCES
Freeman R: Autonomic peripheral neuropathy, *Neurol Clin* 25:277–301, 2007.

Gai WP, Blessing WW: Human brainstem preganglionic parasympathetic neurons localized by markers for nitric oxide synthesis, *Brain* 119:145–1152, 1996.

Griffiths D, Tadic SC, Schaefer W, Resnic NM: Cerebral control of the bladder in normal and urge incontinent women, *Neuroimage* 37:1–7, 2007.

Vernino S, Sandrroni P, Singer W, Low PA: Autonomic ganglia: target and novel therapeutic tool, *Neurology* 70:1926–1932, 2008.

REFERENCES

Kaptchuk TJ, Kelley JM, Conboy LA, et al: Components of placebo effect: randomised controlled trial in patients with irritable bowel syndrome, *BMJ* 336:999–1003, 2008.

Mach T: The brain-gut axis in irritable bowel syndrome – clinical aspects, *Med Sci Monit* 10:RA125–131, 2004.

Yale SH, Musana AK, Kieke A, Hayes J, Glurich I, Chyou P-H: Applying case definition criteria to irritable bowel syndrome, *Clin Med Res* 6:9–16, 2008.

Nerve roots

STUDY GUIDELINES

1 During embryonic development, some immature neurons send out ventral roots while others project along the marginal zone to form fiber tracts. Sensory fibers enter the dorsal horn from the neural crest.
2 In the mature vertebral canal, note disparities of levels, e.g. a collapsed T11 vertebra would crush cord segment L1.
3 Recall that ventral roots S2–4 of cauda equina contain preganglionic parasympathetic fibers vital for bladder and bowel control and that the corresponding posterior roots contain visceral afferents vital for reflexes.
4 Do remember the extradural venous plexus and the harm it can do.
5 It is clinically important to appreciate that a sense of numbness/tingling in the fingers in later life may result from compression of posterior nerve roots!
6 For the commonest and lowest two levels of disk prolapse, the *next* spinal nerve is the one likely to be caught.
7 Make certain that you understand the anatomy of lumbar puncture (spinal tap).

DEVELOPMENT OF THE SPINAL CORD

Cellular differentiation

The neural tube of the embryo consists of a pseudostratified epithelium surrounding the neural canal (Figure 14.1A). Dorsal to the sulcus limitans, the epithelium forms the **alar plate**; ventral to the sulcus it forms the **basal plate**.

The neuroepithelium contains germinal cells which synthesize DNA before retracting to the innermost, **ventricular zone**, where they divide. The daughter nuclei move outward, synthesize fresh DNA, then retreat and divide again. After several such cycles, postmitotic cells round up in the **intermediate zone**. Some of the postmitotic cells are immature neurons; the rest are **glioblasts** which, after further division, become astrocytes or oligodendrocytes. Some of the glioblasts form an ependymal lining for the neural canal.

The microglial cells of the CNS are derived from basophil cells of the blood.

Enlargement of the intermediate zone of the alar plate creates the dorsal horn of gray matter. The dorsal horn receives central processes of dorsal root ganglion cells (Figure 14.1B). As explained in Chapter 1, the ganglion cells derive from the neural crest.

Partial occlusion of the neural canal by the developing dorsal gray horn gives rise to the dorsal median septum and to the definitive central canal of the cord (Figure 14.1C).

Enlargement of the intermediate zone of the basal plate creates the ventral gray horn and the ventral median fissure (Figure 14.1C). Axons emerge from the ventral horn and form the ventral nerve roots.

In the outermost, **marginal zone** of the cord, axons run to and from spinal cord and brain.

Neural cord

The neural tube reaches caudally only to the level of the second lumbar mesodermal somites. Following closure of the posterior neuropore, the ectoderm and mesoderm at the level of the more caudal lumbar and sacral somites blend to form a **neural cord**. This ribbon of cells becomes canalized and links up with the neural tube; it forms the lower end of the spinal cord.

Ascent of the spinal cord (Figure 14.2)

The spinal cord occupies the full length of the vertebral canal until the end of the 12th postconceptual week. The sixth to eighth are marked by regression of the caudal end of the neural tube, to become a neuroglial thread, the **filum terminale**.

After the 12th week, the vertebral column grows rapidly and drags the cord upward. The tip of the cord is at second or third lumbar level at the time of birth. The adult level (first or second lumbar) is attained 3 weeks later.

In consequence of greater ascent of the lower part of the cord compared to the upper part, the spinal nerve roots show an increasing disparity between their segmental levels of attachment to the cord and the corresponding vertebral levels (Figure 14.3).

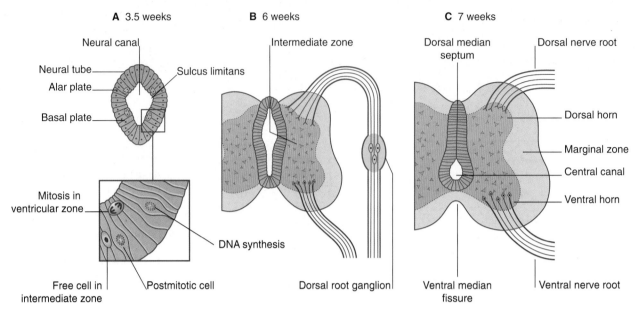

Figure 14.1 (A–C) Cellular differentiation in the embryonic spinal cord.

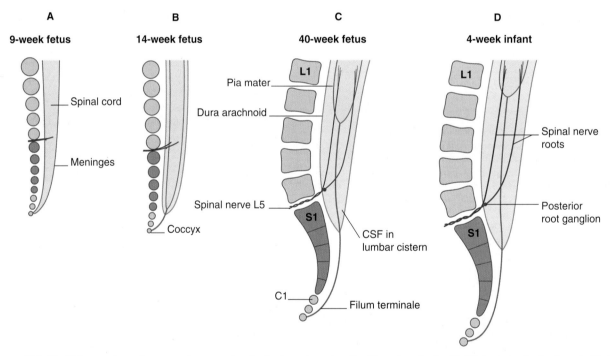

Figure 14.2 (A, B) Regression of coccygeal segments of spinal cord creates the filum terminale. **(C, D)** Ascent of spinal cord. (*Note*: Recent evidence indicates that, as represented here, the number of embryonic coccygeal vertebrae does not exceed three or four.)

Neural arches

During the fifth week, the mesenchymal vertebrae surrounding the notochord give rise to **neural arches** for protection of the spinal cord (Figure 14.4). The arches are initially *bifid* (split). Later, they fuse in the midline and form the vertebral spines.

Conditions where the two halves of the neural arches have failed to unite are collectively known as *spina bifida* (Clinical Panel 14.1).

ADULT ANATOMY

The spinal cord and nerve roots are sheathed by pia mater and float in cerebrospinal fluid contained in the subarachnoid space. The pial **denticulate ligament** pierces the arachnoid and anchors the cord to the dura mater on each side. Outside the dura is the **extradural (epidural) venous plexus** (Figure 14.5), which harvests the vertebral red marrow and empties into the segmental veins (deep cervical, intercostal, lumbar, sacral). These veins are without valves, and reflux of blood from the territory of segmental veins is a *notorious* cause of cancer spread from prostate, lung, breast, and thyroid gland. For example, nerve root compression from collapse of an invaded vertebra may be the presenting sign of cancer in one of these organs.

The respective anterior and posterior nerve roots join at the intervertebral foramina, where the posterior root ganglia are located (Figure 14.5). The arachnoid mater blends with the perineurium of the spinal nerve, and the dura mater blends with the epineurium. The nerve roots carry extensions of the subarachnoid space into the intervertebral foramina.

Below cord level, nerve roots seeking the lower lumbar and sacral intervertebral foramina constitute the **cauda equina** ('horse's tail'). The cauda equina floats in the lumbar

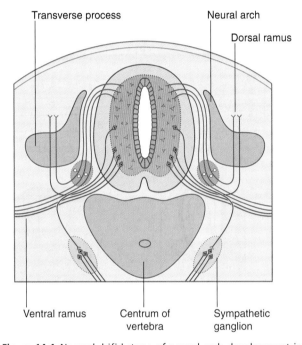

Figure 14.3 Segmental and vertebral levels compared. Spinal nerves 1–7 emerge above the corresponding vertebrae; the remaining spinal nerves emerge below.

Figure 14.4 Normal, bifid stage of neural arch development in an embryo of 8 weeks.

Figure 14.5 Relationships of the sixth cervical spinal nerve.

STUDY GUIDELINES

1 Confirm that the mature spinal cord is not segmented internally.
2 Confirm that anterior horn cells take the form of columns rather than laminae.
3 Appreciate that 'nonconscious sensation' simply means that the ascending afferent impulse activity concerned does not generate any kind of perception.
4 Remember that conscious proprioception is more sensitive than either vision or the vestibular labyrinth in telling us when we are going off balance.
5 Get used to the idea that muscles tell us more than joints do about the position of our limbs in space.
6 It is clinically important to appreciate that one of the two 'conscious' pathways crosses the midline at all levels of the spinal cord, whereas the other crosses all at once, within the brainstem.
7 Appreciate the meaning of the term 'dissociated sensory loss.'

GENERAL FEATURES

The arrangement of gray and white matter at different levels of the spinal cord is shown in Figure 15.1. The cervical and lumbosacral enlargements are produced by expansions of the gray matter required to service innervation of the limbs. White matter is most abundant in the upper reaches of the cord, which contain the sensory and motor pathways serving all four limbs. In the posterior funiculus, e.g., the gracile fasciculus carries information from the lower limb and is present at cervical as well as lumbosacral segmental levels, whereas the cuneate fasciculus carries information from the upper limb and is not seen at lumbar level.

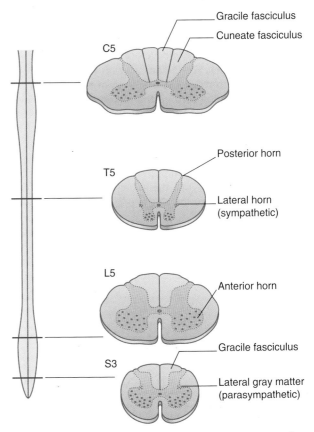

Figure 15.1 Representative transverse sections of the spinal cord.

Although it is convenient to refer to different levels of the spinal cord in terms of numbered segments, corresponding to the sites of attachment of the paired nerve roots, the cord shows no evidence of segmentation internally. The nuclear groups seen in transverse sections are in reality cell columns, most of them spanning several segments (Figure 15.2).

Types of spinal neurons

The smallest neurons (soma diameters 5–20 μm) are *propriospinal*, being entirely contained within the cord. Some are confined within a single segment; others span two or more segments by way of the neighboring **propriospinal tract**. Many of the smallest neurons participate in spinal reflexes. Others are intermediate cell stations interposed between fiber tracts descending from the brain and motor neurons projecting to the locomotor apparatus. Others again are so placed as to influence sensory transmission from lower to higher levels of the CNS.

Medium-sized neurons (soma diameters 20–50 μm) are found in all parts of the gray matter except the substantia

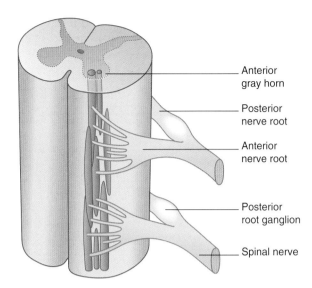

Figure 15.2 Two segments of the spinal cord, showing cell columns in the anterior gray horn.

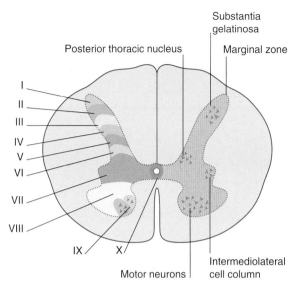

Figure 15.3 Laminae (I–X) and named cell groups at mid-thoracic level.

gelatinosa. Most are *relay (projection) cells* receiving inputs from posterior root afferents and projecting their axons to the brain. The projections are in the form of *tracts*, a tract being defined as a functionally homogeneous group of fibers. As will be seen, the term 'tract' is often used loosely because many projections originally thought to be 'pure' contain more than one functional class of fiber.

The largest neurons of all are the **alpha motor neurons** (soma 50–100 μm) for the supply of skeletal muscles. Scattered among them are small, **gamma motor neurons** supplying muscle spindles. In the medial part of the anterior horn are **Renshaw cells**, which exert tonic inhibition upon alpha motor neurons.

Spinal reflex arcs originating in muscle spindles and tendon organs have been described in Chapter 10, and the withdrawal reflex in Chapter 14.

In thick sections of the spinal cord, the nerve cells exhibit a laminar (layered) arrangement. True lamination is confined to the posterior horn (Figure 15.3), but 10 laminae of Rexed have been defined in the gray matter as a whole in order to correlate findings from animal research in different laboratories.

Spinal ganglia

The spinal or posterior (dorsal) root ganglia are located in the intervertebral foramina, where the anterior and posterior roots come together to form the spinal nerves. Thoracic ganglia contain about 50,0000 unipolar neurons, and those serving the limbs contain about 100,000. The individual ganglion cells are invested with modified Schwann cells called **satellite cells** (Figure 15.4). The common stem axon of each cell bifurcates, sending a centrifugal process into one or other ramus of the spinal nerve (or into the recurrent branch) and a centripetal ('center-seeking') process into the spinal cord. Following stimulation of the peripheral sensory receptors, trains of nerve impulses traverse the point of bifurcation without interruption, although the cell body is also depolarized. The initial segment of the stem axon does not normally generate impulses but it may do so if the adjacent part of the

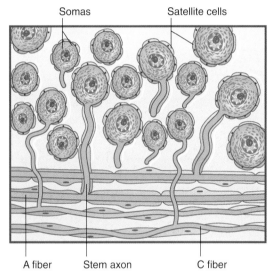

Figure 15.4 Posterior root ganglion. In bottom of figure, note T-shaped bifurcation of stem fibers.

posterior root is compressed, e.g. by a prolapsed intervertebral disc.

Traditionally, the centripetal axons of all spinal ganglion cells have been thought to enter posterior nerve roots. It is now known that many visceral afferents (in particular) enter the cord by way of ventral roots and work their way to the posterior gray horn (Ch. 13). This feature accounts for the frequent failure of *posterior rhizotomy* (surgical section of posterior roots) to relieve pain originating from intra-abdominal cancer.

Central terminations of posterior root afferents (Figure 15.5)

In the *dorsal root entry zone* close to the surface of the cord, the afferent fibers become segregated into medial and lateral

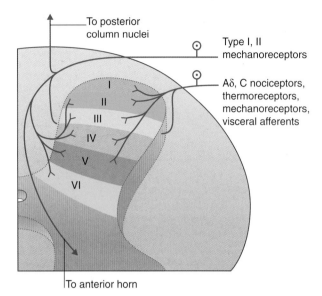

Figure 15.5 Targets of primary afferent neurons in the posterior gray horn.

Figure 15.6 Categories of sensation. [a]Exteroceptors can be categorized as *telereceptors* receiving from a distance (retina and cochlea) and somatic receptors on the body surface (touch, pain, etc.) [b]Enteroceptors (*Gr. enteron*, 'gut') are strictly a subdivision of *interoceptors*, a term signifying all of the viscera. In pathological states they may produce conscious visceral/viscerosomatic sensations.

streams. The medial stream comprises medium and large fibers which divide within the posterior funiculus into ascending and descending branches. The branches swing into the posterior gray horn and synapse in laminae II, III, and IV. The largest ascending fibers run all the way to the posterior column nuclei (gracilis/cuneatus) in the medulla oblongata. These long fibers form the bulk of the gracile and cuneate fasciculi.

The lateral stream comprises small (Aδ and C) fibers which, upon entry, divide into short ascending and descending branches within the **posterolateral tract** of Lissauer. They synapse upon neurons in the marginal zone (lamina I) and in the substantia gelatinosa (lamina II); some fibers synapse upon dendrites of cells belonging to laminae III–V.

ASCENDING SENSORY PATHWAYS

Categories of sensation

In accordance with the flowchart in Figure 15.6, neurologists speak of two kinds of sensation, conscious and nonconscious (unconscious). Conscious sensations are perceived at the level of the cerebral cortex. Nonconscious sensations are not perceived; they have reference to the cerebellum (see later).

Conscious sensations

There are two kinds of conscious sensation: *exteroceptive* and *proprioceptive*. Exteroceptive sensations come from the external world; they impinge either on somatic receptors on the body surface or on telereceptors serving vision and hearing. Somatic sensations include touch, pressure, heat, cold, and pain.

Conscious proprioceptive sensations arise within the body. The receptors concerned are those of the locomotor system (muscles, joints, bones) and of the vestibular labyrinth. The pathways to the cerebral cortex form the substrate for *position sense* when the body is stationary, and for *kinesthetic sense* during movement.

Nonconscious sensations

These also are of two kinds. *Nonconscious proprioception* is the term used to describe afferent information reaching the cerebellum through the spinocerebellar pathways. This information is essential for smooth motor coordination. Second, *interoception* is a little-used term referring to unconscious afferent signals involved in visceral reflexes.

Sensory testing

Routine assessment of *somatic exteroceptive sensation* includes tests for:

- touch, by grazing the skin with the finger tip or a cotton swab
- pain, by applying the point of a pin
- thermal sense, by applying warm or cold test-tubes to the skin.

In alert and cooperative patients, active and passive tests of conscious proprioception can be performed. Active tests examine the patient's ability to execute set-piece activities with the eyes closed:

- in the erect position, stand still, and then 'toe the line' without swaying
- in the seated position, bring the index finger to the nose from the extended position of the arm (finger-to-nose test)
- in the recumbent position, place the heel of the foot on the opposite knee (heel-to-knee test).

Passive tests of conscious proprioception include:

- *Joint sense*. The clinician grasps the thumb or great toe by the sides and moves it while asking the patient to name the direction of movement ('up' or 'down'). Joint sense is mediated in part by articular receptors but mainly by passive stretching of neuromuscular spindles. (If the nerves supplying a joint are anesthetized, or if the joint is completely replaced by a prosthesis, joint sense is only slightly impaired. Alternatively, activation of spindles by means of a vibrator creates the illusion of movement when the relevant joint is stationary.)

- *Vibration sense.* The clinician assesses the patient's ability to detect the vibrations of a tuning fork applied to the radial styloid process or to the shaft of the tibia.

SOMATIC SENSORY PATHWAYS

Two major pathways are involved in somatic sensory perception. They are the *posterior column–medial lemniscal pathway* and the *spinothalamic (anterolateral) pathway*. They have the following features in common (Figure 15.7):

- Both comprise first-order, second-order, and third-order sets of sensory neurons.
- The somas of the first-order neurons, or *primary afferents*, occupy posterior root ganglia.
- The somas of the second-order neurons occupy CNS gray matter on the same side as the first-order neurons.
- The second-order axons *cross the midline* and then ascend to terminate in the thalamus.
- The third-order neurons project from the thalamus to the somatic sensory cortex.

- Both pathways are *somatotopic:* an orderly map of body parts can be identified experimentally in the gray matter at each of the three loci of fiber termination.
- Synaptic transmission from primary to secondary neurons, and from secondary to tertiary, can be modulated (inhibited or enhanced) by other neurons.

Posterior (dorsal) column–medial lemniscal pathway

The first-order afferents include the largest somas in the posterior root ganglia. Their peripheral processes collectively receive information from the largest sensory receptors: Meissner's and Pacinian corpuscles, Ruffini endings and Merkel cell–neurite complexes, neuromuscular spindles, and Golgi tendon organs. The centripetal processes from cells supplying the lower limb and lower trunk give branches to the gray matter before ascending as the **gracile fasciculus (fasciculus gracilis)** to reach the gracile nucleus in the medulla oblongata (Figure 15.8). The corresponding collaterals from the upper limb and upper trunk run in the **cuneate fasciculus (fasciculus cuneatus)** to reach the cuneate nucleus.

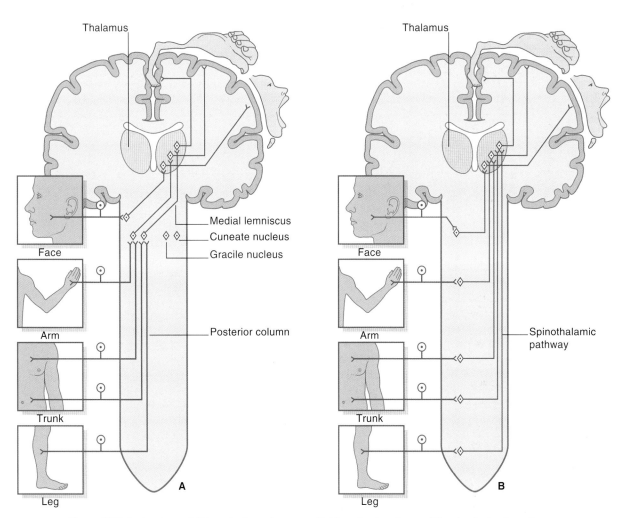

Figure 15.7 Basic plans of **(A)** posterior column–medial lemniscal pathway; **(B)** spinothalamic pathway.

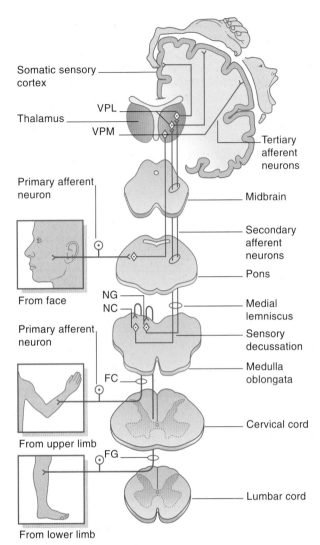

Figure 15.8 The posterior column–medial lemniscal pathway. FC, fasciculus cuneatus; FG, fasciculus gracilis; NC, nucleus cuneatus; NG, nucleus gracilis; VPL, VPM, ventral posterior lateral, ventral posterior medial nuclei of thalamus.

The second-order afferents commence in the posterior column nuclei, namely the **nucleus gracilis** and **nucleus cuneatus**. They pass ventrally in the tegmentum of the medulla oblongata before intersecting their opposite numbers in the great **sensory decussation**. Having crossed the midline, the fibers turn rostrally in the **medial lemniscus**.

The medial lemniscus diverges from the midline as it ascends through the tegmentum of the pons and midbrain. It terminates in the lateral part of the ventral posterior nucleus of the thalamus (**ventral posterolateral nucleus**).

Terminating in the medial part of the same nucleus (**ventral posteromedial nucleus**) is the *trigeminal lemniscus*, which serves the head region.

The third-order afferents project from the thalamus to the somatic sensory cortex (see Ch. 27 for details).

Functions

The chief functions of the posterior column–medial lemniscal pathway are those of *conscious proprioception* and

Figure 15.9 The 'stamp and stick' gait of sensory ataxia.

discriminative touch. Together, these attributes provide the parietal lobe with an instantaneous body image so that we are constantly aware of the position of body parts both at rest and during movement. Without this informational background, the execution of movements is severely impaired.

In humans, disturbance of posterior column function is most often observed in association with demyelinating diseases such as multiple sclerosis. The classic symptom is known as *sensory ataxia*. This term signifies a movement disorder resulting from sensory impairment, in contrast to *cerebellar ataxia*, in which a movement disorder results from a lesion within the motor system. The patient with a severe sensory ataxia can stand unsupported only with the feet well apart and with the gaze directed downward to include the feet. The gait is broad-based, with a stamping action that maximizes any conscious proprioceptive function that remains (Figure 15.9).

Sensory testing in posterior column disease reveals severe swaying when the patient stands with the feet together and the eyes closed. This is *Romberg's sign.* (Inability to 'toe the line' with the eyes closed is *tandem* Romberg's sign.) The finger-to-nose and/or heel-to-knee test may reveal loss of kinesthetic sense. Joint sense and vibration sense may also be impaired.

Note: Romberg's sign may be elicited in patients suffering from vestibular disorders (Ch. 19). In cerebellar disorders, there may be instability of station whether the eyes are open or closed (Ch. 25).

Tactile, painful, and thermal sensations are preserved, but there is impairment of tactile discrimination. The patient has difficulty in discriminating between single and paired stimuli applied to the skin (*two-point discrimination test*); in identifying numbers traced on to the skin by the examiner's finger; and in distinguishing between objects of similar shape but of different textures.

A difficulty in assigning specific functional deficits to posterior column disease is the rarity of pathology affecting the posterior funiculi *alone*. In particular, the posterior part of the lateral funiculus is likely to be involved as well. Post-mortem findings from patients having different degrees of pathology in the posterior and lateral funiculi suggest that kinesthetic sense from the lower limb may be mediated in part by fibers that leave the gracile fasciculus at thoracic level and relay rostrally in the posterior part of the lateral funiculus.

Spinothalamic pathway

The spinothalamic pathway consists of second-order sensory neurons projecting from laminae I–II, IV–V of the posterior gray horn to the contralateral thalamus (Figure 15.10). The cells of origin receive excitatory and inhibitory synapses from neurons of the substantia gelatinosa; these have important 'gating' (modulatory) effects on sensory transmission, as explained in Chapter 24.

The axons of the spinothalamic pathway cross the midline in the anterior commissure at all segmental levels. Having crossed, they run upward in the anterolateral part of the cord. This *anterolateral pathway* (as it is usually called) is divisible into an **anterior spinothalamic tract** located in the anterior funiculus and a **lateral spinothalamic tract** located in the lateral funiculus. The two tracts merge in the brainstem as the **spinal lemniscus**. The spinal lemniscus is joined by trigeminal afferents from the head region, and it accompanies the medial lemniscus to the ventral posterior nucleus of the thalamus, terminating immediately behind the medial lemniscus. Third-order sensory neurons project from the thalamus to the somatic sensory cortex (Ch. 27).

Functions

The functions of the spinothalamic pathway have been elucidated by the procedure known as *cordotomy*, whereby the spinothalamic pathway is interrupted on one or both sides for the relief of intractable pain. For a *percutaneous cordotomy*, the patient is sedated and a needle is passed between the atlas and the axis, into the subarachnoid space. Under radiological guidance, the needle tip is advanced into the anterolateral region of the cord. A stimulating electrode is passed through the needle. If the placement is correct, a mild current will elicit paresthesia (tingling) on the opposite side of the body. The anterolateral pathway is then destroyed electrolytically. Afterwards, the patient is insensitive to *pinprick, heat,* or *cold* applied to the opposite side (Figure 15.11). Sensitivity to *touch* is reduced. The effect commences several segments below the level of the procedure because of the oblique passage of spinothalamic fibers across the white commissure.

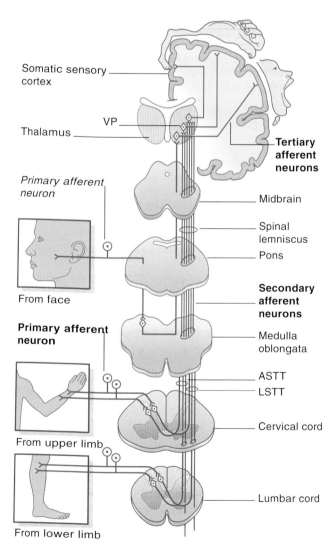

Figure 15.10 The spinothalamic pathway. ASTT, anterior spinothalamic tract; LSTT, lateral spinothalamic tract; VP, ventral posterior nucleus of thalamus.

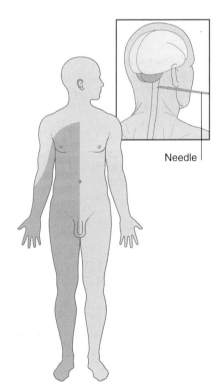

Figure 15.11 Usual extent of analgesia (shaded) following cordotomy at C1–C2 segmental level.

STUDY GUIDELINES

1 This chapter is largely to do with identification of structures in transverse sections of the brainstem. A separate study guide is provided for the sections.
2 Four brainstem decussations should recall those described in Box 3.1.
3 Note that, in magnetic resonance images, brainstem orientation is the reverse of the anatomic convention.

GENERAL ARRANGEMENT OF CRANIAL NERVE NUCLEI

In the thoracic region of the developing spinal cord, four distinct cell columns can be identified in the gray matter on each side (Figure 17.1A, B). In the basal plate, the *general somatic efferent column* supplies the striated muscles of the trunk and limbs. The *general visceral efferent column* contains preganglionic neurons of the autonomic system. In the alar plate, the *general visceral afferent column* receives afferents from thoracic and abdominal organs. A *general somatic afferent* column receives afferents from the body wall.

In the brainstem, these four cell columns can be identified, but they are fragmented, and not all contribute to each cranial nerve. Their connections are as follows.

- *General somatic efferent (GSE) column*. Supplies the striated musculature of the orbit (via the oculomotor, trochlear, and abducens nerves) and tongue (via the hypoglossal nerve).
- *General visceral efferent (GVE) column*. Gives rise to the cranial parasympathetic system introduced in Chapter 13.

The target ganglia are the ciliary, pterygopalatine, otic, and submandibular ganglia in the head, and the vagal ganglia in the thorax and abdomen.
- *General visceral afferent column*. Receives from the visceral territory of the glossopharyngeal and vagus nerves.
- *General somatic afferent column*. Receives from skin and mucous membranes, mainly in trigeminal nerve territory whose most important components are the skin and mucous membranes of the oronasofacial region, and the dura mater.

Three additional cell columns (Figure 17.1C, D) serve branchial arch tissues and the inner ear, as follows.

- *Special visceral (branchial) efferent column*. To branchial arch musculature of face, jaws, palate, larynx, and pharynx (via facial, trigeminal, glossopharyngeal, vagus, and cranial accessory nerves). These striated muscles have visceral functions in relation to food and air intake (hence, *visceral*).
- *Special visceral afferent column*. Receives from taste buds located in the endoderm lining the branchial arches.
- *Special sense afferent column*. Receives vestibular (balance) and cochlear (hearing) from the inner ear.

Figure 17.2 shows the position of the various nuclei in a dorsal view of the brainstem.

In this chapter, details of the internal anatomy of the brainstem accompany nine representative transverse sections and their captions. Connections (direct or indirect) with the *right* cerebral hemisphere have been highlighted in accordance with information to be provided.

BACKGROUND INFORMATION

As stated earlier, exteroceptive and conscious proprioceptive information are transferred (by spinothalamic and dorsal column–medial lemniscal pathways, respectively) from left trunk and limbs to right cerebral hemisphere. It was also explained that corticospinal fibers of the pyramidal tract arising from motor areas of the cerebral cortex supply contralateral anterior horn cells and give a small ipsilateral supply of similar nature, and that those arising from the parietal lobe project to the contralateral posterior gray horn.

The same arrangement holds good for the brainstem. The pyramidal tract fibers terminating in the brainstem are *corticonuclear*. As shown in Figure 17.3, their distribution is predominantly contralateral to somatic and branchial motor nuclei, and entirely contralateral to the somatic sensory nuclei.

Absent from this figure are the three pairs of motor ocular nuclei. Why? Because these do not receive a direct corticonuclear supply. Instead, their predominantly contralateral

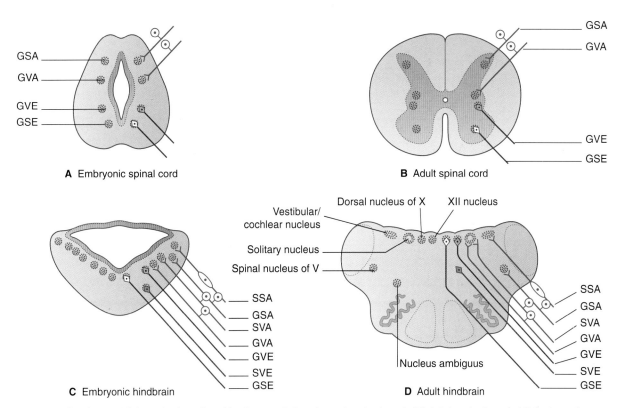

Figure 17.1 Cell columns of the spinal cord and brainstem. **(A)** Embryonic spinal cord. **(B)** Adult spinal cord. **(C)** Embryonic hindbrain. **(D)** Adult hindbrain. *Afferent cell columns*: GSA, general somatic afferent; GVA, general visceral afferent; SSA, special somatic afferent; SVA, special visceral afferent. *Efferent cell columns*: GSE, general somatic efferent; GVE, general visceral efferent; SVE, special visceral efferent.

Figure 17.2 Posterior view of adult brainstem, showing position of cranial nerve cell columns. L, S, I, M, lateral, superior, inferior, medial vestibular nuclei.

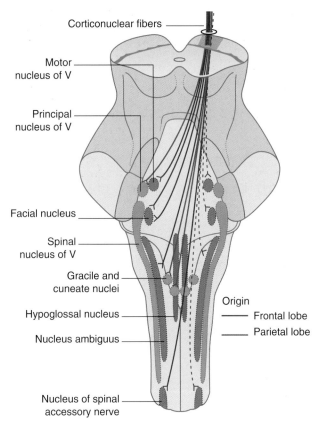

Figure 17.3 Posterior view of brainstem, showing distribution of corticonuclear fibers from the right cerebral cortex.

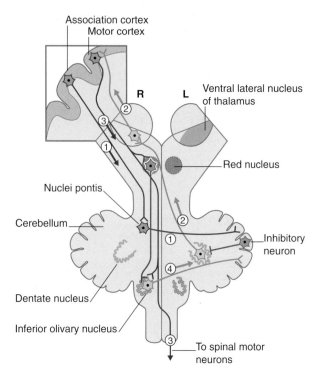

Figure 17.4 Anterior view of the four principal motor decussations of the brainstem. Pathways are numbered in accordance with their sequence of activation in voluntary movements: **(1)** corticopontocerebellar; **(2)** dentatothalamocortical; **(3)** corticospinal; **(4)** olivocerebellar. Also shown is the rubroolivary connection.

supply synapses on adjacent cell groups known as *gaze centers* having the function of synchronizing conjugate (conjoint parallel) movements of the eyes.

For a basic understanding of neural relationships in the brainstem, it is also essential to appreciate hemisphere linkages to the inferior olivary nucleus and to the cerebellum (Figure 17.4).

The general layout of the **reticular formation** (Figure 17.5) is borrowed from a figure in Chapter 24 devoted to this topic. It may be consulted when reading under this heading in successive descriptions.

Figure **17.6** depicts the main components of the **medial longitudinal fasciculus (MLF)**. This fiber bundle extends the entire length of the brainstem, changing its fiber composition at different levels. This figure, too, may be consulted during study of the brainstem sections to be described, following inspection of C1 segment of the spinal cord.

Study guide

The presentation departs from the traditional method, which is to describe photographs or diagrams at successive levels in ascending order without highlights. In the present approach:

1 The various nuclei and pathways are highlighted and labeled on the side having primary affiliation with the right cerebral hemisphere.
2 The nuclei and pathways are color-coded by systems, for example red for motor, blue for sensory, green for connections of cerebellum and reticular formation.

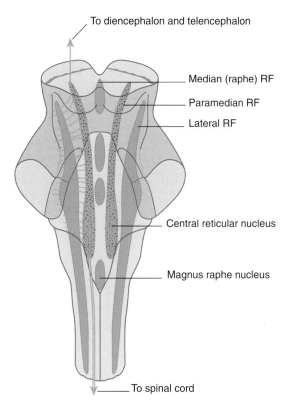

Figure 17.5 Layout of the reticular formation (RF).

3 Highlighting together with color-coding makes it possible to study individual systems in vertical, 'multiple window' mode. The descriptive text related to the brainstem sections enables a logical sequence of study whereby afferent pathways can be followed from below upward to thalamic level (commencing with Figure 17.10), and efferent pathways can be followed from above downward (commencing with Figure 17.19). It must be emphasized that, following study in the vertical mode, a horizontal approach must be undertaken, the location of the various systems to be identified at each level. This is because occlusion of a small artery of supply to the brainstem may affect function in a patch that may include several distinct nuclei or pathways.

At each level, miniature replicas of the diagrams in Figure 17.7 are inserted to assist left–right orientation.

Special note: Readers unfamiliar with the internal anatomy of the brainstem may be disconcerted by the amount of new information contained in the series of sections to be described. It may be reassuring to know that *all* the information will come up again in later chapters. Therefore a sensible approach could be to undertake an initial browse through the sections and to recheck the location of individual items during later reading.

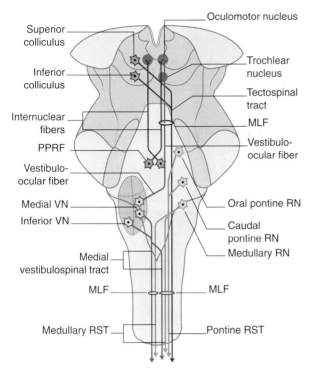

Figure 17.6 Main fiber composition of the medial longitudinal fasciculus (MLF). PPRF, paramedian pontine reticular formation; RN, reticular nucleus; RST, reticulospinal tract; VN, vestibular nucleus.

Overview of three pathways in the brainstem

Figure 17.8 shows the *posterior column–medial lemniscal* and *anterolateral pathways* already described in Chapter 15. Recall that the latter comprises the lateral spinothalamic tract serving pain and temperature, and the anterior spinothalamic tract serving touch. Within the brainstem, the two are combined as the **spinal lemniscus**.

The corticospinal tract, treated in Chapter 16, is shown in Figure 17.9. Also included are corticonuclear projections to the facial and hypoglossal nuclei.

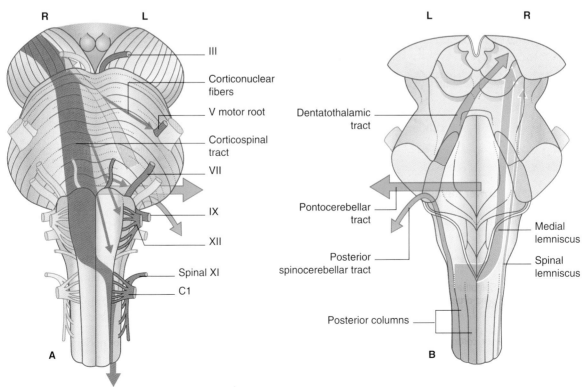

Figure 17.7 (A) Anterior and **(B)** posterior view of brainstem, showing disposition of some major pathways.

C1 SEGMENT OF SPINAL CORD

(Figure 17.10)

Blue The *gracile* and *cuneate fasciculi* constitute the posterior column of the spinal cord on each side. Their axons are ipsilateral central processes of posterior root ganglion cells whose peripheral processes receive information from the large tactile nerve endings in the skin, including Meissner's and Pacinian corpuscles, and from neuromuscular spindles and Golgi tendon organs. The fasciculi terminate in the gracile and cuneate nuclei (Figure 17.12).

The *spinothalamic (anterolateral) pathway comprises* the *anterior* and *lateral spinothalamic tracts.* Unlike those in the posterior column, these two tracts comprise *crossed* axons. As indicated in Figure 15.10, the second-order neurons traverse the anterior white commissure at all segmental levels before ascending to the thalamus.

The *posterolateral tract* of Lissauer contains fine first-order sensory fibers that divide and span several cord segments prior to synapsing in the posterior gray horn.

The *spinal (descending) tract* of the trigeminal nerve contains nociceptive and thermoceptive first-order neurons about to synapse in the posterior gray horn of segments C2 and C3.

Red The large red area on the left side of the cord represents the (crossed) *lateral corticospinal tract.* The *anterior CST* has not yet crossed.

Anterior motor neurons projecting from the anterior gray horn occupy the anterior root of spinal nerve C1 and the uppermost root of the spinal accessory nerve.

The *lateral vestibulospinal tract* (uncrossed) descends in the anterior funiculus to activate antigravity muscles on its own side. *The medial VST* (partly crossed) has emerged from the medial longitudinal fasciculus to activate head-righting reflexes.

Lateral to the anterior gray horn is the autonomic projection from the hypothalamus. Its functions include activation of sacral parasympathetic neurons causing contraction of the bladder and rectum.

Green The *posterior spinocerebellar tract* (from the posterior thoracic nucleus) conveys high-speed nonconscious proprioception from the ipsilateral trunk and limbs, notably from muscle stretch receptors.

The *pontine reticulospinal tract* is descending ipsilaterally to supply motor neurons innervating antigravity muscles. The *medullary reticulospinal tract* supplies flexor motor neurons.

SPINOMEDULLARY JUNCTION

(Figure 17.11)

Blue The gracile and cuneate fasciculi continue to occupy the posterior white column, with the spinal tract and nucleus of the trigeminal nerve alongside. The position of the spinal lemniscus is also unchanged.

Red The dominant feature in this diagram is the *decussation of the pyramids.* Observe the right pyramid: 80% of its fibers cross the midline by decussating with its opposite numbers, to form the left *lateral corticospinal tract*; 10% enter the ipsilateral *anterior corticospinal tract* which will cross lower down; and 10% remain ipsilateral among the fibers of the right lateral CST.

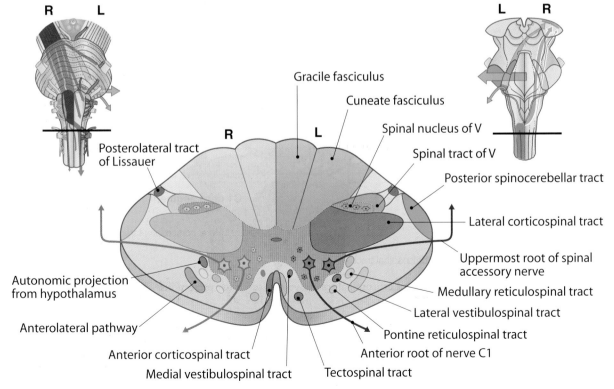

Figure 17.10 C1 segment of spinal cord. (After Noback CR et al. 1996, with permission of Williams & Wilkins.)

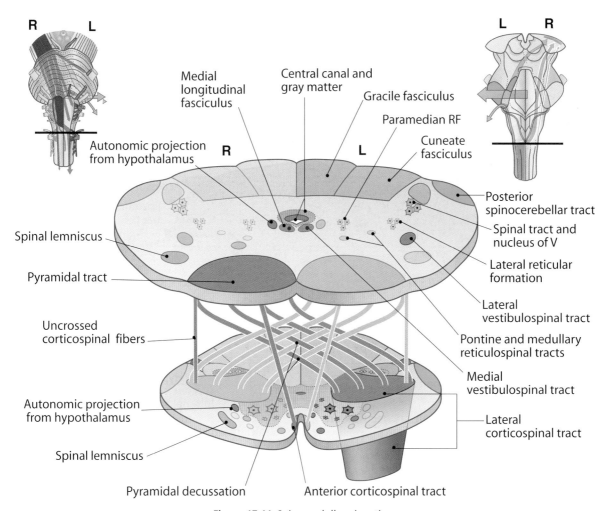

Figure 17.11 Spinomedullary junction.

Within the lateral tegmentum is the lateral vestibulospinal tract. The red spots in the medial longitudinal fasciculi represent the medial vestibulospinal tract, which descends bilaterally within them.

Green The posterior spinocerebellar tract is nearing its point of departure into the inferior cerebellar peduncle. The *paramedian* and *lateral reticular formation* occupy the tegmentum.

MIDDLE OF MEDULLA OBLONGATA

(Figure 17.12)

Blue The left posterior column of the spinal cord ascends to mid-medulla before turning ventrally. The gracile fasciculus synapses in the *gracile nucleus*, the cuneate one in the *cuneate nucleus*. Second-order neurons give rise to *internal arcuate fibers* which cross over in the great *sensory decussation*, then ascend (to thalamus) as the *medial lemniscus*.

The spinal lemniscus contains the (crossed) anterior and lateral spinothalamic tracts.

The vestibulospinal tract is descending from the vestibular nucleus to the spinal cord.

Red The pyramid contains the corticospinal tract prior to the pyamidal decussation; the *hypoglossal nerve* emerges at its lateral edge. Lateral to the XII nucleus is the *dorsal nucleus of vagus nerve*. The *cranial accessory nerve* has emerged from the nucleus ambiguus; it will be incorporated into the vagus below the jugular foramen. The *dorsal longitudinal fasciculus* contains autonomic fibers descending from hypothalamus to spinal cord.

Green The projections from inferior and accessory olivary nuclei to contralateral cerebellar cortex are shown.

The paramedian and lateral reticular formation and the inferior cerebellar peduncle are seen again now.

UPPER PART OF MEDULLA
OBLONGATA (Figure 17.13)

Blue In the mid-region, the medial lemnisci are continuing their ascent to the thalamus. Laterally, we see the *spinal lemniscus*, the *spinal tract and nucleus of the trigeminal nerve*, the *solitary tract and nucleus* (S.t.n.) and the *medial and lateral nuclei of the vestibular nerve*. Sensory fibers of the glossopharyngeal nerve synapse in

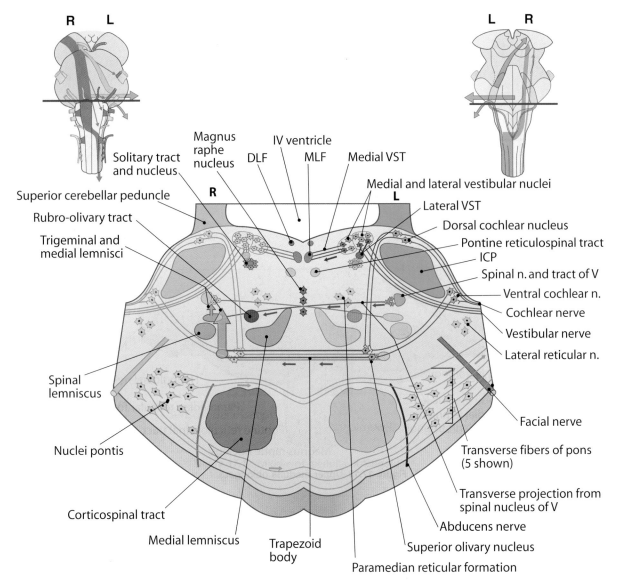

Figure 17.14 Pontomedullary junction.

The *mesencephalic nucleus of the trigeminal nerve* (Mes. n. V) is the *only* unipolar cell group within the CNS. It serves proprioception within the trigeminal area.

Red The *trochlear nerve* is the *only* cranial nerve to decussate (as shown); also the *only* cranial nerve to emerge from the dorsal surface of the brainstem.

The DLF contains autonomic fibers traveling to the spinal cord. The crus of the midbrain contains corticonuclear and corticospinal fibers; the former activate motor cranial nerve nuclei. The *tectospinal tract* is commencing its descent, having crossed from the contralateral superior colliculi. It operates *visuospinal reflexes* whereby the head and trunk are turned in the direction of a source of light.

Green The fronto- and temporopontine fibers are traveling from the corresponding association areas to reach the ipsilateral nuclei pontis.

Brown/gray The anterior tegmentum is occupied by *compact* and *reticular* elements of the *substantia nigra*. The compact part, comprising pigmented dopaminergic neurons, is the source of the *nigrostriatal pathway* to the corpus striatum. The nigrostriatal pathway loses both pigment and cells in those unfortunates bound for *Parkinson's disease* (Ch. 33). The reticular part contains GABAergic neurons.

UPPER MIDBRAIN (Figure 17.18)

The four occupants of the crus cerebri and the substantia nigra are in the same relative positions. So too are the midbrain raphe nucleus and the ventral tegmental and interpeduncular nuclei.

Blue The medial, spinal, and trigeminal lemnisci continue to move dorsally as they near the thalamus. The *spinotectal tract* has emerged from the spinal lemniscus to enter the superior colliculus.

Red At top, the two *tectospinal tracts* have emerged from the superior colliculus and have undergone deccussation. The spinotectal and tectospinal tracts operate the *spinovisual reflex* whereby the eyes and head turn in the direction of

Figure 17.15 Mid-pons.

Figure 17.16 Upper pons.

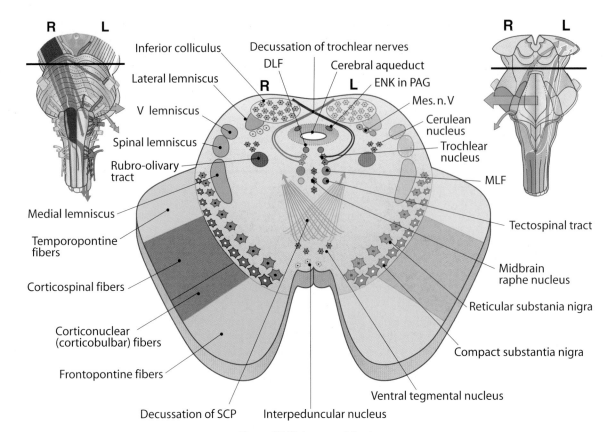

Inferior colliculus
Decussation of trochlear nerves
DLF
Cerebral aqueduct
ENK in PAG
Lateral lemniscus
Mes. n.V
V lemniscus
Cerulean nucleus
Spinal lemniscus
Trochlear nucleus
Rubro-olivary tract
MLF
Medial lemniscus
Tectospinal tract
Temporopontine fibers
Midbrain raphe nucleus
Corticospinal fibers
Reticular substania nigra
Corticonuclear (corticobulbar) fibers
Compact substantia nigra
Frontopontine fibers
Ventral tegmental nucleus
Decussation of SCP
Interpeduncular nucleus

Figure 17.17 Lower midbrain.

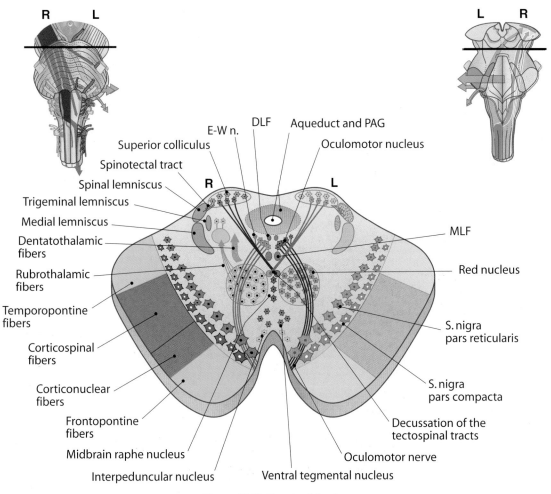

E-W n.
DLF
Aqueduct and PAG
Superior colliculus
Oculomotor nucleus
Spinotectal tract
Spinal lemniscus
Trigeminal lemniscus
Medial lemniscus
MLF
Dentatothalamic fibers
Red nucleus
Rubrothalamic fibers
Temporopontine fibers
S. nigra pars reticularis
Corticospinal fibers
S. nigra pars compacta
Corticonuclear fibers
Decussation of the tectospinal tracts
Frontopontine fibers
Oculomotor nerve
Midbrain raphe nucleus
Ventral tegmental nucleus
Interpeduncular nucleus

Figure 17.18 Upper midbrain.

tactile stimuli. The oculomotor nerves have pierced the red nuclei and substantia nigra to reach the interpeduncular fossa. The *Edinger-Westphal nucleus* (E-W n.) sends preganglionic parasympathetic fibers into the nerves; they activate the ciliary ganglion whose postganglionic fibers cause contraction of the pupillary sphincter and the ciliary muscle.

Green Most dentatothalamic fibers travel direct to the contralateral thalamus. A minority synapse in the red nucleus whence *rubrothalamic* fibers are relayed onward within the *central tegmental tract*.

MIDBRAIN–THALAMIC JUNCTION

(Figure 17.19)

Blue Ascending to the ventral posterior nucleus of thalamus are 3 lemnisci (medial, spinal, trigeminal). Entering the medial (auditory) geniculate nucleus (MGN) of thalamus is the inferior brachium which arose in the inferior colliculus. The lateral (visual) geniculate nucleus (LGN) receives the superior brachium (not seen here).

Red The subthalamic nucleus receives an input from the centromedian nucleus of thalamus and projects to the lentiform nucleus. It may become overactive in Parkinson's disease (cf. Ch. 33). The red nucleus and the contents of the crus cerebri are unchanged.

Green In the dorsal tegmentum, the pretectal nucleus belongs to the visual system. It receives an input from the optic tract and projects to both Edinger-Westphal nuclei, giving rise to bilateral pupillary constriction when a light is shone into one eye (Ch. 23).

Near the midline are the centers for upward and downward gaze. Rarely, a *pinealoma* (pineal gland tumor) may signal its presence by causing *paralysis of upward gaze*.

The superior cerebellar peduncle is aiming for the ventral lateral nucleus of the thalamus. which lies anterior to the ventral posterior nucleus. From there, a final projection will reach the motor cortex and will coordinate ongoing movements.

Green The habenular nuclei are connected across the midline and project via the fasciculus retroflexus to the interpeduncular nucleus, which participates in the sleep–wake cycle (Ch. 34).

ORIENTATION OF BRAINSTEM SLICES IN MAGNETIC RESONANCE IMAGES

(Figure 17.20)

Figure 17.20 shows brainstem slices in magnetic resonance images. Their orientation is the opposite of those in the preceding sections. In photographs and drawings, the convention is to represent anterior structures below. As already mentioned in Chapter 2, in magnetic resonance imaging scans, anterior structures are represented above.

Epilog

Figure 17.21 offers an unlabeled overview of the brainstem sections. Gentle skimmers may opt to photocopy lightly and to crayon pathways.

Figure 17.19 Midbrain–thalamic junction.

Figure 17.20 Magnetic resonance images of **(A)** medulla oblongata, **(B)** pons, and **(C)** midbrain in the standard radiologic orientation. (From a series kindly provided by Professor J. Paul Finn, Director, Magnetic Resonance Research, Department of Radiology, David Geffen School of Medicine at UCLA, California.)

Figure 17.21 Brainstem review.

Core Information

Cell columns

Cranial nerve cell columns and their representations are as follows.

- *General somatic efferent,* represented in the medulla by the hypoglossal nucleus, in the pons by the abducens nucleus, and in the midbrain by the oculomotor and trochlear nuclei.
- *Special visceral efferent,* supplying muscles of branchial arch origin, represented in the medulla by the nucleus ambiguus and in the pons by trigeminal and facial motor nuclei.
- *General visceral efferent,* represented in the medulla by dorsal nucleus of the vagus and in the medulla and in the pons by the salivatory nuclei.
- *General visceral afferent,* represented in the medulla by the inferior solitary nucleus.
- *Special visceral afferent,* represented in the pons by the superior solitary nucleus.
- *General somatic afferent,* represented by trigeminal sensory nuclei: spinal in the medulla, principal sensory in the pons, and mesencephalic in the midbrain.
- *Special sense afferent,* represented at the pontomedullary junction by the cochlear and vestibular nuclei.

Ascending pathways

The gracile and cuneate nuclei send internal arcuate fibers across the midline to form the medial lemniscus, which goes through pons and midbrain to reach the thalamus. The spinal trigeminal nucleus sends fibers across the midline to form the trigeminothalamic tract. The posterior spinocerebellar and cuneocerebellar tracts send their fibers into the ipsilateral inferior cerebellar peduncle, where they mingle with olivocerebellar fibers crossing from the inferior and accessory olivary nuclei. The (crossed) anterior spinocerebellar tract enters the superior cerebellar peduncle; its fibers cross a second time within the cerebellar white matter.

- The spinal lemniscus is formed of the anterior and lateral spinothalamic tracts. It is accompanied first by trigeminothalamic fibers, later by the lateral lemniscus and by fibers crossing from the principal trigeminal nucleus completing the trigeminal lemniscus.
- The cochlear nuclei project fibers across the trapezoid body to form the lateral lemniscus, which ascends to the inferior colliculus. Some fibers synapse instead in a superior olivary nuclear relay to the ipsilateral inferior colliculus. Third-order neurons of the inferior colliculus project via inferior brachium to the medial geniculate body. The medial and superior vestibular

nuclei send fibers to the oculomotor nucleus to execute the vestibuloocular reflex.

- The upper part of the central tegmental tract contains fibers of the ascending reticular activating system.
- In the ventral tegmentum of the midbrain are the pigmented (compact) substantia nigra giving rise to the nigrostriatal pathway, and the ventral tegmental nucleus giving rise to the mesocortical and mesolimbic pathways. The non-pigmented (reticular) nigral neurons are inhibitory.

Descending pathways other than reticulospinal

Corticonuclear fibers from motor areas of the cerebral cortex are distributed preferentially to contralateral motor cranial nerve nuclei excepting the ocular motor slaves of gaze centers. Corticonuclear fibers from sensory areas synapse in contralateral trigeminal and posterior column nuclei and posterior gray horn of spinal cord.

- Prior to the initiation of a voluntary movement on the left side of the body, the left cerebellar hemisphere is notified by discharges from association areas of the right cerebral cortex, along the corticopontocerebellar pathway. The left cerebellum responds via the dentatothalamocortical pathway, to the right primary motor cortex. Then the right pyramidal tract discharges and on its way down notifies the cerebellum a second time by activating the right red nucleus, which in turn activates the right olivocerebellar tract.
- Corticospinal fibers pass through the middle three-fifths of the cerebral crus and through the basilar pons (where they are segregated into bundles by transverse fibers), finally creating the pyramid of the medulla before four-fifths enter the pyramidal decussation.
- The lateral vestibular nucleus gives rise to the lateral vestibulospinal tract having an antigravity function. The medial and inferior vestibular nuclei give rise to the medial vestibulospinal tract involved in head-righting reflexes. The tectospinal tract belongs to the spinovisual reflex arc. The dorsal longitudinal fasciculus contains ipsilateral central autonomic fibers.
- A sleep-related pathway from the septal area reaches the interpeduncular nucleus by way of the habenular nucleus and fasciculus retroflexus.

Reticular formation

In the uppermost midbrain are the upward and downward gaze centers. (The lateral gaze centers

Core Information *(Continued)*

adjoin the abducens nucleus in the pons.) The midbrain also contains an up-going, 'arousal' projection from the cuneiform nucleus, a down-going, pain-suppressant projection from the periaqueductal gray matter, and a locomotor generator, the pedunculopontine nucleus.

The pons contains the noradrenergic, cerulean nucleus, also the oral and caudal pontine reticular nuclei, which send ipsilateral pontine reticulospinal tracts to extensor motor neurons. The medullary reticulospinal tract is partly crossed and supplies flexor motor neurons. Three respiratory reticular nuclei also occupy the medulla.

REFERENCE

Literature references to individual brainstem nuclei and pathways are to be found in the relevant chapters.

REFERENCES

Kautcherov Y, Huang X-F, Halliday G, et al: Organization of human brainstem nuclei. In Paxinos G, Mai JK, editors: *The human nervous system*, ed 2, Amsterdam, 2004, Elsevier, pp 267–320.

Noback CR, et al: *The human nervous system: structure and function*, Baltimore, 1996, Williams & Wilkins.

CHAPTER SUMMARY

Hypoglossal nerve
    Supranuclear supply to the hypoglossal nucleus
Spinal accessory nerve
Glossopharyngeal, vagus, and cranial accessory nerves
    Glossopharyngeal nerve
    Vagus and cranial accessory nerves

CLINICAL PANELS

Supranuclear lesions of the IX, X, and XI cranial nerves
Nuclear lesions of the X, XI, and XII cranial nerves
Infranuclear lesions of the lowest four cranial nerves

STUDY GUIDELINES

Comments on the last four cranial nerves in ascending order:
1. The hypoglossal nerve is straightforward: it is motor to the tongue. The spinal accessory nerve is straightforward: it is motor to the sternomastoid and trapezius.
2. The cranial accessory nerve supplies the intrinsic muscles of larynx and pharynx, and all palatine muscles except tensor palati (supplied by the trigeminal nerve). It is *distributed* by the vagus.
3. The vagus nerve proper is the principal preganglionic parasympathetic nerve. It is also the principal visceral afferent nerve.
4. Main features of the glossopharyngeal nerve are: (a) it provides the afferent limb of the gag reflex; (b) it tells us when we have an inflamed throat; (c) it signals (tastes) bitterness; (d) its carotid branch carries afferents from the carotid sinus, monitoring blood pressure, and from the carotid body, monitoring blood gases; (e) it gives a clinically significant branch to the middle ear.

HYPOGLOSSAL NERVE

The hypoglossal nerve (cranial nerve XII) contains somatic efferent fibers for the supply of the extrinsic and intrinsic muscles of the tongue, except palatoglossus (supplied by the cranial accessory nerve). Its nucleus lies close to the midline in the floor of the fourth ventricle and extends almost the full length of the medulla (Figure 18.1). The nerve emerges as a series of rootlets in the interval between the pyramid and the olive. It crosses the subarachnoid space and leaves the skull through the hypoglossal canal. Just below the skull, it lies close to the vagus and spinal accessory nerves (Figure 18.2). It descends on the carotid sheath to the level of the angle of the mandible, then passes forward on the surface of the hyoglossus muscle where it gives off its terminal branches.

Afferent impulses from about 100 muscle spindles in the same side of the tongue travel from the hypoglossal to the lingual nerve and are then relayed to the mesencephalic nucleus of the trigeminal nerve.

Phylogenetic note

In reptiles, the lingual muscles, the geniohyoid muscle, and the infrahyoid muscles develop together from the uppermost mesodermal somites. The somatic efferent neurons supplying this *hypobranchial muscle sheet* form a continuous ribbon of cells extending from lower medulla to the third cervical spinal segment. In mammals, the hypoglossal nucleus is located more rostrally and its rootlets emerge separately from the cervical rootlets. However, the caudal limit of the hypoglossal nucleus remains linked to the cervical motor cell column by the *supraspinal nucleus*, from which the thyrohyoid muscle is supplied via the first cervical ventral root. In rodents, some of the intrinsic muscle fibers of the tongue receive their motor supply indirectly, from axons which leave the most caudal cells of the hypoglossal nucleus and emerge in the first cervical nerve to join the hypoglossal nerve trunk in the neck. Whether this arrangement holds for primates is not yet known.

Supranuclear supply to the hypoglossal nucleus

The hypoglossal nucleus receives inputs from the reticular formation, whereby it is recruited for stereotyped motor routines in eating and swallowing. For delicate functions including articulation, most of the fibers from the motor cortex cross over in the upper part of the pyramidal decussation; some remain uncrossed and supply the ipsilateral hypoglossal nucleus.

Supranuclear, nuclear, and infranuclear lesions of the hypoglossal nerve are described together with lesions of the accessory nerve (see Clinical Panels 18.1–18.3).

SPINAL ACCESSORY NERVE

The spinal accessory nerve (cranial nerve XI) is a purely motor nerve attached to the uppermost five segments of the spinal cord. The nucleus of origin is a column of α and γ motor neurons in the basolateral anterior gray horn.

The nerve runs upward in the subarachnoid space, behind the denticulate ligament. It enters the cranial cavity through the foramen magnum and leaves it again through the jugular foramen. While in the jugular foramen, it shares a dural sheath with the cranial accessory nerve, but there is no exchange of fibers (Figure 18.3). Upon leaving the cranium, it crosses the transverse process of the atlas and enters the sternomastoid muscle, in company with twigs from roots C2 and C3 of the cervical plexus. It emerges from the posterior border of the sternomastoid and crosses the posterior

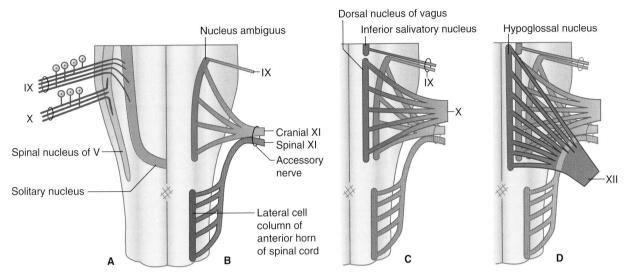

Figure 18.1 (A) Sensory nuclei (left) and motor nuclei (right) serving cranial nerves IX–XII. **(B)** The special visceral efferent cell column giving a contribution to the glossopharyngeal nerve and forming the cranial accessory nerve. **(C)** The general visceral efferent cell column contributing to the glossopharyngeal and vagus nerves. **(D)** The somatic efferent cell column giving rise to the hypoglossal nerve.

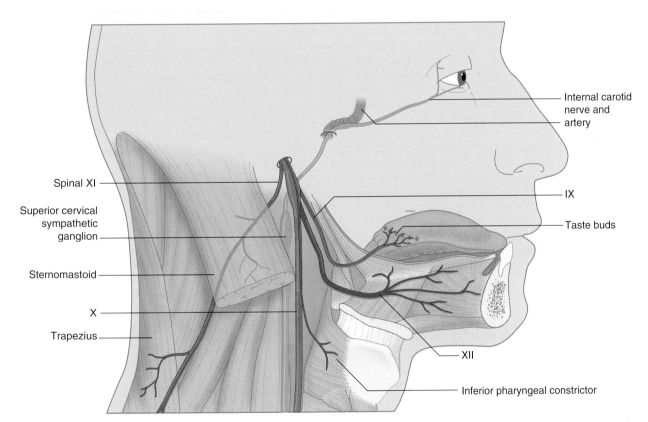

Figure 18.2 Semischematic illustration of the lowest four cranial nerves and the internal carotid branch of the superior cervical ganglion.

triangle of the neck to reach the trapezius. It pierces the trapezius in company with twigs from roots C3 and C4 of the cervical plexus. In the posterior triangle, the nerve is vulnerable, being embedded in prevertebral fascia and covered only by investing cervical fascia and skin.

The spinal accessory nerve provides the extrafusal and intrafusal motor supply to the sternomastoid and trapezius.

The branches from the cervical plexus are proprioceptive in function to the sternomastoid and to the craniocervical part of the trapezius. The thoracic part of the trapezius, which arises from the spines of all the thoracic vertebrae, receives its proprioceptive innervation from the posterior rami of the thoracic spinal nerves. Some of the afferents supplying muscle spindles in the thoracic trapezius do not meet up with

217

Core Information

The static labyrinth comprises the maculae in utricle and saccule. The dynamic labyrinth comprises the semicircular ducts and their cristae. Vestibular bipolar neurons supply all five and synapse in the vestibular nucleus, which is controlled by the flocculonodular lobe of cerebellum. The static labyrinth functions to control balance, via the lateral vestibulospinal tract, by increasing antigravity tone on the side to which the head is tilted. This system is in partnership with proprioceptors and retina in maintaining upright posture. In the absence of good vision, or at night outdoors, a fall is likely if the system has been compromised.

The dynamic labyrinth operates vestibulo-ocular reflexes so as to keep the gaze on target during rotatory movements of the head. For sideways rotation, the main projection is from medial vestibular nucleus to contralateral PPRF which activates VI neurons supplying the lateral rectus muscle and internuclear neurons projecting via the MLF to the contralateral medial rectus. Clinically, this pathway can be activated by the caloric test, which normally elicits nystagmus.

REFERENCES

Angelaki DE, Cullen KE: Vestibular system: the many facets of a multimodal sense, *Ann Rev Neurosci* 31:125–150, 2008.

Barmack NH: Central vestibular system: vestibular nuclei and posterior cerebellum, *Brain Res Bull* 60:511–541, 2003.

Dieterich M, Bense S, Lutz S, Drezega A, Stephan, T, Bartenstein P, Brandt T: Dominance for vestibular cortical function in the non-dominant hemisphere, *Cerebral Cortex* 13:994–1007, 2003.

Fitzpatrick R, McCloskey DI: Proprioceptive, visual and vestibular thresholds for the perception of sway during standing in humans, *J Physiol* 478:173–196, 1994.

Lacour M, Borel L: Vestibular control of posture and gait, *Arch Ital Biol* 131:81–104, 1993.

Landau ME, Barner KC: Vestibulocochlear nerve, *Semin Neurol* 29:66–73, 2009.

Paulesu E, Frackowiak RSJ, Bottini G: Maps of somatosensory systems. In Frackowiak RSJ, Friston KJ, Frith CD, Mazziota JC, editors: *Human brain function*, San Diego, 1997, Academic Press, pp 219–231.

Cochlear nerve

STUDY GUIDELINES

1 Vibrations created by sound waves cross the vestibular membrane to reach the organ of Corti, where cochlear nerve fibers terminate.
2 The central auditory pathway is partly ipsilateral, to the extent that damage on one side does not compromise hearing unduly.
3 Nuclei strung along the brainstem part of the pathway serve to magnify tiny differences in relative intensities of sounds entering the two ears.

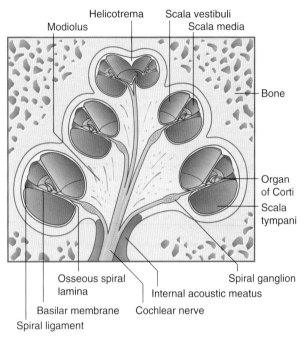

Figure 20.1 The cochlea in section.

AUDITORY SYSTEM

The auditory system comprises the cochlea, the cochlear nerve, and the central auditory pathway from the cochlear nuclei in the brainstem to the cortex of the temporal lobe. The central auditory pathway is more elaborate than the somatosensory or visual pathway. This is because the same sounds are detected by both ears. In order to signal the location of a sound, a very complex neuronal network is in place, with numerous connections (mainly inhibitory) between the two central pathways in order to magnify minute differences in intensity and timing of sounds that exist during normal, binaural hearing.

The cochlea

The main features of cochlear structure are seen in Figures 20.1 and 20.2. The cochlea is pictured as though it were upright, but in life it lies on its side, as shown earlier in Figure 19.1. The central bony pillar of the cochlea (the **modiolus**) is in the axis of the internal acoustic meatus. Projecting from the modiolus, like the flange of a screw, is the **osseous spiral lamina**. The **basilar membrane** is attached to the tip of this lamina; it reaches across the cavity of the bony cochlea to become attached to the **spiral ligament** on the outer wall. The osseous spiral lamina and spiral ligament become

progressively smaller as one ascends the two and one half turns of the cochlea, and the fibers of the basilar membrane become progressively longer.

The basilar membrane and its attachments divide the cochlear chamber into upper and lower compartments. These are the **scala vestibuli** and the **scala tympani**, respectively, and they are filled with perilymph. They communicate at the apex of the cochlea, through the **helicotrema**. A third compartment, the **scala media (cochlear duct)**, lies above the basilar membrane and is filled with endolymph. It is separated from the scala vestibuli by the delicate **vestibular membrane**.

Sitting on the basilar membrane is the **spiral organ** *(organ of Corti)*. The principal sensory receptor epithelium consists of a single row of **inner hair cells**, each one having up to 20 large afferent nerve endings applied to it. The hair cells rest upon **supporting cells**, and there are ancillary cells too. The organ of Corti contains a central **tunnel**, filled with perilymph diffusing through the basilar membrane. On the outer side of the tunnel are several rows of **outer hair cells**, attended by supporting and ancillary cells.

All of the hair cells are surmounted by **stereocilia**. Unlike the vestibular hair cells, they have no kinocilium in the adult state. The stereocilia of the outer hair cells are embedded in the overlying tectorial membrane. Those of the inner hair cells lie immediately below the membrane.

The outer hair cells are contractile (in tissue culture), and they have substantial efferent nerve endings (Figure 20.2).

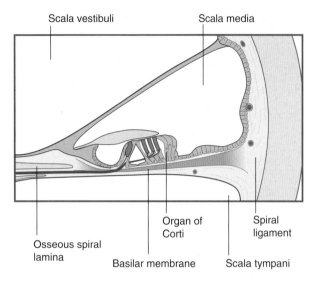

Scala vestibuli   Scala media

Osseous spiral lamina

Organ of Corti

Basilar membrane

Spiral ligament

Scala tympani

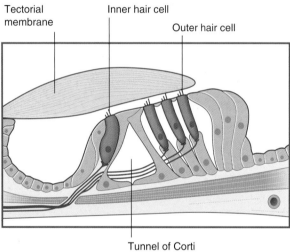

Tectorial membrane

Inner hair cell

Outer hair cell

Tunnel of Corti

Stereocilium

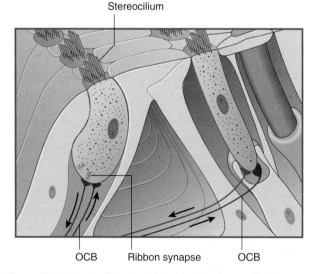

OCB   Ribbon synapse   OCB

Figure 20.2 Organ of Corti at three levels of magnification. Arrows indicate directions of impulse traffic. OCB, fibers of olivocochlear bundle.

In theory, at least, oscillatory movements of outer hair cells could influence the sensitivity of the inner hair cells through effects on the tectorial or basilar membrane.

Sound transduction

The vibrations of the tympanic membrane in response to sound waves are transmitted along the ossicular chain. The footplate of the stapes fits snugly into the oval window, and vibrations of the stapes are converted to pressure waves in the scala vestibuli. The pressure waves are transmitted through the vestibular membrane to reach the basilar membrane. High-frequency pressure waves, created by high-pitched sounds, cause the short fibers of the basilar membrane in the basal turn of the cochlea to resonate and absorb their energy. Low-frequency waves produce resonance in the apical turn where the fibers are longest. The basilar membrane is therefore *tonotopic* in its fiber sequence. Not surprisingly, the inner hair cells have a similar tonotopic sequence. In response to local resonance, the cells become depolarized and liberate excitatory transmitter substance from synaptic ribbons (Figure 20.2).

The nerve fibers supplying the hair cells are the peripheral processes of the bipolar spiral ganglion cells lodged in the base of the osseous spiral lamina.

Cochlear nerve

The bulk of the cochlear nerve consists of the myelinated central processes of some 30,000 large bipolar neurons of the spiral ganglion. Unmyelinated fibers come from small ganglion cells supplying dendrites to the outer hair cells. (Motor fibers do not travel in the cochlear nerve trunk.) The cochlear nerve traverses the subarachnoid space in company with the vestibular and facial nerves, and it enters the brainstem at the pontomedullary junction.

Central auditory pathways

The general plan of the central auditory pathway from the left cochlear nerve to the cerebral cortex is shown in Figure 20.3. The first cell station is the **cochlear nuclei**, where all cochlear nerve fibers terminate upon entry to the brainstem. From here, some second-order fibers project all the way to the opposite **inferior colliculus** by way of the **trapezoid body** and **lateral lemniscus**. The **inferior brachium** links the inferior colliculus to the **medial geniculate body**, which projects to the **primary auditory cortex** in the temporal lobe.

A small but important purely ipsilateral relay passes from the superior olivary nucleus to the higher auditory centers.

Functional anatomy (Figure 20.4)

Cochlear nuclei

The cochlear nuclei comprise dorsal and ventral nuclei, on the surface of the inferior cerebellar peduncle. Many incoming fibers of the cochlear nerve bifurcate and enter both nuclei. The cells in both are tonotopically arranged.

Responses of many cells in the ventral nucleus are called primary-like, because their frequency (firing rate) resembles that of primary afferents. Most of the output neurons project to the nearby superior olivary nucleus.

The cells of the dorsal nucleus are heterogeneous. At least six different cell types have been characterized by their morphology and electrical behavior. Most of the output neurons project to the contralateral inferior colliculus. Individually, they exhibit an extremely narrow range of tonal responses, being 'focused' by collateral inhibition.

Superior olivary nucleus

The superior olivary complex of nuclei is relatively small in the human brain. It contains *binaural neurons* affected by inputs from both ears. Ipsilateral inputs are excitatory to the binaural neurons, whereas contralateral inputs are inhibitory. The inhibitory effect is mediated by internuncial neurons in the **nucleus of the trapezoid body**.

The superior olivary nucleus is responsive to differences in intensity and timing between sounds entering both ears simultaneously. On the side ipsilateral to a sound, stimulation of cochlea and nucleus is earlier and more intense than on the contralateral side. By exaggerating these differences through crossed inhibition, the superior olivary nucleus helps to indicate the spatial direction of incoming sounds. At the same time, the excited nucleus projects to the inferior colliculus of both sides, giving rise to binaural responses in the neurons of the inferior colliculus and beyond.

Lateral lemniscus

Fibers of the lateral lemniscus arise from the dorsal and ventral cochlear nuclei and from the superior olivary nuclei – in each case, mainly contralaterally. The tract terminates in the **central nucleus of the inferior colliculus**. Nuclei within the lateral lemniscus participate in reflex arcs (see later).

Inferior colliculus

Spatial information from the superior olivary nucleus, intensity information from the ventral cochlear nucleus, and pitch information from the dorsal cochlear nucleus are integrated in the inferior colliculus. The main (central) part of the nucleus is laminated in a tonotopic manner. Within each tonal lamina, cells differ in their responses: some have a characteristic 'tuning curve' (they respond only to a particular tone); some fire spontaneously but are inhibited by sound; and some respond only to a moving source of sound.

In addition to projecting to the medial geniculate body (nucleus), the inferior colliculus exerts inhibitory effects on its opposite number through the **collicular commissure** (Figure 20.3). It also contributes to the tectospinal tract.

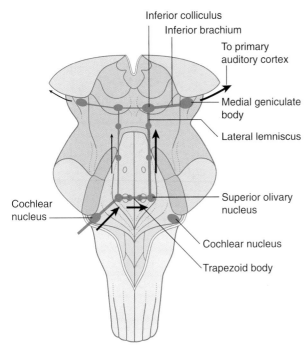

Figure 20.3 Dorsal view of brainstem showing basic plan of central auditory pathways. The strand linking the two inferior colliculi is the collicular commissure.

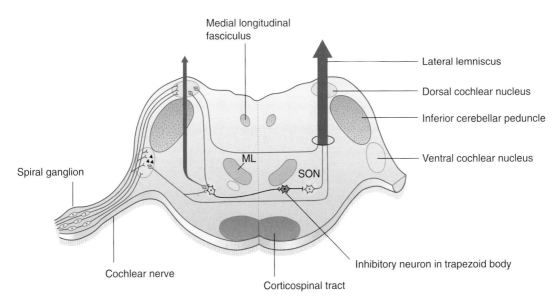

Figure 20.4 Transverse section of lower end of pons showing central connections of cochlear nerve. ML, medial lemniscus; SON, superior olivary nucleus.

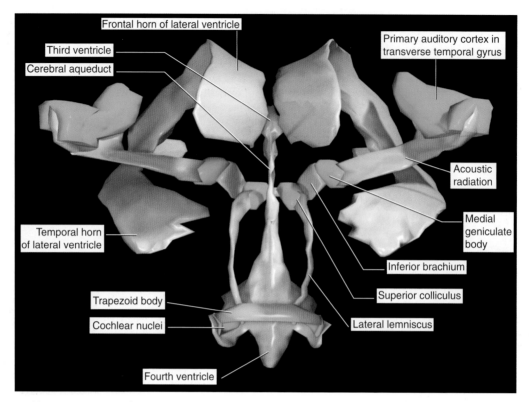

Figure 20.5 Graphic reconstruction of the central auditory pathways from a postmortem brain. (Reproduced from Kretschmann, H-J. and Weinrich, W. *Neurofunctional Systems: 3D Reconstructions with Correlated Neuroimaging: Text and CD-ROM*. New York: Thieme 1998, with kind permission of the authors and the publisher.)

Medial geniculate body

The medial geniculate body is the specific thalamic nucleus for hearing. The main (ventral) nucleus is laminated and tonotopic, and its large (magnocellular) principal neurons project as the **auditory radiation** to the primary auditory cortex (Figure 20.5).

Primary auditory cortex

The upper surface of the temporal lobe shows two or more **transverse temporal gyri**. The anterior one (the **gyrus of Heschl**) contains the **primary auditory cortex** (Figure 20.6). Tonotopic arrangement is preserved in Heschl's gyrus, its posterior part being responsive to high tones and its anterior part to low tones. The auditory cortex responds to auditory stimuli within the *contralateral sound field*. In cats, destruction of a patch of primary cortex on one side produces a *sigoma* or 'deaf spot' in the contralateral sound field. In humans, ablation of the superior temporal gyrus (in the course of tumor removal) does not cause deafness, but it significantly reduces ability to judge the direction and distance of a source of sound.

Brainstem auditory evoked potentials are described in Chapter 31.

Brainstem acoustic reflexes

Collateral branches emerging from the lateral lemniscus form the internuncial linkage for certain reflex arcs:

- Fibers entering the motor nuclei of the trigeminal and facial nerves link up with motor neurons supplying the

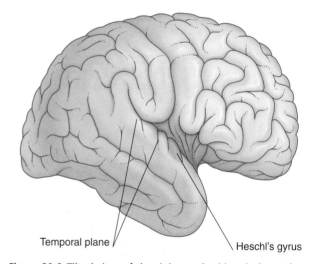

Figure 20.6 Tilted view of the right cerebral hemisphere; the frontal and parietal opercula of the insula have been moved to show the anterior temporal gyrus of Heschl (*blue*).

tensor tympani and stapedius, respectively. These muscles exert a damping action on the ossicles of the middle ear. The tensor tympani is activated by the subject's own voice, the stapedius by external sounds.

- Fibers entering the reticular formation have an important arousal effect, as exemplified by the alarm clock. Sudden loud sounds cause the subject to flinch; this is the 'startle response', mediated by outputs from the reticular formation to the spinal cord and to the motor nucleus of the facial nerve.

Descending auditory pathways

A cascade of descending fibers flows from the primary auditory cortex to the medial geniculate nucleus and inferior colliculus, and from inferior colliculus to superior olivary nucleus. From here the **olivocochlear bundle** emerges in the vestibular nerve and carries efferent, cholinergic fibers to the cochlea along with some for the vestibular labyrinth. The cochlear fibers apply large synaptic boutons to outer hair cells, and small boutons to the afferent nerve endings on inner hair cells.

The primary function of the olivocochlear supply to the outer hair cells is protective: to dampen the basilar membrane's response to dangerously loud noise. Activation of its supply to the inner hair cell nerve endings is thought to enhance the basilar membrane response to sounds requiring attention, e.g. a faint voice in a crowd.

Deafness

Deafness is a widespread problem in the community. About 10% of adults suffer from it in some degree. The cause may lie in the outer, middle, or inner ear, or in the cochlear neural pathway. The two fundamental types of deafness are described in Clinical Panel 20.1.

Clinical Panel 20.1 Two kinds of deafness

All forms of deafness can be grouped into two categories. *Conductive deafness* is caused by disease in the outer ear canal or in the middle ear. *Sensorineural deafness* is caused by disease in the cochlea or in the neural pathway from cochlea to brain.

Common causes of conductive deafness include accumulation of cerumen (wax) in the outer ear, and *otitis media* (inflammation in the middle ear). *Otosclerosis* is a disorder of the oval window in which the spiral ligament of the stapes is progressively replaced by bone. The stapes becomes immobilized, with severe impairment of hearing throughout the full tonal range. Replacement of the stapes by a prosthesis (artificial substitute) often restores normal hearing.

Sensorineural deafness usually originates within the cochlea. The commonest form is the high-frequency hearing loss of the elderly, resulting from deterioration of the organ of Corti in the basal turn. As a result, the elderly have difficulty in distinguishing among high-frequency consonants (d, s, t); vowels, which are low frequency, are quite audible. Therefore the elderly should be addressed distinctly rather than loudly.

Occupational deafness arises from a noisy environment at work. A persistent noise, especially indoors, may eventually lead to degeneration of the organ of Corti in the region corresponding to the particular frequency.

Ototoxic deafness may follow administration of drugs, including streptomycin, neomycin, and quinine.

Infectious deafness may follow more or less complete destruction of the cochlea by the virus of mumps or congenital rubella (German measles).

An important cause of sensorineural deafness in adults is an *acoustic neuroma*. Because the trigeminal and facial nerves may be affected as well as the cochlear and vestibular, this tumor is described in Chapter 22.

Reference
Howarth A, Shone GR: Ageing and the auditory system. *Postgrad Med J* 82:166–171, 2006.

Core Information

The bipolar cochlear neurons occupy the osseous spiral lamina of the modiolus. Their peripheral processes supply hair cells in the organ of Corti. Their central processes end in the cochlear nuclei; from here, a polyneuronal pathway leads mainly through the trapezoid body and lateral lemniscus to the inferior colliculus, but there is a significant ipsilateral pathway too. From the inferior colliculus, fibers run to the medial geniculate body and from there to the primary auditory cortex on the upper surface of the temporal lobe of the brain.

Clinically, deafness is of two kinds: conductive, involving disease in the outer or middle ear; and sensorineural, involving disease of the cochlea (usually) or of central auditory pathways. Hearing is seldom significantly compromised by central pathway lesions because of the bilateral projections to the inferior colliculus and beyond.

REFERENCES

Cooper NP, Cooper JJ: Efferent-mediated control of basilar membrane movement, *J Physiol* 576:49–54, 2006.

Corwin JT, Warchol ME: Auditory hair cells: structure, function, development, and regeneration, *Ann Rev Neurosci* 14:301–333, 1991.

Howarth A, Shone GR: Ageing and the auditory system, *Postgrad Med J* 166–171, 2006.

Raphael Y, Altschuler RA: Structure and innervation of the cochlea, *Brain Res Bull* 60:397–422, 2003.

22 Facial nerve

STUDY GUIDELINES

1 VII is the most commonly paralyzed of all peripheral nerves, owing to the great length of its canal in the temporal bone, where it is at risk of compression when swollen. Because VII supplies the muscles of facial expression, the effects of peripheral facial nerve paralysis are obvious to all.
2 Learn the distinctions between upper and lower motor neuron lesions of VII.
3 Note that VII participates in several important reflex arcs.

FACIAL NERVE

The **facial nerve** supplies the muscles derived from the second branchial arch. These include the muscles of facial expression, and four others mentioned below. It is accompanied during part of its course by the **nervus intermedius** which supplies secretomotor fibers to glands in the eye, nose, mouth, and gustatory fibers to the tongue and palate.

The facial nerve arises from the branchial (special visceral) efferent cell column caudal to the motor nucleus of the trigeminal nerve (Figure 17.2). The **facial nucleus** occupies the lateral region of the tegmentum in the caudal part of the pons (Figures 17.15, 22.1). Before emerging from the brainstem, it loops, as the **internal genu**, around the abducens nucleus, creating the **facial colliculus** in the floor of the fourth ventricle.

The nerve emerges at the lower border of the pons together with the nervus intermedius. Both nerves cross the subarachnoid space in company with the vestibulocochlear nerve, to the internal acoustic meatus. Above the vestibule of the labyrinth, it enters a 7-shaped bony canal having a backward bend at the **external genu** of the facial nerve. Prior to escaping the canal at the stylomastoid foramen, it supplies the stapedius muscle. Upon escape, it supplies the posterior belly of the occipitofrontalis, the stylohyoid, and the posterior belly of the digastric. It then turns forward within the substance of the parotid gland while breaking up into the five named branches to the muscles of facial expression (Figure 22.2).

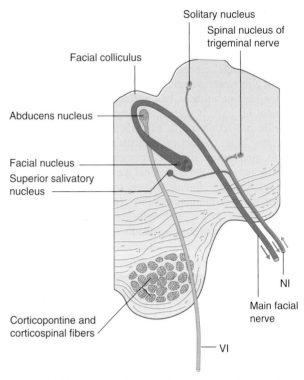

Figure 22.1 Transverse section of the pons, showing the facial nerve and the nervus intermedius (NI).

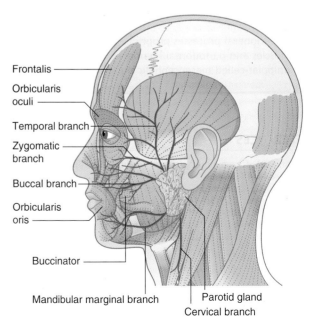

Figure 22.2 Principal extracranial branches of the facial nerve.

Supranuclear connections

All of the cells of the motor nucleus receive a corticonuclear supply from the 'face' area of the contralateral motor cortex. In addition, those to the muscles of the upper face (occipitofrontalis and orbicularis oculi) receive an equal supply from the *ipsilateral* motor cortex. The bilateral supply for the upper facial muscles is reflected in their habitual paired activities in wrinkling the forehead, blinking, and squeezing the eyes closed. The muscles around the mouth, on the other hand, are often activated unilaterally for some expressive purpose. The partial bilateral supply to the facial muscles helps to distinguish a supranuclear from a nuclear or infranuclear lesion of the nerve (Clinical Panel 22.1).

The muscles of facial expression are more responsive to emotional states than any other muscle group. A limbic

---

Clinical Panel 22.1 Lesions of the facial nerve

Supranuclear lesions

The commonest cause of a supranuclear lesion of the seventh nerve is a vascular stroke, in which corticonuclear and corticospinal fibers are interrupted at or above the level of the internal capsule. The usual effect of a stroke is to produce a contralateral motor weakness of the lower part of the face and of the limbs. (The lower part of the face may appear to recover momentarily when participating in a spontaneous smile, as mentioned earlier.) The upper face escapes because of the bilateral supranuclear supply to the upper part of the facial nucleus.

Nuclear lesions

The main motor nucleus may be involved in thrombosis of one of the pontine branches of the basilar artery. As might be anticipated from the relationships depicted in Figure 22.1, the usual result of such a lesion is an *alternating (crossed) hemiplegia*: complete paralysis of the facial and/or abducens nerve on one side combined with motor weakness of the limbs on the opposite side owing to concomitant involvement of the corticospinal tract.

Infranuclear lesions

Bell's palsy is a common disorder caused by a neuritis (possibly viral in origin) of the facial nerve. The inflammation causes the nerve to swell, and conduction is compromised by the close fit of the nerve in its bony canal in the interval between geniculate ganglion and stylomastoid foramen. There may be some initial pain in the ear, but the condition is otherwise painless.

Facial paralysis is usually complete. On the affected side, the patient is unable to raise the eyebrow, close the eye, or retract the lip. The patient may experience *hyperacousis*: ordinary sounds may be unpleasantly loud owing to loss of the damping action of the stapedius muscle.

Tests may reveal blockage of nervus intermedius fibers, with ipsilateral reduced lacrimal and salivary secretions and loss of taste from the anterior part of the tongue.

Four out of five patients recover completely within a few weeks because the nerve has only suffered a conduction block (*neuropraxia*). In the remainder, the nerve undergoes Wallerian degeneration (Ch. 9); recovery takes about 3 months and is often incomplete. During regeneration, some preganglionic fibers of the nervus intermedius may enter the greater petrosal nerve instead of the chorda tympani, with the result that the lacrimal gland becomes active at mealtimes (so-called 'crocodile tears').

Other causes of infranuclear palsy include a patch of demyelination within the pons in the course of multiple sclerosis (Figure CP 22.1.1), tumors in the cerebellopontine angle (Clinical Panel 22.2), middle ear disease, and tumors of the parotid gland. *Herpes zoster oticus* is a rare but well-recognized viral infection of the geniculate ganglion. Severe pain in one ear precedes a vesicular rash in and around the external acoustic meatus. Swelling of the geniculate ganglion may result in a complete facial palsy (*Ramsay Hunt syndrome*).

Figure CP 22.1.1 Complete facial nerve paralysis, patient's right side. The patient has been asked to smile and to look upward. To compare the two sides, cover the left and right halves of the photograph alternately with a card. On the normal side, **(1)** the frontalis muscle has raised the eyebrow, **(2)** the buccinator has retracted the lips, and **(3)** the platysma is in moderate contraction. On the right side, the lower eyelid is drooping due to paralysis of orbicularis oculi.

contribution to the supranuclear supply is to be expected, and indeed two have been identified. One is the **nucleus accumbens** at the base of the forebrain, identified in Figure 33.1. The nucleus accumbens is a ventral part of the basal ganglia, which in turn influence the motor cortex. That circuit is compromised in Parkinson's disease, which is often characterized by a mask-like facies (Ch. 33). The other occupies the *affective area of* the cingulate gyrus (illustrated in Figure 34.10), an emotionally responsive region in the territory of the anterior cerebral artery. It is active during production of a spontaneous smile, and this is of clinical interest, as explained in Clinical Panel 22.1.

Nuclear connections

Five reflex arcs engaging the facial nucleus are listed in Table 22.1. Most important clinically is the corneal reflex.

Corneal reflex

The usual test is to touch the cornea with a cotton wisp. This should elicit a bilateral blink response. The afferent limb of the reflex is the ophthalmic division of the trigeminal nerve (nasociliary branch). The efferent limb is the facial nerve (branch to palpebral element of orbicularis oculi). The reflex can still be elicited following a transection of the spinal tract of the trigeminal nerve (tactotomy, Ch. 21), because the ophthalmic afferents evidently synapse in the principal (pontine) nucleus of the trigeminal. Internuncials projecting from each principal nucleus to both facial nuclei complete the reflex arc.

The corneal reflex may be lost following a lesion of either the ophthalmic or facial nerve. A gradual compression of ophthalmic fibers in the sensory root of the trigeminal nerve may damage corneal neurons selectively. For this reason, the corneal reflex must be tested in patients under suspicion of an acoustic neuroma (Clinical Panel 22.2).

NERVUS INTERMEDIUS

Nervus intermedius aligns with the facial nerve distal to the internal genu. It comprises two sets of parasympathetic and two sets of special sense fibers (Figure 22.3).

The *parasympathetic root* of the nerve arises from the **superior salivatory nucleus** in the pons. This is the motor component of the **greater petrosal** and **chorda tympani** nerves. The greater petrosal synapses in the **pterygopalatine ganglion** ('the ganglion of hay fever'), whose postganglionic fibers stimulate the lacrimal and nasal glands as well as palatine and nasopharyngeal glands. The motor component of chorda tympani synapses in the **submandibular ganglion**, whose postganglionic fibers stimulate the submandibular and sublingual glands.

The *special sense root* of this nerve has unipolar cell bodies in the **geniculate ganglion** of the facial nerve. The peripheral processes of these ganglion cells supply taste buds in the palate via the great petrosal nerve, and taste buds in the anterior two-thirds of the tongue via the chorda tympani. The central processes enter the gustatory part of the solitary nucleus, which also receives fibers from the glossopharyngeal nerve (Ch. 18), as well as the vagus nerve (which carries taste fibers from the epiglottis). From here, second-order neurons project to the thalamus on the *same* side, for relay to the anterior parts of insula and cingulate cortex.

A few cells of the geniculate ganglion supply skin in and around the external acoustic meatus (Clinical Panel 22.1).

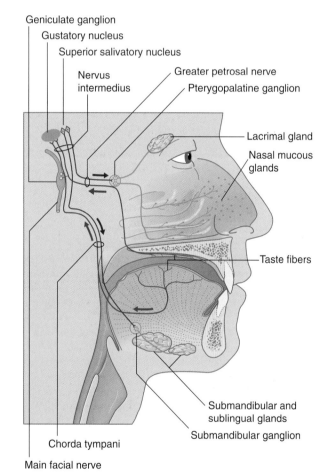

Figure 22.3 The nervus intermedius and its branches. Arrows indicate direction of impulse traffic.

Table 22.1 Brainstem reflexes involving the facial nerve					
	Corneal reflex	**Sucking reflex**	**Blinking to light**	**Blinking to noise**	**Sound attenuation**
Receptor	Cornea	Lips	Retina	Cochlea	Cochlea
Afferent	Ophthalmic nerve	Mandibular nerve	Optic nerve	Cochlear nucleus	Cochlear nucleus
First synapse	Spinal nucleus of trigeminal	Pontine nucleus of trigeminal	Superior colliculus	Inferior colliculus	Superior olivary nucleus
Second synapse	Facial nucleus	Facial nucleus	Facial nucleus	Facial nucleus	Facial nucleus
Muscle	Orbicularis oculi	Orbicularis oris	Orbicularis oculi	Orbicularis oculi	Stapedius

Clinical Panel 22.2 Syndromes of the cerebellopontine angle

The *cerebellopontine angle* is the recess between the hemisphere of the cerebellum and the lower border of the pons. The petrous temporal bone, laterally, completes a triangle having the V nerve at its upper corner and IX and X at its lower corner, and bisected by VII and VIII.

Several kinds of space-occupying lesions may compromise one or more of the nerves. The most frequent is an *acoustic neuroma* (Figure CP 22.2.1), a slow-growing, benign tumor of Schwann cells (*neurolemmoma*). The tumor originates on the

vestibular nerve within the internal acoustic meatus, but the initial symptoms are more often cochlear than vestibular. *An acoustic neuroma must be suspected in every middle-aged or elderly patient presenting with auditory or vestibular symptoms.* Early diagnosis is important because of the difficulty of removing a large neuroma extending into the posterior cranial fossa; also because the cumulative motor and sensory disturbances may not show significant improvement after surgery.

The following is a fairly typical sequence of symptoms and signs in a case escaping early detection:

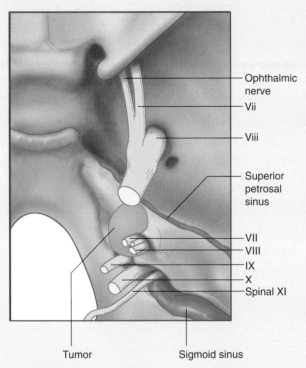

* *Tinnitus* is experienced on the affected side, in the form of a high-pitched ringing or fizzing sound.
* *Deafness* on the affected side is slowly progressive over a period of months or years.
* *Vertigo* occurs episodically. Severe vertigo with nystagmus signifies compression of the brainstem.
* *Loss of the corneal reflex* is an early sign of distortion of the V nerve by a tumor emerging from the internal acoustic meatus into the posterior cranial fossa.
* *Weakness of the masticatory muscles* is a later sign of V nerve involvement. The jaw deviates toward the affected side when the mouth is opened, because the normal lateral pterygoid is unopposed. Wasting of the masseter may be detected by palpation.
* *Weakness of the facial musculature* develops as the VII nerve becomes stretched.
* *Anesthesia of the oropharynx* signifies involvement of the IX nerve.
* *Ipsilateral 'cerebellar signs'* in the arm and leg appear when the cerebellum is compressed.
* *'Upper motor neuron signs'* in the limbs signify compression of the brainstem.
* *Signs of raised intracranial pressure* (headache, drowsiness, papilledema) signify obstruction of cerebrospinal fluid circulation either inside or around the brainstem.

Labels on figure:
Ophthalmic nerve
Vii
Viii
Superior petrosal sinus
VII
VIII
IX
X
Spinal XI
Tumor
Sigmoid sinus

Figure CP 22.2.1 An acoustic neuroma invading the right posterior cranial fossa.

Core Information

Upon leaving its nucleus, the facial nerve whirls around the abducent nerve nucleus, producing the facial colliculus, emerges at the lower border of pons, and at the internal auditory meatus enters a long bony canal opening at the stylomastoid foramen. It supplies the muscles of facial expression, the occipital portion of occipitofrontalis, the stapedius, and the posterior digastric. The upper half of the facial nucleus receives a bilateral supranuclear supply from the motor cortex; the lower half receives only a contralateral supply.

The nervus intermedius travels in part with VII. The superior salivatory nucleus provides the motor components of greater petrosal (for lacrimal and nasal glands by the pterygopalatine ganglion) and chorda tympani (for submandibular and sublingual glands via the submandibular ganglion). The geniculate ganglion of VII has unipolar neurons receiving taste from the palate via greater petrosal nerve and tongue via chorda tympani. A few unipolar neurons supply skin in and around the external acoustic meatus.

REFERENCES

Fischer U, Hess CW, Rosler KM: Uncrossed corticonuclear projections in humans are abundant to facial muscles of the upper and lower face, but may differ between sexes, *J Neurol* 252:21–26, 2005.

Gilchrist JM: Seventh cranial neuropathy, *Semin Neurol* 29:5–13, 2009.

Lang J: Clinical anatomy of the cerebellopontine angle and internal acoustic meatus, *Adv Oto-Rhino-Laryng* 34:8–24, 1984.

Lemon CH, Katz DB: The neural basis of taste, *BMC Neuroscience* 8(S3):1–8, 2007.

Ocular motor nerves

STUDY GUIDELINES

General

Because of the immense diagnostic and therapeutic importance of ocular innervation, and because of its inherent complexity, neuro-ophthalmology has become a branch of medicine in its own right.

It is especially important to appreciate the way in which premotor centers are able to operate bilaterally in order to keep the gaze on target, even when the head is moving.

Particular

1 In addition to nerves III, IV, and VI, the sympathetic supply to the eye is reviewed here because it counterbalances the parasympathetic innervation contained in nerve III.
2 The nerve supply to the six muscles that move the eyeball is straightforward. However, nerve III also supplies the elevator of the upper eyelid.
3 The autonomic supply to the eye is straightforward. For the sympathetic, think of someone being startled awake at night. For the parasympathetic, think of someone eyeing food on a fork.

THE NERVES

The ocular motor nerves comprise the **oculomotor** (III cranial), **trochlear** (IV cranial), and **abducens** (VI cranial) **nerves**. They provide the motor nerve supply to the four

recti and two oblique muscles controlling movements of the eyeball on each side (Figure 23.1). The oculomotor nerve contains two additional sets of neurons: one to supply the levator of the upper eyelid, the other to control the sphincter of the pupil and the ciliary muscle.

The nuclei serving the extraocular muscles (extrinsic muscles of the eye) belong to the somatic efferent cell column of the brainstem, in line with the nucleus of the hypoglossal nerve. The oculomotor nucleus has an additional, parasympathetic nucleus which belongs to the general visceral efferent cell column.

Oculomotor nerve

The nucleus of the third nerve is at the level of the superior colliculus. It is partly embedded in the peri-aqueductal gray matter (Figure 23.2A). It is composed of five individual nuclei for the supply of striated muscles, and one parasympathetic nucleus.

The nerve passes through the tegmentum of the midbrain and emerges into the interpeduncular cistern. It crosses the apex of the petrous temporal bone, pierces the dural roof of the cavernous sinus, runs in the lateral wall of the sinus, and breaks into upper and lower divisions within the superior orbital fissure. The upper division supplies the superior rectus and the levator palpebrae superioris; the lower division supplies the inferior and medial recti and the inferior oblique.

The parasympathetic fibers originate in the **Edinger–Westphal nucleus**. They accompany the main nerve as far as the orbit, then leave the branch to the inferior oblique and synapse in the **ciliary ganglion**. Postganglionic fibers emerge from the ganglion in the **short ciliary nerves**, which pierce

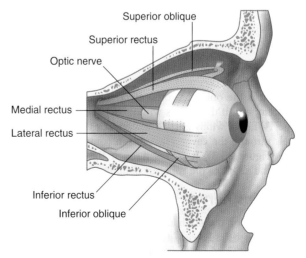

Figure 23.1 Extrinsic ocular muscles.

Core Information

Oculomotor nerve

Somatic efferent fibers of III arise from the main nucleus at superior collicular level. The nerve passes intact through the cavernous sinus and in two divisions through the superior orbital fissure. The upper division supplies superior rectus and levator palpebrae superioris; the lower division supplies inferior and medial recti and inferior oblique.

Parasympathetic fibers emerge from the Edinger–Westphal nucleus, travel with the main nerve, and synapse in the ciliary ganglion for supply of sphincter pupillae and ciliaris.

Paralysis of III is shown by a dilated pupil, followed by ptosis, and later by a divergent squint in addition.

Trochlear nerve

The nucleus of IV is at inferior collicular level. The nerve crosses the midline before emerging below the inferior colliculus. It passes through the cavernous sinus to supply the superior oblique.

Paralysis is characterized by diplopia on looking down.

Abducens nerve

The nucleus is at the level of the facial colliculus in the pons. The nerve runs in the subarachnoid space from lower border of pons to apex of petrous temporal bone, and passes through cavernous sinus and superior orbital fissure supplies lateral rectus.

Paralysis is characterized by convergent squint with inability to abduct the affected eye.

Sympathetic

Muscles stimulated (via α_1 receptors) are dilator pupillae and smooth muscle in the anterior end of the levator palpebrae superioris. Paralysis is characterized by ptosis with a constricted pupil (Horner's syndrome). Muscles inhibited (via β_2 receptors) are sphincter pupillae and ciliaris.

Parasympathetic

Muscles stimulated are the sphincter pupillae and the ciliaris.

Reflex pathways

For the pupillary light reflex: from retina to pretectal nucleus to both Edinger–Westphal nuclei to ciliary ganglion to sphincter pupillae.

For the accommodation reflex: from retina to lateral geniculate body to occipital cortex to Edinger–Westphal nucleus to ciliary ganglion to ciliaris.

Oculomotor controls

Scanning (saccading) is locally activated by six gaze centers. Clinically most important is the PPRF, which operates to pull ipsilateral lateral rectus and contralateral medial rectus conjugately to its own side. Automatic scanning is controlled by the superior colliculi, and voluntary scanning by the frontal eye fields.

Tracking is complex and involves occipital cortex, dynamic labyrinth, cerebellum, superior colliculus, and reticular formation.

REFERENCES

Brazis PW: Isolated palsies of cranial nerves III, IV, and VI, *Semin Neurol* 29:14–28, 2009.

Buttner-Ennever JA: Anatomy of the oculomotor system, *Dev Ophthalmol* 40:1–14, 2007.

Karatas M: Internuclear and supranuclear disorders of eye movements: clinical features and causes, *Eur J Neurol* 16, 2009.

Keane JR: Internuclear ophthalmoplegia, *Arch Neurol* 62:714–717, 2005.

Miley JT, Rodriguez CJ, Hernandez EM, Bundlie SR: Teaching NeuroImage: traumatic internuclear ophthalmoplegia, *Neurology* 70:3–4, 2008.

Moschovakis AK: The neural integrators of the mammalian saccadic system, *Front Biosci* 15:D552–D557, 1997.

Papageorgiou E, Ticini LF, Hardiess G, Schaeffel F, Wiethoelter H, Mallot, HA, Bahlo S, Wilhelm B, Fonthein R, Schiefer U, Karnath H-O: The pupillary light reflex pathway, *Neurology* 70:956–963, 2008.

Tilikete C, Pelisson D: Ocular motor syndromes of the brainstem and cerebellum, *Curr Opin Neurol* 21:22–28, 2008.

Wilhelm H: Neuro-ophthalmology of pupillary function, *J Neurol* 245:573–583, 1998.

Reticular formation

STUDY GUIDELINES

1 The reticular formation has very diverse functions. Some of its nuclear groups have direct access to motor neurons in the brainstem and spinal cord. Others have direct access to autonomic effector nuclei including cardiovascular controls. Some may act simultaneously upon somatic and autonomic nuclei.
2 All of the sensory systems contribute afferents to the reticular formation.
3 Ascending projections of the reticular formation to the forebrain, including the ascending reticular activating system (ARAS), are essential for the state of consciousness.
4 Disturbance of function of aminergic projections from the reticular formation have been correlated with psychiatric states including major depression and schizophrenia.

INTRODUCTION

The reticular formation is phylogenetically a very old neural network, being a prominent feature of the reptilian brainstem. It originated as a slowly conducting, polysynaptic pathway intimately connected with olfactory and limbic regions. The progressive dominance of vision and hearing over olfaction led to localization of sensory and motor functions within the tectum of the midbrain. Direct spinotectal and tectospinal tracts bypassed the reticular formation, which was largely relegated to automatic functions. In mammals, the tectum in turn has been relegated to minor

status with the emergence of very fast pathways linking the cerebral cortex with the peripheral sensory and motor apparatus.

In the human brain, the reticular formation continues to be of importance in automatic and reflex activities, and it has retained its linkages to the limbic system.

ORGANIZATION

The term *reticular formation* refers only to the polysynaptic network in the brainstem, although the network continues rostrally into the thalamus and hypothalamus, and caudally into the propriospinal network of the spinal cord.

The ground plan is shown in Figure 24.1A. In the midline, the *median reticular formation* comprises a series of *raphe nuclei* (*pron.* 'raffay' and derived from the Greek word for seam). The raphe nuclei are the major source of serotonergic projections throughout the neuraxis (see next section).

Next to this is the *paramedian reticular formation*. This part of the network contains *magnocellular* neurons throughout; in the lower pons and upper medulla, some *gigantocellular* neurons also appear, before the network blends with the *central reticular nucleus* of the medulla oblongata.

Outermost is the *lateral, parvocellular* (small-celled) *reticular formation*. Parvocellular dendrites are long and they branch at regular intervals. They have a predominantly transverse orientation, and their interstices are penetrated by long pathways running to the thalamus. The lateral network is mainly afferent in nature. It receives fibers from all of the sensory pathways, including the special senses:

- Olfactory fibers are received through the medial forebrain bundle, which passes alongside the hypothalamus.
- Visual pathway fibers are received from the superior colliculus.
- Auditory pathway fibers are received from the superior olivary nucleus.
- Vestibular fibers are received from the medial vestibular nucleus.
- Somatic sensory fibers are received from the spinoreticular tracts and from the spinal and principal (pontine) nuclei of the trigeminal nerve.

Most parvocellular axons ramify extensively among the dendrites of the paramedian reticular formation. However, some synapse within the nuclei of cranial nerves and act as pattern generators (see later).

The paramedian reticular formation is a predominantly *efferent* system. The axons are relatively long. Some ascend to synapse in the midbrain reticular formation or in the thalamus. Others have both ascending and descending branches contributing to the polysynaptic network. The magnocellular component receives corticoreticular fibers from

Figure 24.1 Reticular formation (RF). **(A)** Subdivisions. **(B)** Aminergic and cholinergic cell groups.

the premotor cortex and gives rise to the pontine and medullary reticulospinal tracts.

Aminergic neurons of the brainstem

Embedded in the reticular formation are sets of aminergic neurons (Figure 24.1B). They include one set producing *serotonin* (5-hydroxytryptamine) and three sets producing *catecholamines*, as listed in Table 24.1.

- The *serotonergic neurons* have the largest territorial distribution of any set of CNS neurons. In general terms, those of the midbrain project rostrally into the cerebral hemispheres; those of the pons ramify in the brainstem and cerebellum; and those of the medulla supply the spinal cord (Figure 24.2). All parts of the CNS gray matter are permeated by serotonin-secreting axonal varicosities. Clinically, enhancement of serotonin activity is part of the treatment for a prevalent condition known as major depression (Ch. 26).
- The *dopaminergic neurons* of the midbrain fall into two groups. At the junction of tegmentum and crus are those of the substantia nigra, which will be considered in Chapter 33. Medial to these, dopaminergic neurons in the **ventral tegmental nuclei** (Figure 24.3) project *mesocortical* fibers to the frontal lobe and *mesolimbic* fibers to the nucleus accumbens in particular (Ch. 34).
- The *noradrenergic neurons* are only marginally less prodigious than the serotonergic ones. About 90% of the somas are pooled in the **cerulean nucleus** (*locus ceruleus*), a 'violet spot' in the floor of the fourth ventricle at the upper end of the pons (Figure 24.4). Neurons of the cerulean nucleus project in *all* directions, as indicated in Figure 24.5.

Table 24.1 Aminergic neurons of the reticular formation

Transmitter	Location
Serotonin	Raphe nuclei of midbrain, pons, medulla
Dopamine	Tegmentum of midbrain
Norepinephrine	Midbrain, pons, medulla
Epinephrine	Medulla

Figure 24.2 Serotonergic projections from the brainstem midline (raphe).

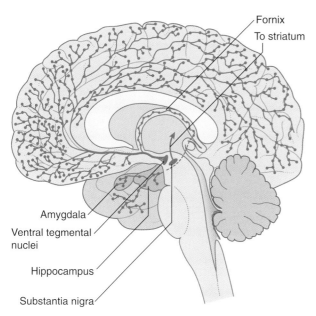

Figure 24.3 Dopaminergic projections from the midbrain.

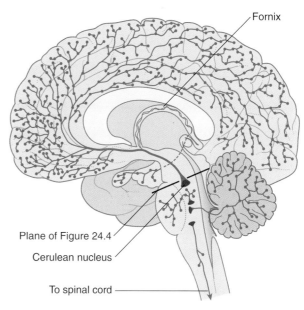

Figure 24.5 Noradrenergic projections from the pons and medulla oblongata.

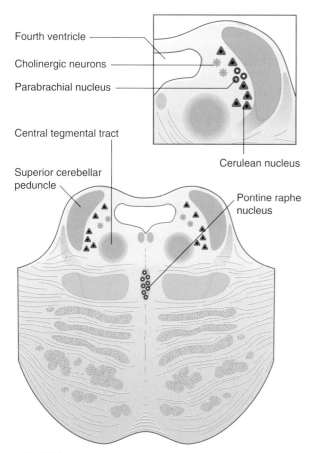

* Acetylcholine
○ Serotonin
▲ Norepinephrine

Figure 24.4 Part of a transverse section through the upper part of the pons, showing elements of the reticular formation.

- *Epinephrine-secreting neurons* are relatively scarce and are confined to the medulla oblongata. Some project rostrally to the hypothalamus, others project caudally to synapse upon preganglionic sympathetic neurons in the spinal cord.

In the cerebral cortex, the ionic and electrical effects of aminergic neuronal activity are quite variable. First, more than one kind of postsynaptic receptor exists for each of the amines. Second, some aminergic neurons liberate a peptide substance also, capable of modulating the transmitter action – usually by prolonging it. Third, the larger cortical neurons receive many thousands of excitatory and inhibitory synapses from local circuit neurons, and they have numerous different receptors. Activation of a single kind of aminergic receptor may have a large or small effect depending on the existing excitatory state.

Although our understanding of the physiology and pharmacology of the monoamines is far from complete, no-one disputes their relevance to a wide range of behavioral functions.

FUNCTIONAL ANATOMY

The range of functions served by different parts of the reticular formation is indicated in Table 24.2.

Pattern generators

Patterned activities involving cranial nerves include:

- Conjugate (in parallel) movements of the eyes locally controlled by premotor nodal points (*gaze centers*) in the midbrain and pons linked to the nuclei of the ocular motor nerves (Ch. 23).
- Rhythmical chewing movements controlled by the supratrigeminal premotor nucleus in the pons (Ch. 21).

Table 24.2 Elements of the reticular formation and their perceived functions

Element	Function
Premotor cranial nerve nuclei	Patterned cranial nerve activities
Pontine locomotor center	Pattern generation
Magnocellular nuclei	Posture, locomotion
Salivatory nuclei	Salivary secretion, lacrimation
Pontine micturition center	Bladder control
Medial parabrachial nucleus	Respiratory rhythm
Central reticular nucleus of medulla oblongata	Vital centers (circulation, respiration)
Lateral medullary nucleus	Conveys somatic and visceral information to the cerebellum
Ascending reticular activating system (ARAS)	Arousal
Aminergic neurons	Sleeping and waking, attention and mood, sensory modulation, blood pressure control

- Swallowing, vomiting, coughing, and sneezing, controlled by separate premotor nodal points in the medulla linked to the appropriate cranial nerves and to the respiratory centers.

Locomotor pattern generators are described in Box 24.1. An overview of gait controls is provided in Box 24.2. Higher-level bladder controls are described in Box 24.3.

The salivatory nuclei belong to the parvocellular reticular formation of pons and medulla. They contribute preganglionic parasympathetic fibers to the facial and glossopharyngeal nerves.

Respiratory control

The respiratory cycle is largely regulated by *dorsal* and *ventral respiratory nuclei* located at the upper end of the medulla oblongata on each side. The dorsal respiratory nucleus occupies the midlateral part of the solitary nucleus. The ventral nucleus is dorsal to the nucleus ambiguus (hence the term *retroambiguus nucleus* in Figure 17.11). A third, *medial parabrachial nucleus*, adjacent to the cerulean nucleus, seems to have a pacemaker function governing respiratory rate (cycles per minute). As will be seen in Chapter 34, stimulation of this nucleus by the amygdala, in *anxiety states*, results in characteristic hyperventilation.

Box 24.1 Locomotor pattern generators

From animal experiments, it has long been agreed that lower vertebrates and lower mammals possess *locomotor pattern generators* in the spinal cord, within the gray matter neurologically connected to each of the four limbs. These *spinal generators* comprise electrically oscillating circuits delivering rhythmically entrained signals to flexor and extensor muscle groups. Spinal generator activity is subject to supraspinal commands from a *mesencephalic locomotor region* (MLR), which in turn obeys commands from motor areas of the cerebral cortex and corpus striatum.

The *MLR* contains the **pedunculopontine nucleus**, close to the superior cerebellar peduncle where this passes along the upper corner of the fourth ventricle to enter the midbrain (Figure 17.16). These nuclei send fibers down the central tegmental tract to the oral and caudal pontine nuclei serving extensor motor neurons and to medullary magnocellular neurons serving flexor motor neurons.

A major focus of spinal rehabilitation is on activation of spinal locomotor reflexes in patients who have experienced injury resulting in partial or complete spinal cord transection. It is now well established that even after complete transection at cervical or thoracic level, a lumbosacral locomotor pattern can be activated by continuous electrical stimulation of the dura mater at lumbar segmental level. The stimulation strongly activates posterior root fibers feeding into the generator in the base of the anterior gray horn. Surface EMG recordings taken from flexor and extensor muscle groups reveal an oscillating pattern of flexor and extensor motor neuron activation, although the pattern

is not identical to the normal one. A normal pattern requires the lesion to be incomplete, with preservation of some supraspinal projection from the pedunculopontine nucleus.

Generation of actual stepping movements is possible in complete lesions if the individual is supported over a moving treadmill belt while the dura is being stimulated, presumably because of the additional cutaneous and proprioceptive inputs to the generator. Muscle strength and stepping speed improve over a period of weeks but not enough to enable unassisted locomotion within a walking frame.

Current research aims at improving the opportunity for supraspinal motor fibers to 'bridge the gap' by clearing tissue debris from the gap and replacing that tissue with a medium having a matrix that will support regenerating axons both physically and chemically.

REFERENCES

Blessing WW: Lower brainstem regulation of visceral, cardiovascular and respiratory function. In Paxinos G, Mai JK, editors: *The human nervous system*, ed 2, Amsterdam, 2004, Elsevier, pp 465–479.

Fouad K, Pearson K: Restoring walking after spinal cord injury, *Progr Neurobiol* 73:107–126, 2004.

Grasso R, Ivanenko YP, Zago M, et al: Distributed plasticity of locomotor pattern generators in spinal cord injured patients, *Brain* 127:1029–1034, 2004.

Jahn K, Deutschlander A, Stephan T, et al: Supraspinal locomotor control in quadriceps and humans, *Prog Brain Res* 171:353–372, 2008.

McCrea DA, Ryback IA: Organization of mammalian locomotor system and pattern generation, *Brain Res Rev* 57:134–146, 2008.

Box 24.2 Overview of gait controls. (Assistance of Professor Tim O'Brien, Director, Gait Laboratory, Central Remedial Clinic, Dublin is gratefully acknowledged.)

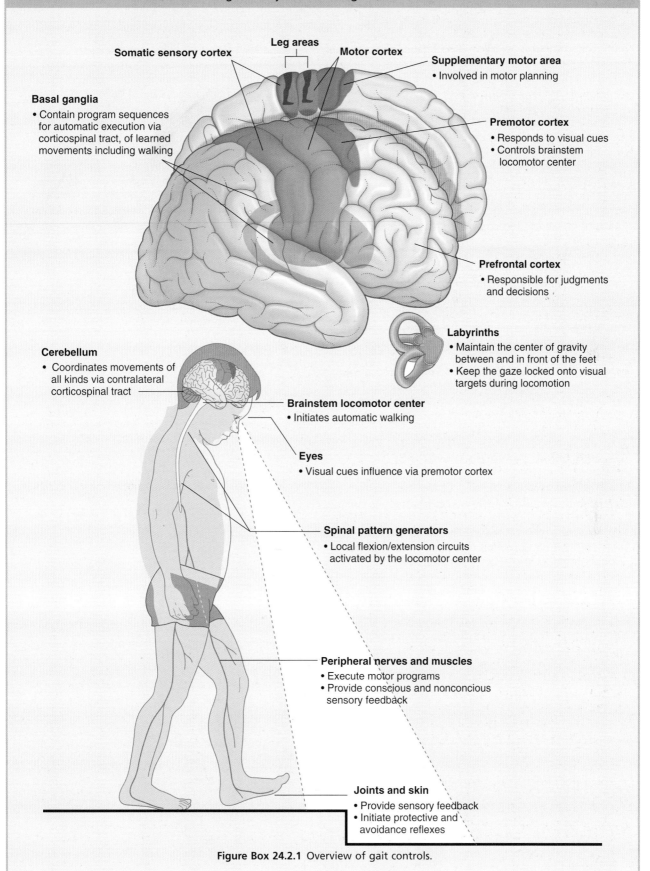

Somatic sensory cortex

Leg areas

Motor cortex

Supplementary motor area
• Involved in motor planning

Basal ganglia
• Contain program sequences for automatic execution via corticospinal tract, of learned movements including walking

Premotor cortex
• Responds to visual cues
• Controls brainstem locomotor center

Prefrontal cortex
• Responsible for judgments and decisions

Labyrinths
• Maintain the center of gravity between and in front of the feet
• Keep the gaze locked onto visual targets during locomotion

Cerebellum
• Coordinates movements of all kinds via contralateral corticospinal tract

Brainstem locomotor center
• Initiates automatic walking

Eyes
• Visual cues influence via premotor cortex

Spinal pattern generators
• Local flexion/extension circuits activated by the locomotor center

Peripheral nerves and muscles
• Execute motor programs
• Provide conscious and nonconcious sensory feedback

Joints and skin
• Provide sensory feedback
• Initiate protective and avoidance reflexes

Figure Box 24.2.1 Overview of gait controls.

Box 24.3 Higher-level bladder controls

The *micturition control center* is in the paramedian pontine reticular formation on each side, with interconnections across the midline. Magnocellular neurons project from here all the way to micturition-related parasympathetic neurons in segments S2–4 of the spinal cord (Figure Box 24.3.1).

Activation of the micturition control center produces not only a rise in intravesical pressure but also relaxation of the external urethral *striated* sphincter, brought about by simultaneous excitation of GABAergic internuncials synapsing in the nucleus of Onuf in sacral segments of the spinal cord (Ch. 13).

More laterally in the pons is the L (lateral) center projecting to Onuf's nucleus. In this context, the micturition control center is referred to as the M (medial) center.

At higher levels, cells in the lateral part of the *right periaqueductal gray matter* (PAG) receive fibers ascending from the sacral posterior gray horn and project excitatory fibers to the insula which generates conscious sensation of normal bladder filling and relays its activity to the medial prefrontal cortex. The lateral PAG also receives an excitatory input from the *right* hypothalamus.

Some spinoreticular projections from the sacral cord excite the L center. Others relay via the thalamus to cells in a part of the *right* **anterior cingulate cortex** (ACCx) known to be active during tasks requiring attention.

This right-sided bias is thought to be related to emotional aspects of micturition.

The micturition cycle

1 When the bladder is half-full, vesical afferents from stretch receptors in the detrusor and in the mucous membrane of the trigone relay this information along spinoreticular fibers reaching pons, midbrain, and insula via thalamus (Figure Box 24.3.2).
2 The insular cortex projects to the *decision center* in the medial prefrontal cortex, keeping it informed about the level of bladder filling.
3 As indicated in Chapter 13, activity in the sympathetic system is stepped up so that *bladder compliance* can be increased (via β_2 receptors). Parasympathetic neurons are silenced by α_2 neuronal interaction.
4 Spinoreticular fibers synapsing in the L nucleus of the pons activate Onuf's nucleus in the sacral cord, thereby raising the tone of the external urinary sphincter.
5 With completion of filling, there is perception of urgency. If time or place is not suitable, part of the medial prefrontal gyrus comes alive. This area puts the ACCx on hold by reducing its level of activity via association-fiber projections to inhibitory internuncials there. Likewise, projections to hypothalamus and midbrain inhibit preoptic area and PAG by activating appropriate internuncials.
6 A final measure, one that cannot be long sustained, is *voluntary contraction of the entire pelvic floor*. The command for this contraction is sent from the prefrontal cortex to the perineal representation on the medial side of the motor cortex in the paracentral lobule.
7 When time and place permit, the medial prefrontal cortex releases its three prisoners. The pelvic floor is allowed to sag in the manner described in Chapter 13, and the hypothalamus joins PAG in activating the M nucleus while inactivating L via inhibitory internuncials.

The right-sided bias of micturition control is consistent with the clinical observation that, among stroke patients of either sex, urinary incontinence is more commonly associated with right-sided lesions of the brain.

Role of monoamines

The motor and sensory spinal cord nuclei serving the bladder are abundantly supplied with serotonergic neurons descending from the magnus raphe nucleus (MRN) in the medulla oblongata. Animal experiments have shown that local applications of 5 HT are excitatory to pelvic sympathetic and sacral anterior horn neurons, inhibitory to pelvic parasympathetic and sacral posterior horn neurons. Distension of the bladder is known to stimulate the MRN (via spinoreticular activation of the periaqueductal gray matter). A quick review of the lower-level bladder controls (Box 13.3) suggests that the MRN sets the general tone in favor of bladder filling.

Noradrenergic fibers descending to the anterior gray horn from the cerulean nucleus potentiate the effect of local glutamate release onto the cells of Onuf's nucleus, thereby enhancing external sphincter tone during the filling phase.

(In real life not all glow simultaneously!)

REFERENCE
Fowler CJ, Griffiths, DJ: A decade of functional brain imaging applied to bladder control, *Neurourol Urodynam* 2009.

The assistance of Professor Mary Pat FitzGerald, Department of Urogynecology, Stritch School of Medicine, Loyola University, Chicago, is gratefully acknowledged.

Box 24.3 *Continued*

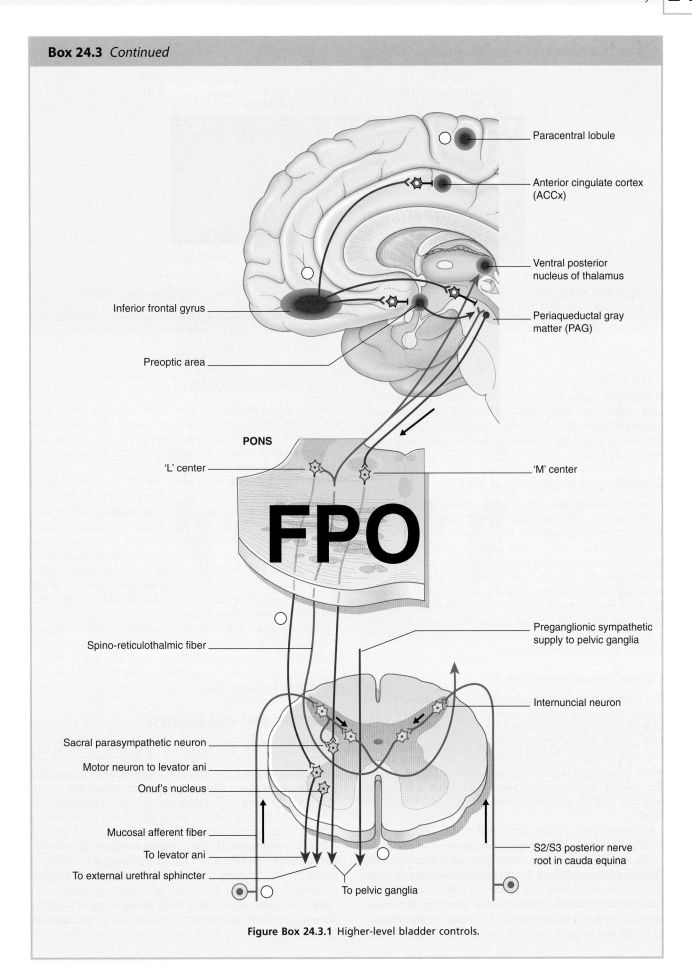

Paracentral lobule

Anterior cingulate cortex (ACCx)

Ventral posterior nucleus of thalamus

Inferior frontal gyrus

Periaqueductal gray matter (PAG)

Preoptic area

PONS

'L' center

'M' center

FPO

Preganglionic sympathetic supply to pelvic ganglia

Spino-reticulothalmic fiber

Internuncial neuron

Sacral parasympathetic neuron

Motor neuron to levator ani

Onuf's nucleus

Mucosal afferent fiber

To levator ani

S2/S3 posterior nerve root in cauda equina

To external urethral sphincter

To pelvic ganglia

Figure Box 24.3.1 Higher-level bladder controls.

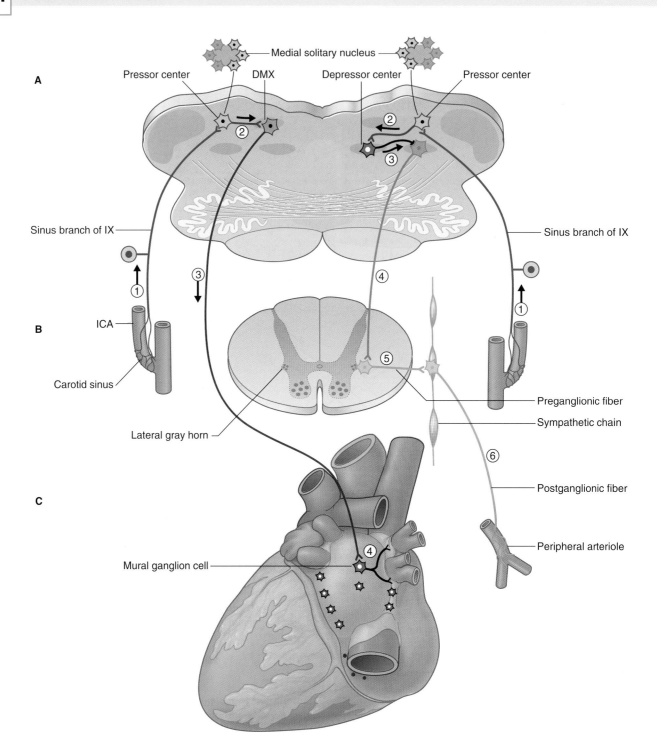

Figure 24.7 Baroreceptor reflexes. **(A)** Upper medulla oblongata. **(B)** Spinal cord segments T1–L3. **(C)** Posterior wall of heart. *Baroreceptor reflex ((left).* **1** Stretch receptors in the carotid sinus excite fibers in the sinus branch of the glossopharyngeal nerve. ICA, internal carotid artery. **2** Baroreceptor neurons of the solitary nucleus respond by stimulating cardioinhibitory neurons in the dorsal (motor) nucleus of the vagus (DMX). **3** Preganglionic, cholinergic parasympathetic vagal fibers synapse upon mural ganglion cells on the posterior wall of the heart. **4** Postganglionic, cholinergic parasympathetic fibers reduce pacemaker activity, thus reducing the heart rate. *Barosympathetic reflex (right).* **1** Carotid sinus stretch receptor afferents excite baroreceptor medial neurons of the solitary nucleus. **2** Baroreceptor neurons respond by exciting the inhibitory neurons of the vasomotor depressor center in the central reticular nucleus of the medulla. **3** Adrenergic and noradrenergic neurons of the pressor center in the lateral reticular nucleus (rostral ventrolateral medulla) are inhibited. **4** Tonic excitation of the lateral gray horn is reduced. **5** and **6** Preganglionic and postganglionic sympathetic tone to peripheral arterioles is reduced, thus lowering the peripheral arterial resistance.

by hypothalamic neurons to form a sleep-inducing substance.

- Cholinergic neurons close to the cerulean nucleus are active during REM sleep and they appear to cause the rapid eye movements by playing upon the ocular motor nuclei.

Ascending reticular activating system

This term refers to the participation of reticular formation neurons in activation of the cerebral cortex, as shown by a change in EEG records from high-amplitude, slow waves to low-amplitude, fast waves during spontaneous arousal from sleep. The strongest candidates for such a role are sets of cholinergic neurons close to the cerulean nucleus (Figure 24.4). In addition to supplying the above-mentioned fibers to the ocular motor nuclei, these neurons project to almost all thalamic nuclei, and they have an excitatory effect upon thalamic neurons projecting to the cerebral cortex.

The **hypothalamus** is an important control center for various body rhythms, including sleep and wakefulness. A second candidate for cortical activation has been found in the hypothalamus, namely the **tuberomammillary nucleus**. This nucleus contains histaminergic neurons having widespread projections to the cerebral cortex (Ch. 26).

Following arousal, the waking-state EEG pattern seems to be sustained by the continuing discharge of the brainstem and hypothalamic neurons mentioned; also by a third set of neurons, embedded in the basal forebrain immediately above the optic chiasm. The third set occupies the **basal nucleus of Meynert** (Ch. 34) projecting cholinergic axons to most parts of the cerebral cortex.

Sensory modulation: gate control

Sensory transmission from primary to secondary afferent neurons (at the levels of the posterior gray horn and posterior column nuclei) and from secondary to tertiary (at the level of the thalamus) is subject to *gating*. The term *gating* refers to the degree of freedom of synaptic transmission from one set of neurons to the next.

Tactile sensory transmission is gated at the level of the posterior column nuclei. Corticospinal neurons projecting from the postcentral gyrus may facilitate or inhibit sensory transmission at this level, as mentioned in Chapter 16.

Nociceptive transmission from the trunk and limbs is gated in the posterior gray horn of the spinal cord. From the head and upper part of the neck, it is gated in the spinal trigeminal nucleus. A key structure in both areas of gray matter is the substantia gelatinosa, which is packed with small excitatory and inhibitory internuncial neurons. The excitatory transmitter is glutamate; the inhibitory one is GABA for some internuncials, enkephalin (an opiate pentapeptide) for others.

Finely myelinated (Aδ) polymodal nociceptive fibers synapse directly upon dendrites of relay neurons of the lateral spinothalamic tract and of its trigeminal equivalent. The Aδ fibers signal sharp, well-localized pain. Unmyelinated, C-fiber nociceptive afferents have mainly indirect access to relay cells, via excitatory gelatinosa internuncials. The C fibers signal dull, poorly localized pain. Most of them contain substance P, which may be liberated as a cotransmitter with glutamate.

Segmental antinociception

Large (A category) mechanoreceptive afferents from hair follicles synapse upon *anterior* spinothalamic relay cells (and their trigeminal equivalents). They also give off collaterals to inhibitory (mainly GABA) gelatinosa cells which synapse in turn upon *lateral* spinothalamic relay cells (Figure 24.8). Some of the internuncials also exert presynaptic inhibition upon C-fiber terminals, either by axo-axonic contacts (which are very difficult to find in experimental material), or by dendro-axonic contacts. Gating of the spinothalamic response to C-fiber activity can be induced by stimulating the mechanoreceptive afferents, thereby recruiting inhibitory gelatinosa cells. This simple circuit accounts for the relief afforded by 'rubbing the sore spot'. It also provides a rationale for the use of *transcutaneous electrical nerve stimulation* (TENS) by physical therapists for pain relief in arthritis and other chronically painful conditions. The standard procedure in TENS is to apply a stimulating electrode to the skin at the same segmental level as the source of noxious C-fiber activity, and to deliver a current sufficient to produce a pronounced buzzing sensation.

Supraspinal antinociception

Magnus raphe nucleus (Figure 24.8)

From the magnus raphe nucleus (MRN) in the medulla oblongata, *raphespinal fibers* descend bilaterally within Lissauer's tract and terminate in the substantia gelatinosa at all levels of the spinal cord. In animals, electrical stimulation of the MRN may produce total analgesia throughout the body, with little effect on tactile sensation. Many fibers of the raphespinal tract liberate serotonin, which excites inhibitory internuncials in the posterior gray horn and spinal trigeminal nucleus. The internuncials induce both pre- and postsynaptic inhibition on the relevant relay cells.

There is evidence that noradrenergic projections to the posterior horn from pons and medulla are also involved in supraspinal antinociception, by a direct inhibitory effect on spinothalamic neurons.

- *Diffuse noxious inhibitory controls.* The MRN is not somatotopically arranged, but it does receive inputs from spinoreticular and trigeminoreticular neurons responding to peripheral noxious stimulation. This anatomical connection accounts for what are called diffuse noxious inhibitory controls. *Painful stimulation of one part of the body may produce pain relief in all other parts.* The arrangement accounts well for the heterotopic relief of pain in acupuncture (Ch. 31), where needles are used to excite nociceptive afferents in the most superficial musculature rather than in the skin.
- *Stimulus-induced analgesia.* MRN is intensely responsive to stimulation of the PAG of the midbrain. This connection has been used to advantage for patients suffering intractable pain: a fine stimulating electrode can be inserted into PAG and wired so that the patient can control the level of self-stimulation.
- *Stress-induced analgesia.* At rest, the PAG projection to the MRN is under tonic inhibition by inhibitory internuncials present within PAG. The internuncials are themselves inhibited by opioid peptides, notably by β-endorphin

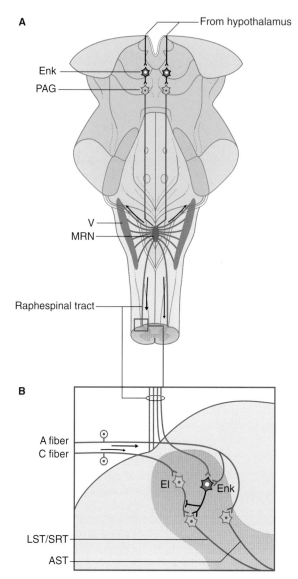

Figure 24.8 Antinociceptive pathways. **(A)** Posterior view of brainstem. **(B)** Right posterior gray horn of spinal cord, viewed from above. The periaqueductal gray matter (PAG) contains an excitatory projection to the magnus raphe nucleus (MRN), and enkephalinergic internuncials (Enk) which exert tonic inhibition upon the projection cells. Inhibitory fibers from the hypothalamus release (*disinhibit*) the excitatory neurons, and MRN responds in turn. The effects within the spinal nucleus of trigeminal (V) and posterior gray horn are the same: serotonin liberated by MRN neurons excites enkephalinergic internuncials which inhibit nociceptive projection cells. The nociceptive pathway at cord level is represented by the C-fiber input to an excitatory internuncial (EI), which in turn excites the lateral spinothalamic or spinoreticular projection cell (LST/SRT) unless this is being inhibited by the enkephalinergic internuncial. Rubbing the sore spot sends impulse trains along A fibers inducing the Enk cell to exert presynaptic inhibition on the EI terminal, and postsynaptic inhibition on the LST/SRT projection cell. Passage of purely tactile information into the anterior spinothalamic tract (AST) is not impeded.

released from a small set of hypothalamic neurons projecting to PAG. In life-threatening situations, where injury may be the price to be paid for escape, PAG may be released (disinhibited) by the hypothalamus. This seems to be the mechanism whereby a bullet wound may be scarcely noticed in the heat of battle. (As will be seen in Ch. 34, excitatory neurons in the PAG may also be stimulated directly by the amygdala, located in the anterior temporal lobe, in fearful situations.)

In addition to the segmental and supraspinal controls of nociceptive transmission from primary to secondary afferents, gating occurs within the thalamus (see Ch. 27).

Furthermore, perception of the aversive (unpleasant) quality of pain seems to require participation of the anterior cingulate cortex (Ch. 34), which is rich in opiate receptors.

Clinical Panel 24.1 Urge incontinence

Urge incontinence is defined as an inability of adult women to control voiding when the storage phase of the micturition cycle is still incomplete. It is characterized by an acute sense of urgency quickly followed by uncontrollable voiding regardless of the circumstances. Hence the term 'overactive bladder' or 'detrusor overactivity'. Many cases have a history of childhood bladder irritability in the form of daytime micturition frequency and/or *nocturnal eneuresis* (bed wetting).

fMRI studies in adult cases reveal increased activity of the right insular cortex, which is considered responsible for the heightened state of bladder awareness, and of the anterior, emotion-related area of the cingulate cortex, consistent with the sense of urgency and fear of imminent voiding.

As mentioned in Chapter 8, G-protein-gated muscarinic receptors, activated by postganglionic fibers from pelvic ganglia, are abundant on the detrusor muscle of the bladder. Accordingly, the drugs of choice are muscarinic receptor antagonists. However,

antimuscarinic side-effects such as dry mouth and constipation may require this therapy to be withdrawn.

Botulinum toxin has been increasingly used to treat detrusor overactivity in recent years. It is known to disrupt the interface between cholinergic synaptic vesicles and target muscle fibers (whether striated or smooth), thereby rendering the synapse ineffective. A flexible cystoscope is passed through the urethra and numerous small Botox injections are inserted into the bladder wall. Twice yearly sessions are standard for the longer term.

REFERENCES

FitzGerald MP, Thom DH, Wassel-Fyr C, et al: Childhood urinary symptoms predict adult overactive bladder symptoms, *J Urol* 175:989–993, 2006.

Griffiths D, Tadic SD: Bladder control, urgency and urge incontinence: evidence from functional brain imaging, *Neurourol Urodynam* 27:466–474, 2008.

Nitti VW: Botulinum toxin for the treatment of idiopathic and neurogenic overactive bladder: state of the art, *Rev Urol* 8:198–208, 2006.

Core Information

Ground plan

The reticular formation extends the entire length of the brainstem, mainly in three cell columns. The lateral, parvocellular column receives afferents from the sensory components of all cranial and spinal nerves. It projects into the paramedian magnocellular reticular formation, which in turn sends long axons to the brain and spinal cord. The median reticular formation contains serotonergic neurons.

Aminergic neurons

Serotonergic neurons of the raphe nuclei project to all parts of the gray matter of the CNS. Dopaminergic neurons project from substantia nigra to striatum and from midbrain ventral tegmental nuclei to prefrontal cortex and nucleus accumbens. Noradrenergic neurons of the cerulean nucleus project to all parts of the CNS gray matter. Epinephrine-secreting neurons of the medulla project to hypothalamus and spinal cord.

Pattern generators

Gaze centers in midbrain and pons control conjugate eye movements; a midbrain locomotor area regulates walking; a pontine supratrigeminal nucleus regulates chewing rhythm, and a pontine micturition center controls the bladder. In the medulla oblongata are

respiratory, emetic, coughing, and sneezing centers, and pressor and depressor centers for cardiovascular control. In addition, the medullary chemosensitive area contains reticular formation neurons sensitive to H^+ ion levels in the cerebrospinal fluid.

Sleeping and wakefulness are influenced by serotonin and norepinephrine neurons, and by cholinergic neurons in the upper pons. The ascending reticular activating system is a physiological concept based on brainstem neuronal networks having an arousal effect on the brain, as seen in EEG traces. An important component is a set of pontine cholinergic neurons having an excitatory effect on thalamocortical neurons.

Antinociception

Segmental antinociception is induced by stimulating A fibers from hair follicles. *Supraspinal antinociception* is a function of the medullary magnus raphe nucleus (MRN), which is activated from hypothalamus and midbrain. Serotonin from MRN terminals in substantia gelatinosa of spinal posterior horn/trigeminal nucleus activates enkephalinergic internuncials that inhibit transmission in spinothalamic/trigeminothalamic neurons.

REFERENCES

Benarroch E: Descending monoaminergic pain modulation, *Neurology* 71: 218–221, 2008.

Benarroch EE: The arterial baroreflex: functional organization and involvement in neurologic disease, *Neurology* 71:1733–1738, 2008.

Bianchi AL, Denavit-Saube M, Champagnet J: Central control of breathing, *Physiol Rev* 75:1–45, 1995.

Edgerton VR, Roy RR: Paralysis recovery in humans and model systems, *Curr Opin Neurobiol* 12:658–667, 2002.

Gonzalez C, Almaraz L, Obeso A, Rigual R: Carotid body chemoreceptors: from natural stimuli to sensory discharges, *Physiol Rev* 74:829–898, 1994.

Rosenfeld JP: Interacting brain components of opiate-activated, descending, pain-inhibitory systems, *Neurosci Behav Rev* 18:403–409, 1994.

Siddall PJ: Pain mechanisms and management, *Clin Exp Pharm Physiol* 22:679–688, 1995.

Cerebellum

STUDY GUIDELINES

1. The cerebellar cortex has much the same microscopic structure throughout.
2. Afferents to the cerebellar cortex enter from spinal cord and brainstem. They are excitatory, whereas the cerebellar cortical outputs are inhibitory, and are exclusively from Purkinje cells.
3. The outputs from the cerebellum as a whole are in general excitatory. This is because they originate from deep, excitatory nuclei which are only partially inhibited by Purkinje cells.
4. Of special research interest are the roles played by the inferior olivary and red nuclei in relation to novel motor programs.
5. Clinically, cerebellar disease is characterized by incoordination of movement, with some differences being evident depending on the mediolateral position of the lesion where this is discrete (e.g. a tumor).

INTRODUCTION

Phylogenetically, the initial development of the cerebellum (in fish) took place in relation to the vestibular labyrinth. With development of quadrupedal locomotion, the anterior lobes (in particular) became richly connected to the spinal cord. Assumption of the erect posture and achievement of a whole new range of physical skills have been accompanied by the appearance of massive linkages between the posterior lobes and the cerebral cortex. In general, cerebellar connections with the labyrinth, spinal cord, and cerebral cortex are arranged such that each cerebellar hemisphere is primarily concerned with the coordination of movements *on its own side*.

The gross anatomy of the cerebellum is described briefly in Chapter 3, where it may be reviewed at this time.

FUNCTIONAL ANATOMY

Phylogenetic and functional aspects can be combined (to an approximation) by dividing the cerebellum into strips, as shown in Figure 25.1. The median strip contains the cortex of the vermis, together with the **fastigial nucleus** in the white matter close to the nodule (Figure 25.2). This strip is the *vestibulocerebellum*; it has two-way connections with the vestibular nucleus. It controls the responses of that nucleus to signals from the vestibular labyrinth. The fastigial nucleus also projects to the gaze centers of the brainstem (Ch. 24).

A paramedian strip, the *spinocerebellum*, includes the paravermal cortex and the **globose** and **emboliform nuclei** (Figure 25.2). The two nuclei are together called the **interposed nucleus**. The spinocerebellum is rich in spinocerebellar connections. It is involved in the control of posture and gait.

The remaining, lateral strip is much the largest and takes in the wrinkled **dentate nucleus** (Figure 25.2). This strip is the *pontocerebellum*, because it receives a massive input from the contralateral nuclei pontis. It is also called the **neocerebellum**, because the nuclei pontis convey information from large areas of the cerebral neocortex (phylogenetically

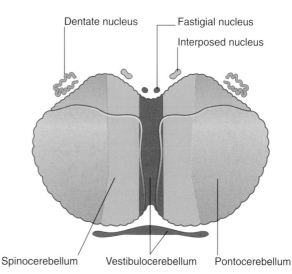

Dentate nucleus   Fastigial nucleus

Interposed nucleus

Spinocerebellum   Vestibulocerebellum   Pontocerebellum

Figure 25.1 Zonation of cerebellum. The central nuclei are represented separately.

Figure 25.2 Transverse section of lower pons and cerebellum showing the position of the central and vestibular nuclei.

the most recent). The neocerebellum is uniquely large in the human brain.

MICROSCOPIC ANATOMY

The structure of the cerebellar cortex is uniform throughout. From within outward, the cortex comprises granular, piriform, and molecular layers (Figure 25.3).

The **granular layer** contains billions of **granule cells**, whose somas are only 6–8 μm in diameter. Their short dendrites receive so-called **mossy fibers** from all sources except the inferior olivary nucleus. Before reaching the cerebellar cortex, the mossy fibers, which are excitatory in nature, give off collateral branches to the central nuclei.

The axons of the granule cells penetrate to the molecular layer where they divide in a T-shaped manner to form **parallel fibers**. The parallel fibers run parallel to the axes of the folia. They make excitatory contacts with dendrites of Purkinje cells.

The granular layer also contains Golgi cells (see later).

The **piriform layer** consists of very large **Purkinje cells**. The fan-shaped dendritic trees of the Purkinje cells are the largest dendritic trees in the entire nervous system. The fans are disposed at right angles to the parallel fibers.

The dendritic trees of Purkinje cells are penetrated by huge numbers of parallel fiber axons of granule cells, each one making successive, one per cell, synapses upon dendritic spines of about 400 Purkinje cells. Not surprisingly, stimulation of small numbers of granule cells by mossy fibers

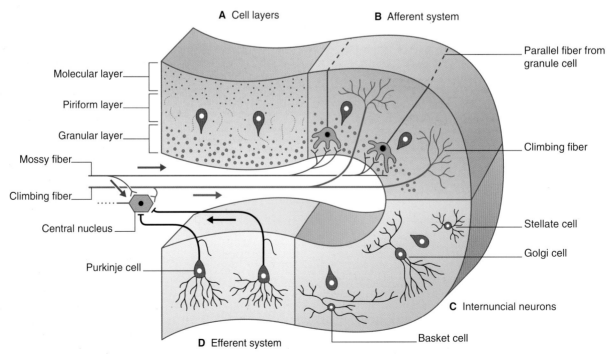

Figure 25.3 Cerebellar cortex. **(A)** Cell layers. **(B)** Afferent systems. **(C)** Internuncial neurons. **(D)** Efferent system.

has a merely facilitatory effect upon Purkinje cells. Many thousands of parallel fibers must act simultaneously to bring the membrane potential to firing level.

Each dendritic tree also receives a single **climbing fiber** from the contralateral inferior olivary nucleus. In stark contrast to the one-per-cell synapses of parallel fibers, the olivocerebellar fiber divides at the Purkinje dendritic branch points and makes thousands of synaptic contacts with dendritic spines. A single threshold pulse applied to one climbing fiber is sufficient to elicit a short burst of action potentials from the client Purkinje cell. Climbing fiber effects on Purkinje cells are so powerful that, for some time after they cease firing, the synaptic effectiveness of bundles of parallel fibers is reduced. In this sense, the Purkinje cells *remember* that they have been excited by olivocerebellar fibers.

The axons of the Purkinje cells are the only axons to emerge from the cerebellar cortex. Remarkably, they are entirely inhibitory in their effects. Their principal targets are the central nuclei. They give off collateral branches also, mainly to Golgi cells.

The **molecular layer** is almost entirely taken up with Purkinje dendrites, parallel fibers, supporting neuroglial cells, and blood vessels. However, two sets of inhibitory neurons are also found there, lying in the same plane as the Purkinje cell dendritic trees. Near the cortical surface are small, **stellate cells**, and close to the piriform layer are larger, **basket cells**. Both sets are contacted by parallel fibers, and they both synapse on Purkinje cells. The stellate cells synapse upon dendritic shafts whereas the basket cells form a 'basket' of synaptic contacts around the soma, as well as forming axo-axonic synapses upon the initial segment of the axon. A single basket cell synapses upon some 250 Purkinje cells.

The final cell type in the cortex is the **Golgi cell**, whose dendrites are contacted by parallel fibers and whose axons divide extensively before synapsing upon the short dendrites of granule cells. The synaptic ensemble that includes a mossy fiber terminal, granule cell dendrites, and Golgi cell boutons is known as a **glomerulus** (Figures 25.4, 25.5).

Spatial effects of mossy fiber activity (Figure 25.6)

As already noted, cerebellar afferents other than olivocerebellar ones form mossy fiber terminals after giving off excitatory collaterals to one of the deep nuclei. The afferents excite groups of granule cells, which in turn facilitate many hundreds of Purkinje cells. Along most of the beam of excitation, known as a *microzone*, the Purkinje cells begin to fire, and to inhibit patches of cells in one of the deep nuclei. At the same time, weakly facilitated Purkinje cells along the edges of the microzone are shut off by stellate and basket cells. As a result, the beam of excitation is sharply focused. The excitation is terminated by Golgi cell inhibition of the granule cells that initiated it. Powerful excitation will last longer because highly active Purkinje cells inhibit underlying Golgi cells through their collateral branches.

REPRESENTATION OF BODY PARTS

Representation of body parts in the human cerebellar cortex is currently under investigation by means of fMRI. These

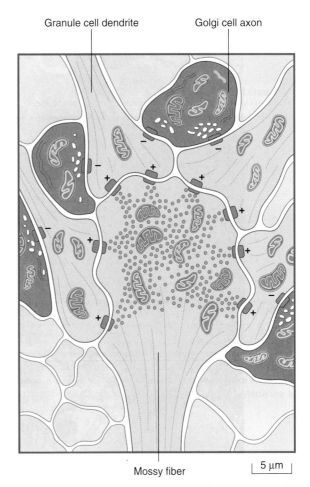

Figure 25.4 A synaptic glomerulus. +/− indicates excitation/inhibition.

investigations, along with some evidence from clinical cases, indicate the presence of somatotopic maps in the anterior and posterior lobes (Figure 25.7).

The maps have been worked out in some detail in laboratory animals during movements. The maps for movement match up with maps of skin, eye, ear, and visceral representation worked out by stimulation of body parts. The expression *fractionated somatotopy* refers to the patchy nature of the representation of body parts. Simple representations like those in Figure 25.7 are likely to be quite inaccurate in view of the vast areas of cortex buried in the fissures.

Figure 25.8, based on PET scans, shows simultaneous activation of the left motor cortex and right cerebellum during repetitive movements of the fingers of the right hand.

See also The Cerebellum and Higher Brain Functions, later.

AFFERENT PATHWAYS

From the muscles and skin of the trunk and limbs, afferent information travels in the posterior spinocerebellar and the cuneocerebellar tract and enters the inferior cerebellar peduncle on the same side. Comparable information from the territory served by the trigeminal nerve enters all three cerebellar peduncles.

Core Information

The cerebellum is primarily concerned with coordination of movements on its own side of the body. Therefore, disease in one cerebellar hemisphere leads to incoordination of limb movements on that side.

The cerebellar cortex contains a thick inner layer of tiny granule cells, a piriform layer of Purkinje cells, and a molecular layer containing granule cell axons and Purkinje dendrites. Granule cells are excitatory to Purkinje cells (via parallel fibers) but Purkinje cells – the only output cells of the cortex – are inhibitory to the central nuclei, which themselves are excitatory. Inhibitory purely cortical neurons are the stellate, basket, and Golgi cells.

The two types of afferents to the cortex are (a) mossy fibers from all sources except the olive – they excite granule cells; and (b) climbing fibers from the olive which powerfully excite Purkinje cells.

The basic input–output circuit is: mossy fibers → granule cells → Purkinje cells → deep nucleus → brainstem or thalamus. Olivocerebellar neurons are most active during novel learning; they elicit poststimulus depression of the Purkinje cell response to mossy fiber activity – a feature surely related to motor learning. The red nucleus is in a position to match the intended input to the cerebellum with the output achieved after passage through the basic circuit.

Functional parts

Vestibulocerebellum comprises vermis and fastigial nuclei, having two-way connections with the vestibular nucleus. It may be affected by midline tumors, yielding nystagmus and truncal ataxia.

Spinocerebellum, next to vermis and including much of the anterior lobe, includes the interposed nucleus. It receives spinocerebellar pathways and it controls posture and gait. Lesions are characterized by ataxia of stance and gait.

Neocerebellum is largest and most lateral, receiving the corticopontocerebellar system. The dentate nucleus projects to the contralateral motor cortex via thalamus, and to the contralateral red nucleus. Lesions result in ipsilateral incoordination, notably of the upper limb, and to faulty phonation and articulation.

REFERENCES

Aumann T: Cerebello-thalamic synapses and motor adaptation, *Cerebellum* 46:69–77, 2002.

Baillieux H, De Smet HJ, Paquier Pf, De Deyn PP, Marien P: Cerebellar neurocognition: insights into the bottom of the brain, *Clin Neurol Neurosurg* 110:763–773, 2008.

Bastian AJ, Thach WT: Structure and function of the cerebellum. In Manto U-B, Pandalfo M, editors: *The cerebellum and its disorders*, Cambridge, 2002, University Press, pp 49–68.

Doyon J, Benali H: Reorganization and plasticity in the adult brain during learning of motor skills, *Curr Opin Neurobiol* 15:161–167, 2005.

FitzGerald MJT: The cerebellum. In Standring S, et al, editors: *Gray's Anatomy*, ed 39, Edinburgh, 2005, Elsevier/Churchill Livingstone, pp 353–368.

Ito M: Cerebellar long-term depression: characterization, signal transduction, and functional roles, *Phys Rev* 8:1143–1195, 2001.

Middleton FA, Strick PL: Cerebellar output channels. In Schmahmann JD, editor: *The cerebellum and cognition: international review of neurobiology* (vol 41), San Diego, 1997, Academic Press, pp 255–271.

Nitschke MF, Kleinschmidt A, Wessel K, Frahm J: Somatotopic motor representation in the human anterior cerebellum, *Brain* 119:1023–1029, 1996.

Schmahmann JD, Sherman JC: The cerebellar cognitive affective syndrome, *Brain* 121:561–579, 1998.

Topke H, Mescheriakov S, Boose A, Kunz R, Hetrich I, Seydel L, Dichgans J, Rothwell J: A cerebellar-like terminal and postural tremor induced in normal man by transcranial magnetic stimulation, *Brain* 125:1551–1562, 1999.

Visser JE, Carpenter MG, van der Kooij, Bloem BR: The clinical utility of posturography, *Clin Neurophysiol* 119:2424–2436, 2008.

Wood J, Glickstein M: The anatomy of the cerebellum, *Trends Neurosci* 21:370–375, 1998.

Hypothalamus

STUDY GUIDELINES

1 Hypothalamic neuroendocrine cells fulfill the basic criteria both for neurons and for endocrine cells. Small neuroendocrine cells control release of hormones by the purely endocrine cells of the anterior pituitary gland into the cavernous sinus. Large ones have their terminals in the posterior pituitary, where they release hormones into the cavernous sinus directly.

2 Some neurons confined to the hypothalamus are involved in control of body temperature, food and fluid intake, and sleep. Others, involved in attack and defense responses and memory, are controlled by the limbic system.

Figure 26.1 Hypothalamic nuclei and hypophysis, viewed from the right side. DMN, dorsomedial nucleus; DN, dorsal nucleus; MB, mammillary body; PN, posterior nucleus; PVN, paraventricular nucleus; TN, tuberomammillary nucleus; VMN, ventromedial nucleus. The lateral hypothalamic nucleus is shown in *pink*.

INTRODUCTION

The hypothalamus develops as part of the limbic system, which is concerned with preservation of the individual and of the species. Therefore it is logical that the hypothalamus should have significant controls over basic survival strategies, including reproduction, growth and metabolism, food and fluid intake, attack and defense, temperature control, the sleep–wake cycle, and aspects of memory.

Most of its functions are expressed through its control of the pituitary gland and of both divisions of the autonomic nervous system.

GROSS ANATOMY

The hypothalamus occupies the side walls and floor of the third ventricle. It is a bilateral, paired structure. Despite its small size – it weighs only 4 g – it has major functions in homeostasis and survival. Its homeostatic functions include

control of the body temperature and the circulation of the blood. Its survival functions include regulation of food and water intake, the sleep–wake cycle, sexual behavior patterns, and defense mechanisms against attack.

Boundaries

The boundaries of the hypothalamus are as follows (see Figures 26.1 and 26.2):

• *Superior*: the **hypothalamic sulcus** separating it from the thalamus.

277

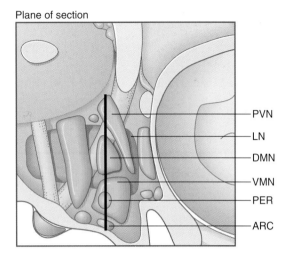

Plane of section

- PVN
- LN
- DMN
- VMN
- PER
- ARC

Table 26.1 Hypothalamic nuclei

Posterior	Middle	Anterior
Posterior	Paraventricular	Preoptic
Mammillary	Dorsomedial	Supraoptic
Tuberomammillary	Lateral	Suprachiasmatic
Dorsal	Ventromedial	
	Arcuate	

involving placement of lesions. Named nuclei in the three regions are listed in Table 26.1.

In the coronal plane, the hypothalamus can be divided into *lateral*, *medial*, and *periventricular* regions. The full length of the lateral region is occupied by the **lateral hypothalamic nucleus**. Merging with the lateral nucleus is the **medial forebrain bundle**, carrying aminergic fibers to the hypothalamus and to the cerebral cortex.

FUNCTIONS

Hypothalamic control of the pituitary gland

The arterial supply of the pituitary gland comes from hypophyseal branches of the internal carotid artery (Figure 26.3). One set of branches supplies a capillary bed in the wall of the infundibulum. These capillaries drain into **portal vessels** which pass into the adenohypophysis (anterior lobe). There they break up to form a second capillary bed which bathes the endocrine cells and drains into the cavernous sinus.

The neurohypophysis receives a direct supply from another set of hypophyseal arteries. The capillaries drain into the cavernous sinus, which delivers the secretions of the anterior and posterior lobes into the general circulation.

Secretions of the pituitary gland are controlled by two sets of **neuroendocrine cells**. Neuroendocrine cells are true neurons in having dendrites and axons and in conducting nerve impulses. They are also true endocrine cells because they liberate their secretions into capillary beds (Figure 26.4). With one exception (mentioned below), the secretions are peptides, synthesized in clumps of granular endoplasmic reticulum and packaged in Golgi complexes. The peptides are attached to long-chain polypeptides called *neurophysins*. The capillaries concerned are outside the blood–brain barrier, and are fenestrated.

The somas of the neuroendocrine cells occupy the *hypophysiotropic area* in the lower half of the preoptic and tuberal regions. Contributory nuclei are the **preoptic**, **supraoptic**, **paraventricular**, **ventromedial**, and **arcuate** (infundibular). Two classes of neurons can be identified: **parvocellular** (small) **neurons** reaching the median eminence, and **magnocellular** (large) **neurons** reaching the posterior lobe of the pituitary gland.

The parvocellular neuroendocrine system

Parvocellular neurons of the hypophysiotropic area give rise to the **tuberoinfundibular** tract, which reaches the infundibular capillary bed. Action potentials traveling along these neurons result in calcium-dependent exocytosis of *releasing hormones* from some and *inhibiting hormones* from others,

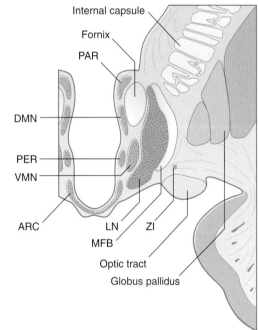

Internal capsule
Fornix
PAR
DMN
PER
VMN
ARC
LN   ZI
MFB
Optic tract
Globus pallidus

Figure 26.2 Hypothalamic nuclei, and related neural pathways, in a coronal section. ARC, arcuate nucleus; DMN, dorsomedial nucleus; LN, lateral nucleus; MFB, medial forebrain bundle; PAR, paraventricular nucleus; PER, periventricular nucleus; VMN, ventromedial nucleus; ZI, zona incerta.

- *Inferior*: the **optic chiasm**, **tuber cinereum**, and **mammillary bodies**. The tuber cinereum shows a small swelling, the **median eminence**, immediately behind the **infundibulum** ('funnel') atop the pituitary stalk.
- *Anterior*: the lamina terminalis.
- *Posterior*: the tegmentum of the midbrain.
- *Medial*: the third ventricle.
- *Lateral*: the internal capsule.

Subdivisions and nuclei

In the sagittal plane, it is customary to divide the hypothalamus into three regions: *anterior* (supraoptic), *middle* (tuberal), and *posterior* (mammillary). The descriptive use of 'regions' has been convenient for animal experiments

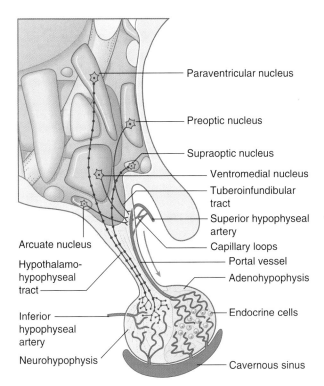

Figure 26.3 Hypothalamic neuroendocrine cells. The blood supply to the hypophysis, including the endocrine cells of the adenohypophysis, is also shown (arrow indicates direction of blood flow in the portal system).

Figure 26.4 Morphology of a peptide-secreting neuroendocrine cell.

for transport to the adenohypophysis in the portal vessels. The cell types of the adenohypophysis are stimulated/inhibited in accordance with Table 26.2. In the left-hand column, the only non-peptide parvocellular hormone is the prolactin-inhibiting hormone, which is *dopamine*, secreted from the arcuate (infundibular) nucleus.

The releasing/inhibiting hormones are not wholly specific: they have major effects on a single cell type, and minor effects on one or two others.

Multiple controls exist for parvocellular neurons of the hypophysiotropic area. The controls include: depolarization by afferents entering from the limbic system and from the reticular formation; hyperpolarization by local-circuit GABA neurons, some of which are sensitive to circulating hormones; and inhibition of transmitter release by opiate-releasing internuncials, which are numerous in the intermediate region of the hypothalamus. The picture is further complicated by the fact that opiates and other modulatory peptides may be released into the portal vessels and activate receptors on the endocrine cells of the adenohypophysis. *Stress* causes increased secretion of ACTH, which in turn stimulates the adrenal cortex to raise the plasma concentration of glucocorticoids, including cortisol. Normally, cortisol exerts a negative feedback effect by exciting inhibitory hypothalamic neurons having glucocorticoid receptors. In patients suffering from major depression, this feedback system fails (Clinical Panel 26.1).

The magnocellular neuroendocrine system

Magnocellular neurons in the supraoptic and paraventricular nuclei give rise to the **hypothalamohypophyseal tract**, which

Table 26.2 Hypothalamic parvocellular releasing/inhibiting hormones (RH/IH)

RH/IH	Anterior lobe hormone
Corticotropin RH	ACTH
Thyrotropin RH	Thyrotropin
Growth hormone RH	Growth hormone
Growth hormone IH	Growth hormone
Prolactin RH	Prolactin
Prolactin IH	Prolactin
Gonadotropic hormone RH	FSH/LH

descends to the neurohypophysis (posterior lobe) (Figure 26.3). Minor contributions to the tract are received from opiatergic and other peptidergic neurons in the periventricular region of the hypothalamus, and from aminergic neurons of the brainstem.

Two hormones are secreted by separate neurons located in both the supraoptic and paraventricular nuclei: *antidiuretic hormone* (*vasopressin*) and *oxytocin*. Axonal swellings containing the secretory granules for these hormones make up nearly half the volume of the neurohypophysis. The largest swellings, called Herring bodies, may be as large as

CHAPTER SUMMARY
Thalamus
    Thalamic nuclei
    Thalamic peduncles
Epithalamus

STUDY GUIDELINES
1. The thalamus is an assembly of largely independent nuclear groups.
2. Six *specific (relay)* nuclei are reciprocally connected to motor/sensory areas of the cerebral cortex.
3. Four *association* nuclei are reciprocally connected to association areas of the cortex.
4. *Non-specific* nuclei (two described here) are not concerned with any specific motor or sensory function.

THALAMUS

The thalamus is the largest nuclear mass in the entire nervous system. It is a prominent feature in MRI scans in each of the three planes in which slices are taken. The afferent and efferent connections of the main nuclear groups are listed in Table 27.1. The connections are so diverse that the thalamus cannot be said to have a unitary function.

As noted in Chapter 2, the two thalami lie at the center of the brain. Their medial surfaces are usually linked across the third ventricle and their lateral surfaces are in contact with the posterior limb of the internal capsule. The upper surface of each occupies the floor of a lateral ventricle. The under-aspect receives sensory and cerebellar inputs as well as an upward continuum of the reticular formation.

Thalamic nuclei

All thalamic nuclei except one (the reticular nucleus) have reciprocal excitatory connections with the cerebral cortex. The Y-shaped **internal medullary lamina** of white matter divides the thalamus into three large cell groups: *medial dorsal, anterior,* and *lateral* (Figure 27.1A). The lateral group comprises *dorsal and ventral nuclear tiers*. At the back of the thalamus are the **medial** and **lateral geniculate bodies**. The **external medullary lamina** separates the thalamus from the shell-like **reticular nucleus**.

The thalamic nuclei are categorized into three functional groups: *specific* or *relay nuclei, association nuclei,* and *non-specific nuclei*.

Specific nuclei

The specific or relay nuclei are reciprocally connected to specific motor or sensory areas of the cerebral cortex. They comprise the nuclei of the ventral tier and the geniculate bodies (nuclei). Their afferent and efferent connections are indicated in Figure 27.1B.

The **anterior nucleus** receives the mammillothalamic tract and projects to the cingulate cortex. It is involved in a limbic circuit and has a function in relation to memory (Ch. 34).

The **ventral anterior nucleus** (VA) receives afferents from the globus pallidus, and it projects to the prefrontal cortex.

Table 27.1 Thalamic nuclei and their connections

Type	Nucleus	Afferents	Efferents
Specific (or relay)	Anterior	Mammillothalamic tract, hippocampus	Cingulate gyrus
	Ventral anterior (VA)	Globus pallidus	Prefrontal cortex
	Ventral lateral (VL)		
	VL – anterior part	Globus pallidus	Supplementary motor area
	VL – posterior part	Cerebellum	Motor cortex
	Ventral posterior (VP)		
	Ventral posteromedial (VPL)	Somatic afferents from trunk and limbs	Somatic sensory cortex
	Ventral posterolateral (VPM)	Somatic afferents from the head region	Somatic sensory cortex
	Medial geniculate body	Brachium of the inferior colliculus	Primary auditory cortex
	Lateral geniculate body	Optic tract, (Superior colliculus?)	Primary visual cortex
Association	Lateral dorsal (LD)	Hippocampus	Cingulate cortex
	Mediodorsal (or Dorsomedial, DM)	Prefrontal cortex, olfactory, limbic	Prefrontal cortex
	Lateral posterior (LP)	Superior colliculus, primary visual, auditory and somatosensory cortex	Parietal association cortex
	Pulvinar		
Non-specific	Intralaminar (centromedian, parafascicular, others)	Reticular formation, basal ganglia, limbic system	Cerebral cortex, corpus striatum
	Reticular	Thalamus and cortex	Thalamus

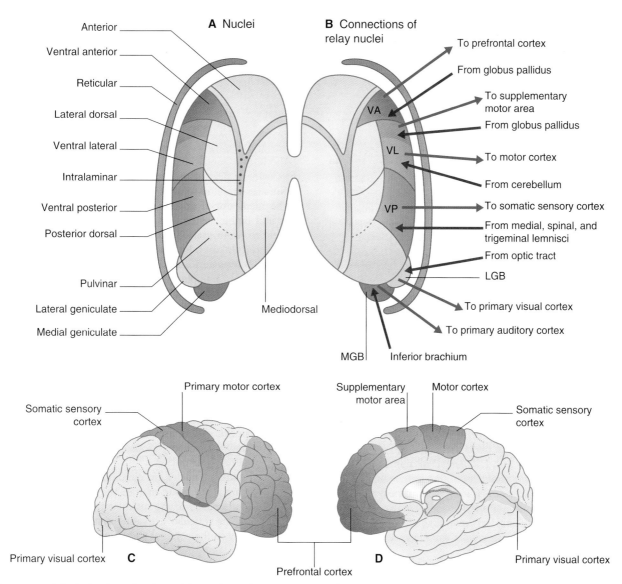

Figure 27.1 (A) Thalamic nuclei viewed from above. **(B)** Connections of the specific (relay) nuclei. LGB, MGB, lateral and medial geniculate bodies; VA, ventral anterior nucleus; VL, ventral lateral nucleus; VP, ventral posterior nucleus. **(C)** Lateral and **(D)** medial surface of hemisphere showing cortical areas receiving projections from the relay nuclei.

The anterior part of the **ventral lateral nucleus** (VL) receives afferents from the globus pallidus and projects to the supplementary motor area. The posterior part of VL is the principal target of the contralateral superior cerebellar peduncle, which originates in the dentate nucleus of the cerebellum; the posterior VL projects to the motor cortex.

The **ventral posterior nucleus** (VP) receives all of the fibers of the medial, spinal, and trigeminal lemnisci (Figure 27.2). It projects to the somatic sensory cortex (SI). A smaller projection is sent to the second somatic sensory area (SII) at the foot of the postcentral gyrus (see Ch. 29).

The VP is somatotopically arranged, as indicated in Figure 27.3. The portion of the nucleus devoted to the face and head is called the **ventral posterior medial nucleus** (VPM), that for the trunk and limbs the **ventral posterior lateral nucleus** (VPL). Modality segregation is a feature of both nuclei, with proprioceptive neurons most anterior, tactile neurons in the

midregion, and nociceptive neurons at the back. The nociceptive region is sometimes called the *posterior nucleus*.

There is no evidence in the VP of an antinociceptive mechanism comparable to that found in the substantia gelatinosa region of the spinal cord and spinal trigeminal nucleus. An unexplained disorder, the *thalamic syndrome*, may follow a vascular lesion that disconnects the posterior thalamic nucleus from the somatic sensory cortex. In this condition, a period of complete sensory loss may occur on the contralateral side of the body, to be replaced by bouts of severe pain occurring either spontaneously or in response to tactile stimuli. (See also Ch. 35, *central poststroke pain*.)

The **medial geniculate body** (medial geniculate nucleus) is the thalamic nucleus of the auditory pathway. It receives the inferior brachium from the inferior colliculus (which carries auditory signals from both ears, Ch. 20), and it projects to the primary auditory cortex in the superior temporal gyrus.

> ### Core Information
>
> **Thalamus**
> The internal medullary lamina divides the thalamus anatomically into mediodorsal, anterior, and lateral nuclear groups, the lateral being separable into dorsal and ventral tiers. The thalamus may be divided functionally into specific, association, and non-specific nuclear groups.
>
> Of the specific nuclei:
>
> - the anterior receives the mammillothalamic tract and projects to the cingulate cortex
> - the anterior part of ventral lateral receives inputs from globus pallidus and projects to supplementary motor area, whereas the posterior part receives from contralateral cerebellum and projects to motor cortex
> - ventral posterior receives the somatic sensory pathways and projects to the somatic sensory cortex
> - the medial geniculate nucleus receives inferior brachium and projects to the primary auditory cortex
> - the lateral geniculate nucleus receives from the optic tract and projects to the primary visual cortex.
> - ventral anterior receives inputs from globus pallidus and projects to prefrontal cortex
>
> Of the association nuclei:
>
> - the mediodorsal is reciprocally connected to all parts of the prefrontal cortex
> - the lateral posterior–pulvinar complex receives from the superior colliculus and projects to the parietal association cortex.
>
> Of the non-specific nuclei:
>
> - the intralaminar nucleus receives inputs from the reticular formation and projects widely to the cerebral cortex, also to the corpus striatum
> - the reticular nucleus (external to the thalamus proper) receives excitatory collaterals from all thalamocortical and corticothalamic neurons, and returns inhibitory fibers to all nuclei within the thalamus. Its best known function is generation of rhythmical electrical oscillations characteristic of early sleep. Reciprocal connections between thalamus and cortex travel in four thalamic peduncles which become incorporated into the corona radiata.
>
> **Epithalamus**
> The epithalamus includes the pineal gland, the habenula, and the stria terminalis.

REFERENCES

Alitto HJ, Usry WM: Corticothalamic feedback and sensory processing, *Curr Opin Neurobiol* 13:440–445, 2003.

Benarroch E: The midline and intralaminar thalamic nuclei, *Neurology* 71:944–949, 2008.

Hall AJ, Lomber SG: Auditory cortex projections target the peripheral field representation of primary visual cortex, *J Exp Neurol* 190:413–430, 2008.

Ohye C: Thalamus. In Paxinos G, editor: *The human nervous system*, ed 2, San Diego, 1990, Academic Press, pp 439–468.

Pinault D: The thalamic reticular nucleus: structure, function and concept, *Brain Res Rev* 46:1–31, 2004.

Visual pathways

STUDY GUIDELINES

1   The great length of the visual pathways makes them vulnerable to disease at widely separate locations. The pattern of visual defect differs in accordance with the site of damage.
2   Visual defects can often be detected by merely wiggling a finger in different parts of the visual field of each eye in turn.
3   The most important item of anatomic information concerns the representations of the visual fields at successive steps along the visual pathways.

INTRODUCTION

The visual pathways are of outstanding importance in clinical neurology. They extend from the retinas of the eyes to the occipital lobes of the brain. Their great length makes them especially vulnerable to demyelinating diseases such as multiple sclerosis; to tumors of the brain or pituitary gland; to vascular lesions in the territory of the middle or posterior cerebral artery; and to head injuries.

The visual system comprises the retinas, the visual pathways from the retinas to the brainstem and visual cortex, and the cortical areas devoted to higher visual functions. The retinas and visual pathways are described in this chapter. Higher visual functions are described in Chapter 29.

RETINA

The retina and the optic nerves are part of the central nervous system. In the embryo, the retina is formed by an outgrowth from the diencephalon called the optic vesicle (Ch. 1). The optic vesicle is invaginated by the lens and becomes the two-layered optic cup.

The outer layer of the optic cup becomes the pigment layer of the mature retina. The inner, nervous layer of the cup gives rise to the retinal neurons.

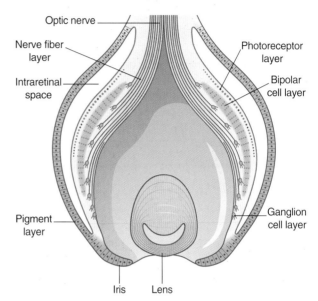

Figure 28.1 Embryonic retina. *Green* and *red* represent rods and cones, respectively.

Figure 28.1 shows the general relationships in the developing retina. The nervous layer contains three principal layers of neurons: **photoreceptors**, which become applied to the pigment layer when the intraretinal space is resorbed; **bipolar neurons**; and **ganglion cells** which give rise to the optic nerve and project to the thalamus and midbrain.

Note that the retina is *inverted*: light must pass through the layers of optic nerve fibers, ganglion cells, and bipolar neurons to reach the photoreceptors. However, at the point of most acute vision, the **fovea centralis**, the bipolar and ganglion cell layers lean away all around a central pit (fovea), and light strikes the photoreceptors directly (see Foveal Specialization, later). In the mature eye, the fovea is about 1.5 mm in diameter and occupies the center of the 5 mm wide **macula lutea** ('yellow spot') where many of the photoreceptor cells contain yellow pigment. The fovea is the point of most acute vision and lies in the *visual axis* – a line passing from the center of the visual field of the eye, through the center of the lens, to the fovea (Figure 28.2). To *fixate* or *foveate* an object is to gaze directly at it so that light reflected from its center registers on the fovea.

The axons of the ganglion cells enter the optic nerve at the **optic papilla** (*optic nerve head*), which is devoid of retinal neurons and constitutes the physiological 'blind spot'.

The visual fields of the two eyes overlap across two-thirds of the total visual field. Outside this *binocular field* is a *monocular crescent* on each side (Figure 28.3). During passage through the lens, the image of the visual field is reversed, with the result that, e.g., objects in the left part of the binocular visual field register on the right half of each

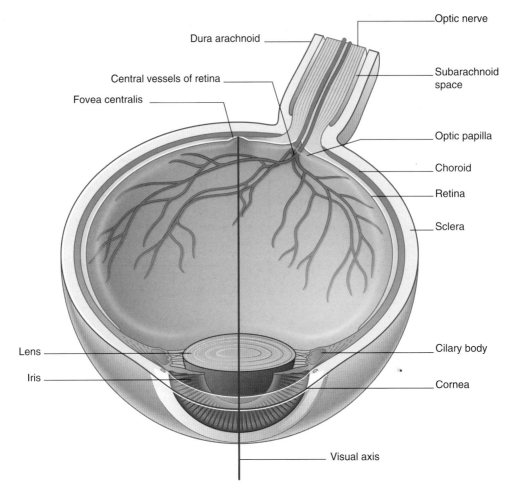

Figure 28.2 Horizontal section of the right eye, showing the visual axis.

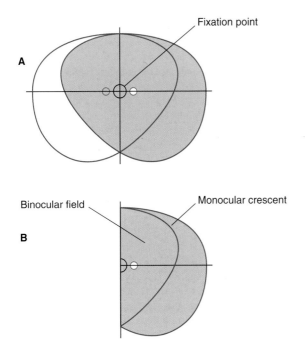

Figure 28.3 (A) Visual fields. Both eyes are targeted on the fixation point. The visual field of the right eye is shaded. **(B)** The right visual field. The *white spot* represents the blind spot of the right eye.

retina, and objects in the upper part of the visual field register on the lower half. This arrangement is preserved all the way to the visual cortex in the occipital lobe.

From a clinical standpoint, it is essential to appreciate that *vision is a crossed sensation*. The visual field on one side of the visual axis registers on the visual cortex of the opposite side. In effect, the right visual cortex 'sees' the left visual field. Only half of the visual information crosses in the optic chiasma, for the simple reason that the other half has already crossed the midline in space.

Visual defects caused by interruption of the visual pathway are always described *from the patient's point of view*, i.e. in terms of the visual fields, and not in terms of retinal topography.

Structure of the retina

In addition to the serially arranged photoreceptors, bipolar cells, and ganglion cells shown in Figure 28.1, the retina contains two sets of neurons arranged transversely: **horizontal cells** and **amacrine cells** (Figure 28.4). A total of eight layers are described for the retina as a whole.

Action potentials are generated by the ganglion cells, providing the requisite speed for conduction to the thalamus and midbrain. For the other cell types, distances are very short and passive electrical charge (electrotonus) is sufficient for

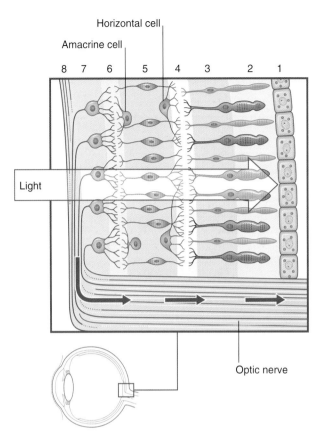

Figure 28.4 The layers of the retina. (1) Pigment layer; (2) photoreceptor layer; (3) outer nuclear layer; (4) outer plexiform layer; (5) inner nuclear layer; (6) inner plexiform layer; (7) ganglion cell layer; (8) nerve fiber layer.

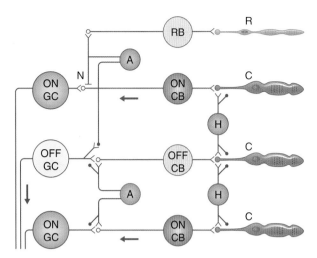

Figure 28.5 Retinal circuit diagram. (Adapted from Massey and Redburn, 1987.) A, amacrine cell; C, cone; CB, cone bipolar neuron; GC, ganglion cell; H, horizontal cell; N, nexus (gap junction); R, rod; RB, rod bipolar.

intercellular communication, whether by gap-junctional contact or transmitter release.

Photoreceptors

The photoreceptor neurons comprise **rods** and **cones**.

Rods function only in dim light and are not sensitive to color. They are scarce in the outer part of the fovea and absent from its center. Cones respond to bright light, are sensitive to color (received in the form of electromagnetic wavelength energy) and to shape, and are most numerous in the fovea.

Each photoreceptor has an outer and an inner segment and a synaptic end-foot. In the outer segment, the plasma membrane is folded to form hundreds of membranous discs which incorporate visual pigment (rhodopsin) formed in the inner segment. The synaptic end-foot makes contact with bipolar neurons and horizontal cell processes in the outer plexiform layer.

A surprising feature of the photoreceptors is that they are hyperpolarized by light. During darkness Na^+ channels are opened, creating sufficient positive electrotonus to cause leakage of transmitter (glutamate) from the end-feet. Illumination causes the Na^+ channels to close.

Cone and rod bipolar neurons

Cone bipolar neurons

Cone bipolar neurons are of two types. ON bipolars are switched on (depolarized) by light, being inhibited by

transmitter released in the dark. They converge onto ON ganglion cells. OFF bipolars have the reverse response and converge onto OFF ganglion cells (Figure 28.5).

Rod bipolar neurons

Rod bipolar neurons are all hyperpolarized by light. They activate ON and OFF ganglion cells indirectly, by way of amacrine cells (Figure 28.5).

Horizontal cells

The dendrites of horizontal cells are in contact with photoreceptors. The peripheral dendritic branches give rise to axon-like processes which make inhibitory contacts with bipolar neurons.

The function of horizontal cells is to inhibit bipolar neurons outside the immediate zone of excitation. The excited bipolars and ganglion cells are said to be on-line; the inhibited ones are off-line.

Amacrine cells

Amacrine cells have no axons. Their appearance is octopus-like, the dendrites all emerging from one side of the cell. Dendritic branches come into contact with bipolar neurons and ganglion cells.

More than a dozen different morphological types of amacrine cells have been identified, as well as several different transmitters, including acetylcholine, dopamine, and serotonin. Possible functions include contrast enhancement and movement detection. For the rods, they convert large numbers of rods from OFF to ON with respect to ganglion cells.

Ganglion cells

The ganglion cells receive synaptic contacts from bipolar neurons in the inner plexiform layer. The typical response of ganglion cells to bipolar activity is 'center-surround'. An ON ganglion cell is excited by a spot of light, and inhibited by a surrounding annulus (ring) of light. The inhibition is caused by horizontal cells. OFF ganglion cells give the reverse response.

Coding for color

There are three types of cone with respect to spectral sensitivity. One is sensitive to red, one to green, and one to blue. Groups of each type are connected to ON or OFF ganglion cells.

The characteristic response of ganglion cells is one of *color opponency*:

- Ganglion cells that are on-line for green are off-line for red.
- Ganglion cells that are on-line for red are off-line for green.
- Ganglion cells that are on-line for blue are off-line for yellow, i.e. for green and red cones acting together.

Coding for black and white

White light is a mixture of green, red, and blue. In bright conditions, it is encoded by the three corresponding cones, all of them converging onto common ganglion cells. Both ON and OFF ganglion cells are involved in black-and-white vision, just as in color vision.

In very dim conditions, e.g. starlight, only rod photoreceptors are active, and objects appear in varying shades of gray. The rods are subject to the same rules as cones, showing center-surround antagonism between white and black, and being connected to ON or OFF ganglion cells.

Most rod and cone ganglion cells are small (parvocellular or 'P'), having small receptive fields and being responsive to color and shape. A minority are large (magnocellular or 'M'), having large receptive fields and being especially responsive to movements within the visual field.

Foveal specialization

The relative density of cones increases progressively, and their size diminishes progressively, from the edge of the fovea inwards (Figure 28.6). The central one-third of the fovea, little more than 100 μm wide and known as the **foveola**, contains only *midget* cones. Two special anatomical features assist the foveal cones in general, and the midget cones in particular, in transducing the maximum amount of information concerning the form and color values of an object under direct scrutiny. First, the more superficial layers of the retina lean outward from the center, and their neurites are exceptionally long, with the result that the outer two-thirds of the foveola are little overlapped by bipolar cell bodies and the inner third is not overlapped at all; light reflected from the object strikes the cones of the foveola without any diffraction. Second, fidelity of central transmission is enhanced by one-to-one synaptic contact between the midget cones and *midget* bipolar neurons, and between these and *midget* ganglion cells. Outside the foveola, the amount of cone-to-bipolar-to-ganglion cell convergence increases progressively.

CENTRAL VISUAL PATHWAYS

Optic nerve, optic tract

The optic nerve is formed by the axons of the retinal ganglion cells. The axons acquire myelin sheaths as they leave the optic disc.

The number of ganglion cells varies remarkably between individuals, from 800,000 to 1.5 million. Since every ganglion cell contributes to the optic nerve, the number of axons in the optic nerve is correspondingly variable.

The retinal ganglion cells are homologous with the sensory projection neurons of the spinal cord. The optic nerve is homologous with spinal cord white matter, and is *not* a peripheral nerve. As explained in Chapter 9, true peripheral nerves, whether cranial or spinal, contain Schwann cells and collagenous sheaths, and are capable of regeneration. The optic nerve contains neuroglial cells of central type (astrocytes and oligodendrocytes) and is not capable of regeneration in mammals. In addition, the nerve is invested with meninges containing an extension of the subarachnoid space – a feature largely responsible for the changed appearance of the fundus oculi when the intracranial pressure is raised (*papilledema*, Ch. 4).

At the optic chiasm, fibers from the nasal hemiretina (medial half-retina) enter the contralateral optic tract, whereas those from the temporal (lateral) hemiretina remain uncrossed and enter the ipsilateral tract.

As already noted in Chapter 26, some optic nerve fibers enter the suprachiasmatic nucleus of the hypothalamus. This connection has been invoked to account for the beneficial effect of bright artificial light, for several hours per day, in the treatment of wintertime depression.

Each optic tract winds around the midbrain and divides into a medial and a lateral root.

Medial root of optic tract

The medial root contains 10% of the optic nerve fibers. It enters the side of the midbrain. It contains four distinct sets of fibers:

1 Some fibers, mainly from retinal M cells, enter the superior colliculus and provide for automatic scanning, e.g. reading this page.
2 Some fibers are relayed from the superior colliculus to the pulvinar of the thalamus; they belong to the extrageniculate pathway to the visual association cortex (Ch. 29).
3 Some fibers enter the pretectal nucleus and serve the pupillary light reflex (Ch. 23).
4 Some fibers enter the parvocellular reticular formation, where they have an arousal function (Ch. 24).

Lateral root of the optic tract and lateral geniculate body

The lateral root of the optic tract terminates in the lateral geniculate body (LGB) of the thalamus. The LGB shows six cellular laminae, three of which are devoted to crossed fibers and three to uncrossed fibers. The two deepest laminae (one for crossed and one for uncrossed fibers) are magnocellular and receive axons from retinal 'M' ganglion cells concerned with detection of *movement*. The other four are parvocellular and receive the axons of 'P' cells concerned with *particulars*, namely visual detail and color.

The circuitry of the LGB resembles that of other thalamic relay nuclei, and includes inhibitory (GABA) terminals derived from internuncial neurons and from the thalamic reticular nucleus. (The portion of the reticular nucleus serving

Figure 28.6 (**A**) Horizontal section of the right eyeball at the level of the optic disk and fovea centralis. (**B**) Enlargement from (A). Recurrent axons sweep around the fovea as shown in C. (**C**) Surface view of fovea centralis and neighboring retina. Cones have been omitted at intervals to show the 'chain' sequence of neurons. BCL, bipolar cell layer; GCL, ganglionic cell layer.

Figure 28.10 Pathway from the visual field of the left eye to the primary visual cortex. T denotes the temporal (outer) half of the left visual field; N denotes the nasal (inner) half of the left visual field.

In the left retina and optic nerve (ON), the neural representation of the image is reversed side to side. It is also inverted top to bottom. The right retina and optic nerve are inactive because this eye is shielded.

At the optic chiasm (OC) the axons forming the nasal half of the left optic nerve cross the midline and form the medial half of the right optic tract (OT). Those forming the lateral half of the nerve form the lateral half of the left optic tract. Each set synapses in the corresponding lateral geniculate body (LGB).

The optic radiations (OR) are fan-like (cf. Figure 28.7), with the axons carrying the foveal input initially in the middle of the fan.

As they approach the occipital pole, the foveal axons (red) in both hemispheres move to the back and enter the posterior part of the primary visual cortex (PVC). Note the striped pattern of delivery to the cortex on both sides. The blank intervals between are the same width and contain the axons and cortex responsible for the visual field of the *right* eye. SC, superior colliculus.

Clinical Panel 28.1 Lesions of the visual pathways

The following points arise in testing the visual pathways:

- The patient may be unaware of quite extensive blindness – sometimes even of a hemianopia.
- Large visual defects can often be detected by simple confrontation, as follows. The patient covers one eye at a time, and focuses on the examiner's nose. The examiner, seated opposite, looks the patient in the eye while bringing one or other hand into view from various directions, with the index finger wiggling.
- In a blind area, the patient does not see blackness; the patient does not see anything.
- Visual defects are described from the patient's viewpoint, in terms of the visual fields.
- Possible sites of injury to the visual pathways are shown in Figure CP 28.1.1. The effects produced correspond to the numbers in the following list:

Lesions	Field defects
1 Partial optic nerve	Ipsilateral scotoma[a]
2 Complete optic nerve	Blindness in that eye
3 Optic chiasm	Bitemporal hemianopia
4 Optic tract	Homonymous[b] hemianopia
5 Meyer's loop	Homonymous upper quadrantanopia
6 Optic radiation	Homonymous hemianopia
7 Visual cortex	Homonymous hemianopia
8 Bilateral macular cortex	Bilateral central scotomas

[a]Patch of blindness.
[b]Matching.

Notes on the numbered lesions

1 Eccentric lesions of the optic nerve produce scotomas in the nasal or temporal field of the affected eye. *When a young adult presents with a scotoma, multiple sclerosis must always be suspected.*
2 Total conduction blockage may follow head injury.
3 Compression of the middle of the chiasm is most often caused by an adenoma (benign tumor) of the pituitary gland.
4 Lesions of the optic tract are rare. Although homonymous (matching) visual fields are affected, the outer, exposed half of the tract tends to be more affected than the inner half, and the hemianopia is then described as incongruous.
5 Meyer's loop may be selectively caught by a tumor in the temporal lobe.
6 Lesions involving the optic radiation include tumors arising in the temporal, parietal, or occipital lobe. The visual fields of both eyes tend to be affected to an equal extent (*congruously*). Tumors impinging on the radiation from below produce an upper quadrantic defect at first, whereas tumors impinging from above produce a lower quadrantic defect. The stem of the radiation occupies the retrolentiform part of the internal capsule and is often compromised for some days by edema, following hemorrhage from a branch of the middle cerebral artery (classic stroke, Ch. 35).
7 Thrombosis of the posterior cerebral artery produces a homonymous hemianopia. The notches in field chart no. 7 represent macular sparing. Sparing of the macular hemifields is inconstant.
8 Bilateral central scotomas are most often caused by a backward fall with occipital contusion.

Visual fields

Figure CP 28.1.1 Visual field defects following various lesions of the visual pathways.

REFERENCE
Remington LA: *Clinical anatomy of the visual system*, ed 2, 2005, Butterworth-Heinemann.

Core Information

The embryonic retina is an outgrowth of the diencephalon. The embryonal optic cup is composed of an outer, pigment layer, an inner, nervous layer, with an intraretinal space between. The nervous layer contains three sets of radially disposed neurons, viz. photoreceptors, bipolar cells, and ganglion cells, and two tangential sets, viz. horizontal cells and amacrine cells. Except at the fovea centralis, light must pass through the other layers to reach the photoreceptors. The visual image is inverted and reversed by the lens. Two-thirds of the visual field are binocular, the outer one-sixth on each side being monocular. Visual defects are described in terms of visual fields.

Rod photoreceptors function in dim light and are absent from the fovea. Cones are most numerous in the fovea; they are responsive to shape and have three kinds of sensitivity to color. Ganglion cell responses are concentric, showing center-surround color opponency.

M ganglion cells are relatively large, are movement detectors, and project their axons to the two magnocellular layers of the lateral geniculate body (LGB). P ganglion cells signal particular features of the image as well as color and project to the four parvocellular layers of LGB. LGB is binocular, receiving signals from the contralateral nasal hemiretina (via the optic chiasm) and from the ipsilateral temporal hemiretina. Both sets of axons arrive by the optic tract, which also gives offsets to the midbrain for lower-level visual reflexes.

The geniculocalcarine tract (optic radiation) arises from M and P cells of the LGB and swings around the side of the lateral ventricle to reach the primary visual cortex, in the walls of the calcarine sulcus.

Distinctive visual field defects occur following damage at any of the five major components of the visual pathway (optic nerve, optic chiasm, optic tract, optic radiation, visual cortex).

REFERENCES

Karten HJ, Keyser KT, Brecha NC: Biochemical and morphological heterogeneity of retinal ganglion cells. In Cohen B, Bodis-Wollner I, editors: *Vision and the brain*, New York, 1990, Raven Press, pp 19–33.

Massey SC, Redburn DA: Transmitter circuits in the vertebral retina, *Prog Neurobiol* 28:55–96, 1987.

Rees G: The anatomy of blindsight, *Brain* 131:1414–1415, 2008.

Sadun AA, Glaser JS, Bose S: Anatomy of the visual sensory system. In Tasman W, editor: *Duane's clinical ophthalmology* (vol 2), Philadelphia, 2005, Lippincott, Williams and Wilkins, pp 1–23.

Selhorst JB, Chen Y: The optic nerve, *Semin Neurol* 29:29–35, 2009.

Treue S: Visual attention: the where, what, how and why of saliency, *Curr Opin Neurobiol* 13:428–432, 2003.

Wilhelm H: The pupil, *Curr Opin Neurol* 21:36–42, 2008.

Zou Q, Long X, Zuo X, et al: Functional connectivity between the thalamus and visual cortex under eyes closed and eyes open conditions: a resting-state fMRI study, *Hum Brain Mapp* 30:3066–3078, 2009.

Cerebral cortex

STUDY GUIDELINES

1 The cerebral cortex is the part of the body that makes us truly human. Its structure is enormously complex, and assignment of functions to different parts is made difficult, and often unrealistic, by the multiplicity of interconnections.
2 Sensory, motor, and cognitive areas of the cortex are taken in turn.
3 Although damage often leads to permanent disability, the *plasticity* of the cortex is of special interest to all concerned with neurorehabilitation. Examples are taken from sensory and motor areas.

STRUCTURE

The cerebral cortex, or *pallium* (*Gr.* 'shell'), varies in thickness from 2 to 4 mm, being thinnest in the primary sensory areas and thickest in the motor and association areas. More than half of the total cortical surface is hidden from view in the walls of the sulci. The cortex contains about 50 billion

neurons; about 500 billion neuroglial cells; and a dense capillary bed.

Microscopy reveals the cortex to have both a laminar and a columnar structure. The general cytoarchitecture varies in detail from one region to another, permitting the cortex to be mapped into dozens of histologically different 'areas'. Although considerable progress has been achieved in relating these to specific functions, the 'areas' are merely nodal points having widespread connections with other parts of the brain.

Laminar organization

A laminar (layered) arrangement of neurons is apparent in sections taken from any part of the cortex. Phylogenetically old elements, including the *paleocortex* of the uncus (concerned with olfaction), and the *archicortex* of the hippocampus in the medial temporal lobe (concerned with memory), are made up of three cellular laminae, whereas six laminae are seen in the **neocortex** (*neopallium*) covering the remaining 90% of the brain.

Cellular laminae of the neocortex (Figure 29.1)

I   The **molecular layer** contains the tips of the apical dendrites of pyramidal cells (see below), and the most distal branches of axons projecting to the cortex from the intralaminar nuclei of the thalamus.
II The **outer granular layer** contains small pyramidal and stellate cells.
III The **outer pyramidal layer** contains medium-sized pyramidal cells and stellate cells.
IV The **inner granular layer** contains stellate cells receiving afferents from the thalamic relay nuclei. Stellate cells are especially numerous in the primary somatic sensory cortex, primary visual cortex, and primary auditory cortex. The term *granular cortex* is applied to these areas. In contrast, the primary motor cortex contains relatively few stellate cells in lamina IV and is called *agranular cortex*.
V   The **inner pyramidal layer** contains large pyramidal cells projecting to the corpus striatum, brainstem, and spinal cord.
VI The **fusiform layer** contains modified pyramidal cells projecting to the thalamus.

Columnar organization (Figure 29.1)

In the somatic sensory cortex, the neurons were discovered (in monkeys) to be arranged functionally in terms of *columns* 50–100 μm in diameter extending radially through all laminae. Within each column, all of the cells are modality-specific. For example, a given column may respond to

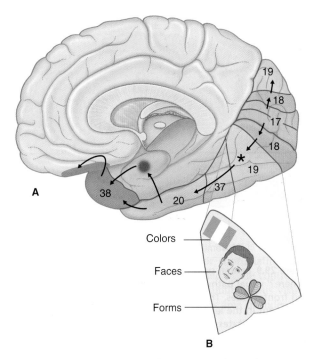

Figure 29.10 (A) Medial view of right hemisphere, showing the 'What?' pathway. The asterisk marks the visual identification area within the fusiform gyrus on the inferior surface. Ventral area 19 is enlarged in **(B)**.

- Relatively medial is the *color recognition area*, essential for recognition of all colors except black and white. A state of *achromatopsia* may occur following a sustained fall in blood pressure within both posterior cerebral arteries, caused, e.g., by an embolus blocking the top of the parent basilar artery. Such patients see everything only in black and white (gray scale).

Recognition of individual objects and faces is a function of the anterior part of the 'What?' pathway in the *inferotemporal cortex* (area 20) and in the cortex of the temporal pole (area 38). These two areas are engaged during identification of, for example, *Mary's* face or *my* dog. Failure of facial recognition (*prosopagnosia*) is a frequent and distressing feature of Alzheimer disease (Ch. 34), where the patient may cease to recognize family members despite retaining the sense of familiarity of common objects.

Threatening sights or faces cause areas 20 and 38 to activate the *amygdala*, especially in the right (emotional) hemisphere; the right amygdala in turn activates the fear-associated *right orbitofrontal cortex* (see Ch. 30).

How are visual association areas activated, e.g. in execution of a decision to look for an apple in a bowl of mixed fruit, or for a particular word in a page of text? In PET studies, the frontal lobe is active whenever attention is being paid to a task at hand. The DLPFC is particularly active during visual tasks involving form and color. During visual searching, the role of the frontal lobe seems to be to activate memory stores within the visual association areas, so that the relevant memories are held on-line during the search. The anterior part of the cingulate cortex is also active.

The V1–V5 nomenclature

Specialists in vision research use the following designations in relation to cortical visual processing:

V1 equates with Brodmann area 17.
V2 and V3 equate with Brodmann areas 18 and 19, respectively.
V4 includes the three sets of identification modules in the fusiform gyrus (anteromedial Brodmann area 19).
V5 equates with the movement detection modules in the lateral occipital cortex (anterolateral Brodmann area 19).

Auditory cortex (areas 41, 42, 22)

The *primary auditory cortex* occupies the anterior transverse temporal gyrus of Heschl, described in Chapter 20. Heschl's gyrus corresponds to areas 41 and 42 on the upper surface of the superior temporal gyrus. Columnar organization in the primary auditory cortex takes the form of *isofrequency stripes*, each stripe responding to a particular tonal frequency. Higher frequencies activate lateral stripes in Heschl's gyrus, lower frequencies activate medial stripes. Because of incomplete crossover of the central auditory pathway in the brainstem (Ch. 20), *each ear is represented bilaterally*. In experimental recordings, the primary cortex responds equally well from both ears in response to monaural stimulation but the contralateral cortex is more responsive during simultaneous binaural stimulation.

The auditory association cortex corresponds to area 22, for speech perception (considered in Ch. 32). Visual and auditory data are brought together in the polymodal cortex bordering the superior temporal sulcus (junction of areas 21 and 22).

Excision of the entire auditory cortex (in the course of removal of a tumor) has no obvious effect on auditory perception. The only significant defect is loss of *stereoacusis*: on testing, the patient has difficulty in appreciating the direction and the distance of a source of sound.

MOTOR AREAS

Primary motor cortex

The primary motor cortex (area 4) is a strip of agranular cortex within the precentral gyrus. It gives rise to 60–80% (estimates vary) of the pyramidal tract (PT). The remaining PT fibers originate in the premotor and supplementary motor areas and in the parietal cortex, as illustrated in Chapter 16.

There is an inverted somatotopic representation of contralateral body parts except the face, with relatively large areas devoted to the hand, circumoral region, and tongue (Figure 29.7). The hand area can usually be identified as a backward projecting knob 6–7 cm from the upper margin of the hemisphere.

Ipsilateral body parts are also represented in the somatotopic map, ipsilateral motor neurons being supplied by the 10% of PT fibers that remain uncrossed.

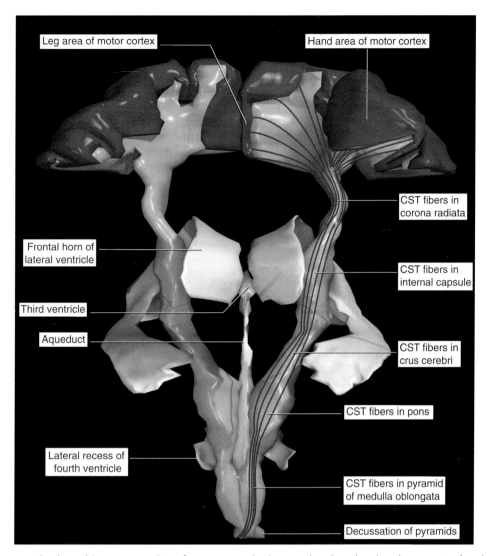

Figure 29.11 Computerized graphic reconstruction of postmortem brain; anterior view showing the precentral gyri, and the relationships of the corticospinal tracts (CST) to the ventricular system. Some corticospinal fibers have been added to the original. (Reproduced from Kretschmann, H-J. and Weinrich, W. *Neurofunctional Systems: 3D Reconstructions with Correlated Neuroimaging: Text and CD-ROM.* 1998 New York: Thieme, with kind permission of the authors and publisher.)

A computerized graphic reconstruction of the motor cortex and corticospinal tracts from a postmortem brain is shown in Figure 29.11.

Direct stimulation of the human motor cortex indicates that the cell columns control *movement direction*. Individual PT fibers are known to branch extensively as they approach the anterior gray horn, and to terminate on motor neuronal dendrites in nuclei serving several different muscles. The pattern of distribution of PT fibers is directed toward *movement synergy*, which in this context means the simultaneous contraction of all of the muscles concerned, with a bias among them suited to the task at hand. The act of picking up a pen, e.g., requires a moderate contraction of opponens pollicis as prime mover, a matching level of contraction of the portion of flexor digitorum profundus providing the tendon to the terminal phalanx of the index finger, and lesser levels of contraction of adductor and flexor brevis pollicis.

Steadying the upper limb as a whole during any kind of manipulative activity is a function of the premotor cortex (see later).

Plasticity in the motor cortex

In monkeys and in lower mammals, small lesions of the motor cortex produce an initial paralysis of the corresponding body part, followed within a few days (sometimes within hours) by progressive recovery. The recovery is attributable to a change of allegiance of cell columns close to the lesion, which take on the missing motor function. Instead of inflicting a lesion, it is possible to enlarge the motor territory of a patch of cortex merely by injecting a GABA antagonist drug locally into the cortex. Expansion of motor territories at spinal cord level is already provided for by extensive overlap of projections from area 4 to the motor cell columns in the ventral gray horn.

Sources of afferents to the primary motor cortex

1 *The opposite motor cortex*, through the corpus callosum. The strongest commissural linkages are between matching cell columns that control the vertebral and abdominal musculature. This is to be expected since these muscle groups routinely act bilaterally in maintaining the upright position of the trunk and head. The weakest commissural linkages are between cell columns controlling the distal limb muscles, where the two sides tend to act independently.

2 *Somatosensory cortex. Cutaneous* cell columns in areas 1, 2, and 3 feed forward via short association fibers. Linkages for the hand are especially numerous; the distance is short because the hand areas of the motor and somatic sensory cortex mainly occupy the corresponding walls of the central sulcus. *Proprioceptive* cell columns in area 3a receive afferent relays from the annulospiral endings of muscle spindles; they send short association fibers to the corresponding motor columns for execution of the long-loop stretch reflex (Ch. 25).

3 *Contralateral dentate nucleus.* The cerebellum assists in the selection of appropriate muscles for synergic activities, and in the timing and strength of their contractions.

4 *Supplementary motor area.*

Premotor cortex

The premotor cortex (PMC, area 6 on the lateral surface of the hemisphere) is about six times larger than the primary motor cortex. It receives cognitive inputs from the frontal lobe in the context of motor intentions, and a rich sensory input from the parietal lobe (area 7) incorporating tactile and visuospatial signals. It is especially active when motor routines are run in response to visual or somatic sensory cues, e.g. reaching for an object in full view or identifying an object out of sight by manipulation. The PMC is usually active bilaterally if at all. One explanation is the need for interhemispheric transfer of motor plans through the corpus callosum. It is also the case that the PMC has a major projection to the brainstem nuclei that give origin to the reticulospinal tracts (and a minor one to the pyramidal tract). Lesions confined to the human PMC are rare, but they are characterized by postural instability of the contralateral shoulder and hip. A significant function of the PMC therefore seems to be that of bilateral postural fixation, e.g. to fixate the shoulders during bimanual tasks and to stabilize the hips during walking. The PMC may contribute to recovery of function in cases of pure motor hemiplegia (Ch. 35) following a vascular lesion confined to the corticospinal tract within the corona radiata. The PMC shows increased activity on PET scans following such a lesion; the corticoreticulospinal pathway descends anterior to the corticospinal tract.

Supplementary motor area

In contrast to the PMC's responsiveness to external cues, the supplementary motor area (SMA, area 6 on the medial surface of the hemisphere) responds to *internal cues*. In particular, it is involved in *motor planning*, as exemplified by the fact that SMA is activated by the frontal lobe (DLPFC) the moment we *intend* to make a movement, even if the movement is not performed. The principal function of SMA seems to be that of preprogramming movement sequences that have already been built into motor memory. It functions in collaboration with a motor loop passing through the basal ganglia (Ch. 33) and projects to area 4 as well as contributing directly to the pyramidal tract. Unilateral lesions of SMA are associated with *akinesia* (inability to initiate movement) of the contralateral arm and leg. Bilateral lesions are accompanied by total akinesia, including akinesia for speech initiation.

Cortical eye fields

Figure 29.12 illustrates six *cortical eye fields* involved in scanning movements (saccades). Their connections and functions are summarized in Table 29.1.

Figure 29.12 Areas of cerebral cortex involved in saccadic movements. 1. Supplementary eye field, 2. Frontal eye field, 3. Parietal eye field, 4. Visual association cortex.

Dorsolateral prefrontal cortex

This is a higher-level cognitive center engaged in assessment of the visual scene, in decisions about making voluntary saccades and in voluntary repression of reflexive saccades. (*Voluntary* saccades result from internally generated decisions. *Reflexive* saccades are automatic responses to objects appearing in the peripheral visual field. Strictly speaking, reflexive saccades should be called *responsive*; they are not true reflexes, being amenable to voluntary suppression.)

Cingulate cortex

Participates with DLPFC in decision-making, and in assessing the emotional significance, or *valence*, of visual targets.

Supplementary eye field

Occupies the anterior part of the supplementary motor area, and is engaged in motor planning, especially when multiple saccades are required.

Frontal eye field (FEF)

Initiates voluntary saccades in response to one or more of the three inputs listed. Both clinical and experimental (monkey) observations indicate that:

- The FEFs are tonically active, bilaterally.
- Increased activity in the midregion of the FEF on one side causes a horizontal saccade toward the contralateral visual hemispace (a *contraversive saccade*).
- Increased activity in the upper region on one side produces an obliquely downward contraversive saccade; bilateral upper region activation causes both eyes to look straight down.
- Increased lower region activity has corresponding effects with respect to upward gaze.

Parietal eye field (PEF)

Initiates reflexive saccades and prompts FEF to initiate voluntary saccades. PEF is also involved in spatial perception by generating a map of the visual scene.

For prefrontal cortex and frontal lobe dysfunction, see Chapter 32.

Table 29.1 Cortical eye fields

Eye field	Afferents from	Efferents to	Function
Dorsolateral prefrontal cortex (DLPFC)	Visual association areas	Ipsilateral FEF, SEF, SC and CCx	Voluntary saccades
Cingulate cortex (CCx)	DLPFC, FEF, SEF	Ipsilateral FEF and SC	Assessment of emotional significance
Supplementary eye field (SEF)	DLPFC, PEF, area 22	Ipsilateral FEF and SC	Motor planning
Frontal eye field (FEF)	DLPFC, FEF, PEF	Contralateral PPRF, ipsilateral CCx and SC	Voluntary saccades
Parietal eye field (PEF)	'Where' visual pathway, pulvinar and DLPFC	Ipsilateral FEF and SC	Reflexive saccades
Area 22	Auditory association cortex, PEF	Ipsilateral SC	Saccades to source of sound

SC, superior colliculus; PPRF, paramedian pontine reticular formation.
Note: *The left PPRF pulls the eyes to the left. The right SC also pulls the eyes to the left, because of a crossed projection from it to the left PPRF.*

Clinical Panel 29.1 Stiff person syndrome

An unusual but well-recognized condition, known as *stiff person syndrome (SPS)*, is associated with the presence of circulating antibodies to glutamic acid decarboxylase. A state of rigidity, with superimposed muscle spasms, is produced by co-contraction of prime movers and antagonists of the trunk and limbs. Normally the upper motor neurons are held in check by tonic activity of nearby GABAergic neurons, and a residue of liberated but unutilized GABA drifts into the cerebrospinal fluid from the brain extracellular space.

In SPS patients, CSF samples show this residue to be significantly reduced. Some areas of the cortex are affected more than others, and the clinical effects relate to GABA deficiency in the upper half of the precentral gyrus.

REFERENCE
Levy LM, Levy-Reis I, Fujii M, Fujii M, Dalakis M: Brain γ-aminobutyric acid changes in stiff-person syndrome, *Arch Neurol* 62:970–974, 2005.

Core Information

The cerebral cortex has both a laminar and a columnar organization. The two basic cell types are pyramidal and stellate. Pyramidal cells occupy laminae II, III, V, and (as fusiform cells) lamina VI. Lamina IV is rich in spiny stellate cells. Small pyramidal cells link the gyri within the hemisphere; medium-sized pyramidal cells link matching areas of the two hemispheres; the largest ones project to thalamus, brainstem, and spinal cord. Spiny stellate cells are excitatory to pyramidal cells, smooth ones are inhibitory. Columnar organization takes the form of cell columns 50–100 μm wide.

The somatic sensory cortex contains an inverted representation of body parts. Important inputs come from the ventral posterior nucleus of thalamus; important outputs go to the primary motor and inferior parietal cortex. The primary visual cortex receives the geniculocalcarine tract. Cellular responses of differing complexity depend upon convergence of simpler on to more complex cell types. The visual association areas are characterized by feature extraction, e.g. motion, color, shape. Form and color extraction continues into the cortex on the underside of the temporal lobe, motion into the posterior parietal lobe. The primary auditory cortex occupies the upper surface of the superior temporal gyrus and the auditory association cortex is lateral to it.

The primary motor cortex occupies the precentral gyrus. It gives rise to most of the pyramidal tract, the body parts being represented upside down. Its main inputs are from somatosensory cortex, cerebellum (via the ventral posterior nucleus of thalamus), and the premotor and supplementary motor areas. The premotor area operates mainly in response to external cues, the supplementary motor area in response to internally generated cues. Under control of the dorsolateral prefrontal cortex, four distinct cortical areas are involved, in different contexts, in producing contraversive saccades.

REFERENCES

Barbeau EJ, Taylor MJ, Regis J, et al: Spatiotemporal dynamics of face recognition, *Cereb Cortex* 18:997–1009, 2008.

Behrmann M, Geng JJ, Shomstein S: Parietal cortex and attention, *Curr Opin Neurobiol* 14:210–217, 2004.

Burke MR, Barnes GR: Brain and behavior: a task-dependent eye movement study, *Cereb Cortex* 18:126–135, 2008.

Crowley, JC, Katz LC: Ocular dominance development revisited, *Curr Opin Neurobiol* 12:104–109, 2002.

DeFelipe J: Chandelier cells and epilepsy, *Brain* 122:1807–1822, 1999.

Edeline J-M: Learning-induced physiological plasticity in the thalamocortical sensory systems, *Progr Neurobiol* 57:165–224, 1999.

Garoff RJ, Slotnick SD, Shacter DL: Neural origins of specific and general memory: the role of the fusiform cortex, *Neuropsychologia* 43:847–859, 2005.

Ghose GM: Learning in mammalian sensory cortex, *Curr Opin Neurobiol* 14:513–518, 2004.

Grefkes C, Fink GR: The functional organization of the intraparietal sulcus in humans and monkeys, *J Anat* 207:3–17, 2005.

Im K, Lee J-M, Lyttelton O, et al: Brain size and cortical structure in the human brain, *Cereb Cortex* 18:2181–2191, 2008.

Kretschmann H-J, Weinrich W: *Neurofunctional systems: 3D reconstructions with correlated neuroimaging: text and CD-ROM*, New York, 1998, Thieme.

Munoz DP: Commentary: saccadic movements: overview of neural circuitry, *Neuroreport* 13:2325–2330, 2002.

Passingham D, Sakai K: The prefrontal cortex and working memory: physiology and brain imaging, *Curr Opin Neurobiol* 14:163–168, 2004.

Penfield W, Rasmussen T: *The cerebral cortex of man*, New York, 1960, Hafner.

Pollen DA: Fundamental requirements for primary visual perception, *Cereb Cortex* 18:1191–1198, 2008.

Posner MI, Raichle ME: Images of the brain. In Posner MI, Raichle ME, editors: *Images of the mind*, New York, 1994, Scientific American Library, pp 57–82.

von Economo G, Koskinas GN: In Triarhou LC, editor: *Atlas of cytoarchitectonics of the adult human cerebral cortex*, Basel, 2009, Karger.

Zilles K, Palomero-Gallagher N, Schleicher A: Transmitter receptors and functional anatomy of the cerebral cortex, *J Anat* 205:417–432, 2004.

Zou Q, Long X, Zuo X, Zuo Q, et al: Functional connectivity between the thalamus and visual cortex under eyes closed and eyes open conditions: a resting-state fMRI study, *Human Brain Mapping* 30:3066–3078, 2009.

Electroencephalography

STUDY GUIDELINES

The EEG is an important neurological tool, for three main reasons:

1 It is central to the study of the physiology of sleep and the pathophysiology of sleep disorders.
2 It is essential for analysis of seizures and for monitoring progress during their treatment.
3 It is a valuable aid to localization of space-occupying lesions including brain tumors.

We suggest you review the amino acid transmitters in Chapter 8 before reading about drug therapy in the Clinical Panels.

NEUROPHYSIOLOGICAL BASIS OF THE EEG

Since its initial development, EEG has remained a unique tool for the study of cortical function and a valuable supplement to history, physical examination, and information gained by radiological studies.

When small metallic disc electrodes are placed on the surface of the scalp, oscillating currents of 20–100 μV can be detected and are referred to as an *electroencephalogram (EEG)*. Their origin is a direct consequence of the additive effect of groups of cortical pyramidal neurons being arranged in radial (outward-directed) columns. The columns relevant here are those beneath the surface of the cortical gyri. As the membrane potentials of these columns fluctuate, an electrical dipole (adjacent areas of opposite charge) develops. The dipole results in an electrical *field potential* as current flows through the adjacent extracellular space as well as intracellularly through the neurons (Figure 30.1). It is the extracellular component of this current that is recorded in the EEG and variations in both the strength and density of the current loops result in its characteristic sinusoidal waveform.

The oscillations of the EEG, measured in microvolts (μV) are thought to be generated by reciprocal excitatory and inhibitory interactions of neighboring cortical cell columns.

TECHNIQUE

After careful preparation of the skin of the scalp to ensure good contact, electrodes are affixed in a placement that is in conformity with the *10–20 International System of Electrode Placement,* when the scalp is divided into a grid in accordance with Figure 30.2.

By defining a consistent placement of electrodes, direct comparison to follow-up studies is feasible, as is a method to compensate for differences in head size. Each electrode placement allows it to preferentially record over a cortical surface area of approximately 6 cm^2. The nomenclature employed to define each electrode position combines a letter with a number, as shown in the figure.

Actual EEG recordings are made from all sites simultaneously. The potential difference between electrode pairs is recorded (as a rule) and this is displayed as a separate individual graph or channel. Often other physiological recordings are performed at the same time (e.g. an electrocardiograph and/or a surface EMG).

If varying pairs of electrodes are used, the *montage* (output) is termed *bipolar* (Figure 30.3A). If they have one recording site in common (auricle, or mastoid area), it is called *referential* (Figure 30.3B).

Figure 30.4 provides a complete set of normal tracings.

TYPES OF PATTERN

Normal EEG rhythms

Awake state EEG

The EEG demonstrates prominent changes both with the level of alertness and during the various stages of sleep. Each of these patterns is specific and is taken into account during the EEG interpretation. A routine EEG study will usually take 30–45 minutes and will include recordings made during wakefulness and during early stages of sleep, since specific abnormalities (especially epileptiform ones) may only be detected during the sleep portion of the recording.

In the alert awake state (Figure 30.5A), the pattern is described as *desynchronized* because the waveforms are quite irregular. The *background frequency* is usually around 9.5 Hz. A *beta frequency* of more than 14 Hz may be superimposed over anterior head regions.

In a relaxed state with the eyes closed, rhythmic waveforms appear in the *alpha frequency* (8–14 Hz), notably over the parieto-occipital area (Figure 30.5B).

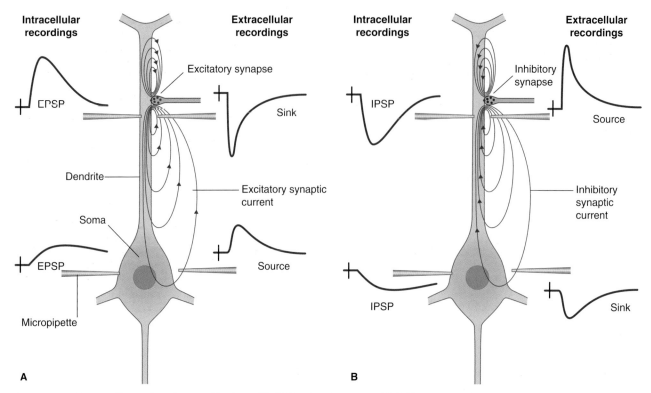

Figure 30.1 Diagram illustrating the contribution of individual excitatory and inhibitory synaptic currents to the extracellular field potentials. Micropipettes are being used to sample intracellular and extracellular events. **(A)** *Intracelluar recordings* show that the excitatory synapse generates a rapid EPSP (excitatory postsynaptic potential) at the synaptic site on the dendrite and a slower and smaller EPSP at the soma. *Extracellular recordings* show that the *source* (positive) of excitatory synaptic current flows outward through the membrane of proximal dendrite and soma, and inward (the *sink*) at the synaptic site. **(B)** An inhibitory synapse is seen to have the opposite effect. The IPSP (inhibitory postsynaptic potential) is associated with a current source at the synaptic site and a sink along the proximal dendrite and soma.

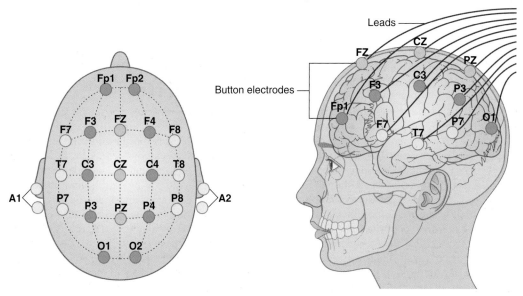

Figure 30.2 Deployment of surface electrodes on the scalp. *Letters:* Fp, frontopolar; F, frontal; T, temporal; P, parietal; C, coronal; O, occipital; Z, midline. *Numbers:* Odd numbers, left side; even numbers, right side. A1, A2 are reference electrode positions (see text).

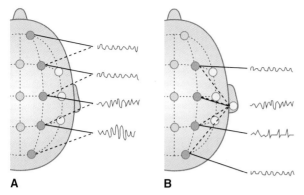

Figure 30.3 (A) Bipolar recording. A succession of adjacent pairs of electrodes is used. Only four sample tracings are shown. **(B)** Referential recording. The reference electrode is attached to the ear in this example. Again only four sample tracings are shown.

Figure 30.5 EEG in the awake state. **(A)** Subject is alert with eyes open. Beta waves are seen in Fp2–F4 and F4–C4. **(B)** Subject is relaxed with eyes closed. An eyeblink artifact is seen in the Fp2–F4 tracing. Alpha waves are seen in P4–O2. The beta waves are characterized by low amplitude and high frequency, the alpha waves by rhythmic waxing and waning.

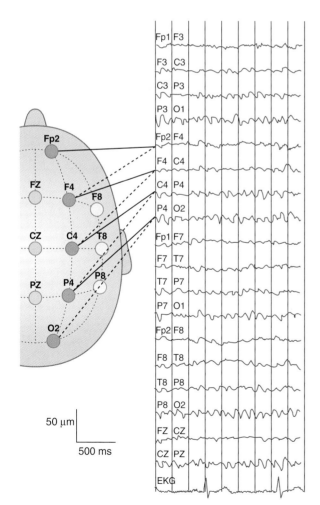

Figure 30.4 A complete set of normal tracings is shown, tagged in accordance with the nomenclature in Figure 30.2. (An electrocardiogram [EKG] has been taken simultaneously.) Note the low amplitude of the waves (20 μV or less) and their high frequency in this 2-second sample.

Normal sleep EEG

Glossary

- **REM sleep** Dreamy light sleep accompanied by *rapid eye movements*; also called *paradoxical sleep* because of EEG resemblance to the awake state.
- **NREM sleep** *Non–rapid eye movement* sleep (stages 1–3); stage 3 is also called *slow wave sleep*.

People normally pass through three to five sleep cycles per night. The sequence of events is summarized in Figure 30.5. Alpha rhythm becomes apparent (on occipital leads) during quiet rest with eyes closed.

By general agreement, sleep proper is associated with slow-wave patterns in the EEG. There is a rapid descent through stage 1, characterized by a steady theta rhythm, into stage 2, characterized by theta waves interrupted by sinusoidal waveforms called *sleep spindles,* and by occasional *K complex* spikes. Stage 3 is characterized by slow, *delta* waves – hence the term *slow wave sleep* for that stage (Figure 30.6).

It is generally agreed that the waxing and waning of cortical activity during slow wave sleep has its origin in the thalamus, where the relay nuclei projecting to the cortex also enter a rhythmic discharge mode during slow wave sleep. This rhythm is characterized by a succession of hyperpolarized states alternating with depolarized states exhibiting bursts of firing. The vigorous firing is triggered by momentary opening of voltage gated calcium channels. The *transient* (momentary) opening accounts for the term *T-channels* applied to these.

As described in Chapter 27, thalamocortical projections pass through an inhibitory shell in the form of the thalamic reticular nucleus, with reciprocal connections to parent relay cells as shown in Figure 27.4. Burst firing excites the reticular nucleus, which in turn causes the relay neurons to become hyperpolarized by opening the GIRK potassium channels (Figure 8.11).

The rhythmic waxing and waning of thalamic neurons is attributed to a pulsatile discharge pattern inherent to the cells of the reticular nucleus. Exaggeration of the normal

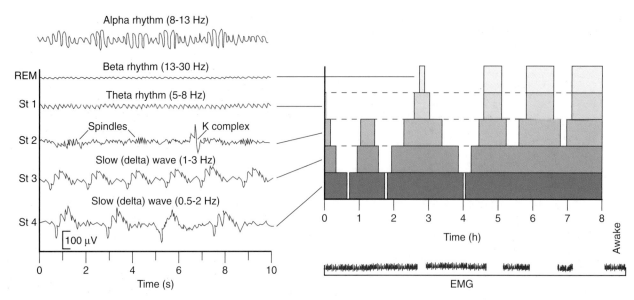

Figure 30.6 Typical 8-hour sleep and EEG patterns. Note that the REM (rapid eye movement) period (in pink) is not one of the official four sleep stages despite being routinely referred to as REM sleep. The EMG trace shows that skeletal muscles are 'paralyzed' during REM sleep.

spike and wave pattern is found in a common form of epilepsy known as 'absence' seizures (see later).

After about an hour's sleep the stage 2 wave pattern is repeated and is succeeded by a longer period of slow wave sleep. Up to a minute may then be spent in REM sleep, a dream state accompanied by:

- visual imagery
- rapid eye movements generated by the extraocular muscle contractions
- electromyographic silence in the musculature of trunk and limbs
- an EEG beta rhythm characteristic of the waking state – hence the term *paradoxical sleep*.

REM sleep is the dominant state during the final two cycles in the 8 hours spent in bed. Although the significance of dreams is a matter of endless debate, activation of the visual cortex is brought about by the *PGO pathway*, from pontine reticular formation to lateral geniculate body to occipital cortex. In individuals blind from birth, dreams have a purely auditory content, perhaps associated with activation of the lateral geniculate body.

In the clinic, because of the brief time that an EEG is recorded, a patient does not often cycle through REM sleep patterns. It should be noted that in normal circumstances REM sleep almost never occurs during the *first* descent into sleep. Should it do so, the strange sleep disorder called *narcolepsy* should come to mind (Clinical Panel 30.1).

It should also be mentioned that volunteers awakened during REM sleep do not invariably report a dream; and that dreaming occasionally happens during NREM sleep.

EEG activation procedures

In order to check for susceptibility to seizures, a routine EEG includes a brief period of hyperventilation and another of photic stimulation using strobe (flickering) light at varying frequencies (Figure 30.7).

Figure 30.7 In normal subjects, stroboscopic lighting induces matching spikes in occipital recordings. Many epileptic patients are at risk of generalized tonic-clonic seizures caused by forward spread of strobe effects. (Adapted from Binnie, 1988.)

Maturation of wave format

Accurate interpretation of printouts necessitates familiarity on the part of the electroencephalographer with those patterns which are age-specific and hence represent normal maturational stages of development. Earliest recordings, from premature babies, show only intermittent electrical activity which is asynchronous between the hemispheres. Continuous symmetrical activity emerges during childhood, with increasingly distinctive wakeful and sleeping patterns. During early teenage years the adult EEG pattern is established.

Abnormal EEG rhythms

Focal abnormalities without seizures

Focal slowing

Focal slowing, in the form of delta waves (Figure 30.8), indicates presence of a mass or lesion of some kind.

Clinical Panel 30.1 Narcolepsy

Narcolepsy (Gr. 'sleep seizure') is a sleep disorder characterized by daytime sleep attacks. These attacks form part of the *narcoleptic syndrome*. The complete syndrome has characteristic features:

- An irresistable desire to sleep, for periods of up an hour, several times during the day. This is accompanied by *sleep paralysis,* at either the beginning or the end of an attack, where the patient is in a state of complete awareness but is unable to even open the eyes, for 1–2 minutes.
- *Hypnogogic* (Gr. 'accompanying sleep') *hallucinations* at sleep onset, characterized by striking visual imagery. The hallucinations are a distorted version of REM sleep.
- During the awake state, there occur brief episodes of muscle paralysis, known as *cataplexy,* a term used to signify sudden paralysis, triggered by emotion, notably by surprise of any kind. Cataplexy occurs in three out of four patients and may range from mild (e.g. dropping the head or jaw, dropping something held in the hand) to severe, with collapse due to flaccid paralysis of the trunk and limbs with consciousness fully preserved. Occasionally, cataplexy may be the *only* presenting symptom.

The 'distorted REM' nature of narcolepsy appears obvious from the occurrence of the two kinds of

paralysis during the awake state rather than during the vivid dream period. Narcolepsy has a familial incidence and may be an immune disorder. It can be very distressing: the patient may be accused of laziness or incompetence at work and is at risk of accidents when driving a car or merely crossing the street.

The key problem is a diminution of gray matter in the walls of the hypothalamus associated with scant production of the excitatory peptide *orexin (hypocretin)* by a group of neurons in the lateral hypothalamus. Orexin receptors are normally present on the histaminergic neurons of the tuberomammillary nucleus (TMN). As mentioned in Chapter 26, the TMN projects widely to the cerebral cortex and maintains the awake state by activating H_1 receptors on cortical neurons. The drug *modafinil* is now a medication used to treat narcolepsy, perhaps by decreasing GABA-mediated neurotransmission. The current conventional approach is to reduce sleep attacks by means of noradrenergic drugs such as amphetamine in low dosage, and/or monoamine oxidase inhibitors; both of these prolong the action of norepinephrine released by the cerulean nucleus, and reduce REM sleep.

REFERENCE

Kim SJ, Lyoo IK, Lee YS, Lee J-Y, Yoon SJ, Kim JE, Kim JH, Hong SJ, Jeong D.-U.: Gray matter deficits in young adults with narcolepsy, *Acta Neurol Scand* 119:61–67, 2009.

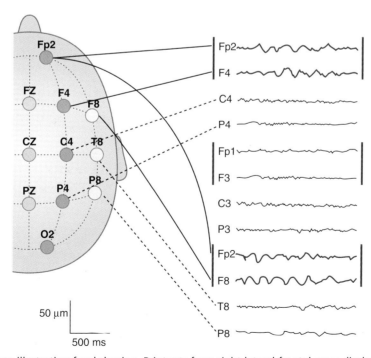

Figure 30.8 Bipolar montage illustrating focal slowing. Printouts from right lateral frontal areas display delta waves in this 60-year-old female suffering from headache and drowsiness for several months without overt physical signs. Coronal MRI slices showed compression of the right lateral ventricle. Surgery revealed the cause to have been an astrocytoma. (Analogous tracings from the left frontal area are normal.)

Focal spike or sharp wave discharges may show a patch of *phase reversal* between adjacent electrodes (Figure 30.9). In the frontal or parietal regon, this is suggestive of an ictal focus; in the occipital it is associated with visual impairment.

Phase reversal

Focal spike or *sharp wave discharges* are occasionally seen over localized areas of the cortex. Both appear as abrupt events, individual spikes lasting 80–100 ms and sharp waves 100–200 ms. Such discharges project to the surface with a negative polarity and the point of *phase reversal* between adjacent electrodes defines their EEG localization (Figure 30.9). In anterior temporal and frontal areas they may be indicative of an *ictal focus*, a term denoting a locus of origin of seizures. In the occipital region any correlation is usually with visual impairment.

Generalized abnormalities without seizures

Disorders that cause generalized dysfunction within cortical or subcortical structures result in a diffuse pattern of abnormalities on EEG. Such disorders include hypoglycemia, hypoxia, and dementia. This can be manifested by replacement of normal background frequency by diffuse slowing. Disorders involving the white matter of the brain are more often associated with delta waves and are often polymorphic (of variable appearance and less sinusoidal).

Seizures

See Clinical Panel 30.2

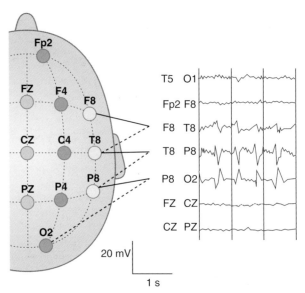

Figure 30.9 Phase reversal. This patient suffered from primary focal seizures. Phase reversal between the T8 and P8 electrodes suggests an ictal focus located in the right posterior temporal lobe.

Clinical Panel 30.2 Seizures

Next to cerebrovascular disease, seizures (epileptic attacks) are the most common group of problems encountered in clinical neurology. Some 3% of the population suffer two or more attacks during their lifetime.

The term 'seizure' or 'ictus' refers to a transient alteration of behavior brought about by abnormal burst-firing of neurons in the cerebral cortex. The 'interictal period' is the time interval between seizures.

Seizures are categorized as follows:

A complex seizure has an ictal focus of origin, usually in the temporal lobe. It spreads to induce a secondarily generalized tonic-clonic seizure. In this context, seizures that are generalized from the start are called *primary generalized tonic-clonic seizures.*

Generalized seizures
Generalized, tonic–clonic seizures (formerly known as *grand mal* seizures) are characterized by sudden onset of unconsciousness. The individual is 'struck down'. The body stiffens, for up to a minute (tonic stage), and then exhibits jerky movements of all four limbs, and chewing movements of the mouth for about another minute (clonic stage). Usually, a third minute is spent in more relaxed unconsciousness. EEG recordings taken at the onset of this kind of *ictus* (attack) show simultaneous bilateral burst-firing all over the cortex (Figure CP 30.2.1).

In those at risk, hyperventilation, or photic stimulation by strobe lighting (Figure 30.7), can precipitate tonic-clonic attacks.

Absence seizures (formerly, *petit mal*) are characterized by a generalized, 3 Hz spike-and-wave activity (Figure CP 30.2.2). These seizures usually occur between the ages of 4 and 14.

Clinical Panel 30.2 *Continued*

Figure CP 30.2.1 Characteristic 'frenzied' pattern of a tonic-clonic seizure.
(A) End of interictal period.
(B) Generalized seizure pattern involving all electrode positions.
(C) In less than 1 second, the seizure pattern is 'scribbled' by generalized tonic muscle spasm.
(D) Immediate postictal period, with slow waveform pattern throughout.
(E) Resumption of normal waveforms.

The typical case is a child who, upon relaxing after some physical or mental activity, passes through 'blank' periods (absences) of 10–30 seconds, usually with detectable twitching of muscles of the face or fingers. Dozens of such episodes may occur over a period of several hours, often so mild that low-level activities such as walking are not interrupted. The child is unaware of individual episodes, which may occur a hundred or more times in one day. The 'blank' periods are brought about by prolonged inhibitory postsynaptic potentials on sensory thalamic relay neurons generated by thalamic reticular neurons made hyperactive by corticothalamic excitatory discharges.

Focal (partial) seizures
Note: The term 'partial' refers to seizure origin in a particular lobe (focus) of the brain and not to seizures confined to one part of the body. Complex partial seizures can become generalized.

Simple focal seizures are almost always motor or sensory. Loci of origin are as shown in Table CP 30.2.1.

A *jacksonian seizure* (named after neurologist John Hughlings Jackson) involves sequential activation of adjacent areas of the motor cortex, e.g ankle, knee, hip, shoulder, elbow, hand, lips, tongue, larynx. A jacksonian seizure may be followed by weakness/ paralysis of the affected limb(s) for a period of hours or days; it is known as *Todd's paralysis*.

(Continued)

Clinical Panel 30.2 *Continued*

Benign rolandic epilepsy, a relatively common disorder in childhood, has an ictal focus of origin in front of or behind the fissure of Rolando (central sulcus). *Motor attacks* originate in front of the rolandic fissure and usually involve only the contralateral arm or leg or face, although some become jacksonian. *Somatosensory attacks* (Figure CP 30.2.3) originate behind the fissure and are described in Table CP 30.2.1.

Table CP 30.2.1 Loci of origin of simple focal seizures	
Motor	Movement of any part of the motor homunculus, sometimes with aphasia
Somatosensory	Contralateral nunbness/ tingling of face, fingers or toes
Primary visual cortex	Flashes of light or patches of darkness in contralateral visual field
Visual association cortex	Twinkling-light images in contralateral visual field
Basal occipitotemporal junction	Formed visual images of people or places, sometimes accompanied by sounds
Superior temporal gyrus (unusual)	Tinnitus, sometimes garbled word sounds

Figure CP 30.2.2 (A) Absence seizure. This episode was recorded over a period of 4 seconds. The spike-and-slow wave pattern is bilateral and generalized. In this patient the pattern is rather faster than usual. **(B)** The spike-and-slow-wave prototype.

Figure CP 30.2.3 Simple partial seizure originating in the right somatic sensory cortex (R) and expressed by 'pins-and-needles' along the left arm. There is some spread to to the left sensory cortex (L). (Refer to Figure 30.2 for R and L electrode positions.)

Clinical Panel 30.2 *Continued*

A diagnosis of benign rolandic epilepsy requires EEG confirmation while the child is quietly asleep during an interictal period. Here, a normal background montage is interrupted by high-voltage spikes that occur at short intervals in the area of the ictal focus. Frequency of attacks dwindles during maturation and the EEG becomes normal by the 16th year.

Complex focal seizures are synonymous with *temporal lobe epilepsy*. They will be taken up in Chapter 34 following a description there of the relevant areas of the temporal lobe.

Drug therapy
Anticonvulsant drugs, administered in appropriate amounts, control about half of all seizures completely and another quarter almost completely. The drugs are of a broadly predictable nature. Most of them either reduce glutamatergic activity or enhance GABA-mediated inhibitory processes. For tonic-clonic and complex partial seizures, some current drugs of choice are:

- *Glutamate antagonists: phenytoin* and *carbamazepine* (Tegretol), reduce high-frequency repetitive firing by blocking glutamate ionotropic receptors (Ch. 8), making their ion channels less permeable to sodium and/or calcium.
- *GABA agonists: benzodiazepines* and *barbiturates* enhance the hyperpolarizing effect of GABA on glutamate neurons, as illustrated in Figure 8.7. *Sodium valproate* blocks the transaminase enzyme which converts GABA to glutamate within adjacent astrocytes (Ch. 8), thereby extending GABA's time in the synaptic cleft.

The most widely used and most effective drug for absence seizures is *ethosuximide*. Ethosuximide is a specific T-channel blocker. At appropriate dosage, excitability of thalamic relay neurons is sufficiently reduced to prevent them entering burst-firing mode.

REFERENCES
Dichter MA: Emerging concepts in the pathogenesis of epilepsy and eleptogenesis, *Arch Neurol* 66:443–447, 2009.
Oliviero A, Della Marca G, Tonali PA, Pilato E, Saturno E, Dileone M, Versace V, Mennuni G, Di Lazzaro V: Functional involvement of the cerebral cortex in human narcolepsy, *J Neurol* 252:56–61, 2005.
Smith SJM: EEG in the diagnosis, classification, and management of patients with epilepsy, *J Neurol Neurosurg Psychiatry* 76(Suppl II): ii2–ii7, 2005.
Steriade M: Sleep, epilepsy and thalamic reticular nucleus, *Trends Neurosci* 28:317–324, 2005.

Core Information

The oscillations recorded in the electroencephalogram are produced by excitatory and inhibitory postsynaptic potentials collectively produced by cortical cell columns. The grid-like standard arrangement of the recording elecrodes permits overall sampling of electrical activity in a manner that is applicable to both children and adults.

Sleep
The awake state EEG displays a desynchronized (irregular) background frequency, sometimes with a beta frequency of 9.5 Hz superimposed in frontal montages. During quiet rest with eyes closed, alpha rhythms (8–15 Hz) appear in parieto-occipital tracings. Stage 1 of sleep exhibits theta rhythm at 5–8 Hz. During stage 2, theta rhythm is interrupted by sleep spindles and K complex spikes. Stages 3 and 4 are characterized by 'slow wave sleep' in the delta range (3 Hz or less). The final four sleep cycles are capped by 'paradoxical sleep' associated with wake-type desynchronization, rapid eye movements (REM), and dreams with high visual content.

Narcolepsy is a sleep disorder characterized by an irresistible desire to sleep for up to an hour several times during the day, by hypnogogic hallucinations at sleep onset, by cataplexy (momentary muscle paralysis), and sleep paralysis at beginning or end of an attack.

Abnormal EEG rhythms
Focal abnormalities without seizures include focal slowing and phase reversal. Generalized abnormalities without seizures include hypoglycemia, hypoxia, and dementias, any of which may replace normal background activity by diffuse slowing expressed in theta frequency. Disorders involving cerebral white matter may be expressed by delta activity with polymorphic interference.

Seizures
Seizures are of two broad kinds: *generalized*, manifested by either tonic-clonic or absence attacks; and *focal* (partial), where consciousness is preserved during simple motor or sensory attacks but lost during complex attacks. Complex focal seizures refer to temporal lobe epilepsy.

Anticonvulsant drugs have one or more effects. Most enhance GABA-mediated inhibitory activity; some inhibit glutamate activity by either inhibiting glutamate synthesis or by blocking sodium channels at glutamatergic nerve terminals.

REFERENCES

Binnie CD: Electroencephalography. In Laidlaw J, Richins A, Oxley J, editors: *A textbook of epilepsy*, Edinburgh, 1988, Churchill Livingstone, pp 236–306.

Grigg-Damberger M: Normal sleep: impact of age, circadian rhythms, and sleep debt, *Continuum: Lifelong Learning in Neurology* 13:31–84, 2007.

Nestler EJ, Hyman SE, Malenka RC: Sleep, arousal and attention. In *Molecular neuropharmacology: a foundation for clinical neuroscience*, New York, 2001, McGraw-Hill, pp 409–432.

Siegel JM: The neurobiology of sleep, *Semin Neurol* 29:277–296, 2009.

Smith PE: The bare essentials: epilepsy, *Neurology in Practice* 8:195–202, 2008.

Staunton H: Mammalian sleep, *Naturwissenschaften* 92:203–220, 2005.

STUDY GUIDELINES

1 'Sensory evoked potentials' are the waveforms detected by specific EEG recording electrodes in response to different kinds of peripheral sensory stimulation. The objective is to assess the integrity of central sensory pathways.
2 'Motor evoked potentials' are elicited in skeletal muscles by magnetic stimulation of the motor cortex. The main clinical objective is to ascertain the conduction velocity of the corticospinal tract.

   A physiological observation of general interest revealed by this technique is that acquisition of a particular motor skill can be accelerated by mental rehearsal.

SENSORY EVOKED POTENTIALS

The term *sensory evoked potentials* is used to define the response of the CNS to specific sensory stimulation. In clinical neurophysiology the specific stimuli relate to vision, hearing, and cutaneous sensations.

   A difficulty with these evoked potentials is that their low amplitudes, of 20 μV or even less, render them undetectable in routine EEG recordings because of the background wave pattern. Advantage is taken of the regularity of the response to repeated stimuli of the same type. With repetitive stimulation followed by computer averaging, irregular backround rhythms cancel each other out and the evoked potentials can be clearly seen.

   The three basic kinds of sensory evoked potentials are described as *visual, auditory* and *somatosensory.*

Visual evoked potentials

The speed and amplitude of impulse conduction in the visual pathway are tested by the technique known as *pattern reversal* or *pattern shift*. With one eye covered at a time, the patient stares at a spot in the center of a screen illuminated in a black-and-white checkerboard pattern. Once or twice per second the pattern is reversed (to white and black), over a period of 100 repetitions. Averaging is performed on the first 500 ms of data from a bipolar recording at the occipital and parietal midline EEG sites (OZ and PZ).

   The wave peak of interest is called P100. In healthy subjects it is a positive deflection 100 ms poststimulus (Figure 31.1). In the clinical example shown, taken from a patient with a presumptive diagnosis of multiple sclerosis, the normal P100 wave from the right-eye test indicated that both optic tracts and both optic radiations were clear. The P100 wave from the left eye was both delayed and of reduced amplitude, suggesting presence of one or more plaques of myelin degeneration in the left optic nerve. (*Note:* On screen and in printouts, it is now customary for the waveforms to be 'flipped', with positive responses registering as upward deflections.)

   Conduction defects caused by demyelination are more often expressed in the form of *latency delays* of the kind shown, than in the form of amplitude abnormalities.

   In the absence of any evidence for MS elsewhere, an abnormal P100 from one eye may be caused by an ocular disease such as glaucoma or by compression or ischemia of the optic nerve.

   Bilateral abnormal P100 recordings can indicate pathology in one or both optic radiations. In such a situation, it is usual to take recordings from electrode pairs placed a few centimeters to one side of the midline and then a few centimeters to the other side. Should the (say) right optic radiation be at fault, any P100 abnormality is likely to be more pronounced in recordings from that side of the midline.

Brainstem auditory evoked potentials

Remarkably, it is possible to follow the sequence of electrical events in the auditory pathway, step by step, from cochlea to primary auditory cortex. Following placement of temporal scalp recording electrodes, 0.1 ms click sounds are presented at approximately 10 Hz to each ear in turn through conventional audiometric earphones. Click intensity is adjusted to 65–70 decibels above click hearing threshold for the ear being tested. The contralateral ear is 'masked' by white noise.

   A sequence of seven averaged-out waves (I–VII) constitutes the BAER (brainstem auditory evoked response). They are accounted for in the caption to Figure 31.2.

   Pathology anywhere along the auditory pathway results in reduction or abolition of the wave above that level. *The technique is the most sensitive screening test available for acoustic neuroma.* A diagnostic feature here is *I–III latency separation.* (*Latency* refers to the time interval between stimulus and response; *separation* refers to extension of the interval between waves I and III, caused by delay during passage along the affected cochlear nerve during a characteristically reduced amplitude wave II.)

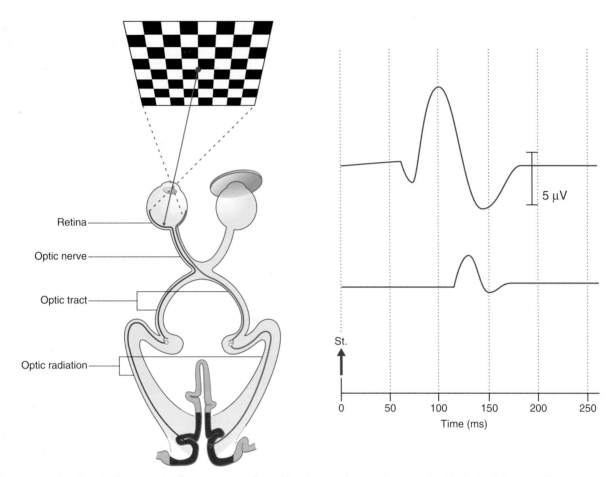

Figure 31.1 Visual evoked potentials. The patient's right eye has been tested and is now shielded. The left eye is fixated on the spot in the center of the checkerboard during pattern reversal episodes. The pattern from the right eye is normal, showing a positive deflection at 100 ms poststimulus. In the recording from the left eye the P100 is both delayed and reduced in amplitude. The combined results indicate presence of a lesion in the left eye or left optic nerve.

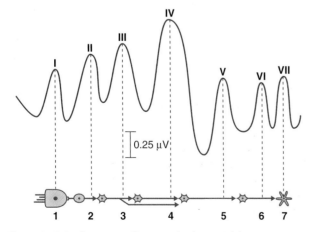

Figure 31.2 Brainstem auditory evoked potentials. Sources of evoked potentials: **1** distal cochlear nerve (cochlear hair cells); **2** cochlear nerve (proximal); **3** from cochlear nucleus; **4** from lateral lemniscus; **5** from inferior colliculus (inferior brachium); **6** from medial geniculate body (auditory radiation); **7** primary auditory cortex.

In about 30% of patients who have multiple sclerosis (MS) with no clinical evidence of brainstem lesions, the BAER is abnormal. Most frequent abnormalities are reduced amplitude of wave V and overall slowing of conduction indicated by increased interwave intervals.

Another clinical application of the BAER technique is the assessment of cochlear function in infants under suspicion of congenital deafness.

Assessment of brainstem auditory evoked potentials is also important in the medicolegal domain, to assess veracity of claims of deafness induced by environmental noise in industry.

Evidence for a 'Where' auditory pathway

When recording electrodes are specifically deployed over the temporoparietal region, and brief sounds are emitted from loudspeakers placed in the left and right visual fields, a cortical response can be detected over the posterior part of the temporal plane, close to the temporoparietal junction. The right posterior temporal plane **gives** a stronger response, suggesting a right-sided dominance for auditory as well as visual space analysis.

Somatosensory evoked potentials

Somatosensory evoked potentials are the waveforms recorded at surface landmarks en route from the point of stimulation of a peripheral nerve to the contralateral somatic sensory cortex. The rate and amplitude of impulse conduction provide valuable information about the status of myelinated nerve fibers in both peripheral nerves and central pathways.

The nerve of choice for stimulation in the upper limb is the median at the wrist, in the lower limb the common peroneal at the knee. Repetitive electrical pulses are delivered to the nerve through a surface or needle electrode. The larger myelinated fibers are stimulated. Computer averaging is required to distinguish the stimulated responses from background noise, notably within the CNS. In the example shown in Figure 31.3, impulse traffic along the median nerve is detected by a sequence of active electrodes attached to the skin for the purpose of recording speed and amplitude of nerve conduction in sequential segments. as follows:

1 over the brachial plexus, to assess the median nerve segment extending from wrist to anterior triangle of neck;
2 over the spine of vertebra C2, for the segment 1 plus transit through nerve roots and ipsilateral posterior column (fasciculus cuneatus);
3 over the contralateral scalp at some distance away from the somatic sensory cortex, to 'pick up' stimulus traffic ascending the medial lemniscus;
4 directly over the hand area of the somatic sensory cortex, to detect activity in the thalamocortical projection.

In the various peripheral neuropathies mentioned in Chapter 9 the first segment (wrist to brachial plexus) reveals slowing, usually with a reduction of amplitude. The second segment (brachial plexus to nucleus gracilis) may be affected in the first few milliseconds of its time course as a result of posterior nerve root compression by osteophytes in patients with cervical spondylosis. A little later, the curve may be affected by posterior column disease (Ch. 15). Abnormality in the third segment (contralateral medial lemniscus) is found in 9 out of 10 patients suffering from MS in the presence of sensory symptoms, and in 6 out of 10 in the absence of sensory symptoms.

MOTOR EVOKED POTENTIALS

Motor evoked potentials are motor unit action potentials (MUAPs) detected in surface EMG recordings following controlled excitation of the corticospinal tract. The technique was mentioned in Chapter 18 because it revealed that the pyramidal tract pathway to sternomastoid spinal motor neurons is essentially crossed, rather than being ipsilateral as previously thought. The most frequent objective is to determine *central motor conduction time* along the corticospinal tract. The procedure is both safe and painless. It uses a subtraction approach comparable in principle to that used to determine peripheral nerve conduction times (Figure 31.3).

The procedure is known as *transcranial magnetic stimulation* (TMS). Figure 31.4 illustrates the concept in action. Stimulation is by means of a magnet in the form of a circular coil about 10 cm in diameter. To stimulate the pyramidal cells of the corticospinal tract supplying left anterior horn motor neurons, the magnet is hand held a little to the right side of the vertex and the patient maintains the selected limb muscle (biceps brachii in this example) in a state of slight contraction. A few very brief (200 ms) currents are pulsed at an intensity comfortably above the threshold required to elicit a twitch. The patient feels only a small 'tap' sensation on the scalp. The procedure is then repeated with the magnet touching the skin of the neck overlying the spine of vertebra C5, again eliciting a 'tap' sensation. It is generally agreed that the second pulse depolarizes the axons of anterior nerve roots exiting the vertebral canal.

The latencies and amplitudes of the compound motor action potentials (CMAPs) are measured. The right biceps can then be activated in the same manner. The same procedure can be performed for the lower limb, the spinal stimulus being delivered in the lumbar region.

In neurophysiology units, central motor conduction time is estimated where there is reason to suspect the presence of plaques of multiple sclerosis in the white matter of brain or spinal cord; and where muscle wasting in the arms and/or legs leads to suspicion that upper as well as lower motor neurons may be degenerating; and in patients where moderate muscle weakness on one side, associated with brisk tendon reflexes, raises suspicion of a stroke.

Motor training

A remarkable degree of plasticity in the healthy motor cortex has been demonstrated by TMS studies. Figure 31.5 represents outcomes of five-finger piano-playing exercises. A small magnetic coil was used over the scalp to locate the modules primarily involved in flexion and extension of the fingers of the right hand. This small scalp area was marked in three sets of volunteers, and the baseline size was measured for each subject. Group A *imagined* doing the five-finger exercise for 2 hours per day for 5 days; Group B *did* the exercises for the same periods; Group C did not participate in any way prior to attempting the task once on day 5. As indicated in the figure, merely thinking about performance led to a major increase in the number of modules that activated the fingers when stimulated on days 3 and 5. Group B – the actual performers – showed the greatest increase of participating motor modules. The performance skills on day 5 were substantially better in Group B than Group A, and Group A's performance was better than that of Group C.

There is general agreement that dramatic alterations such as those shown in this group experiment are best explained in terms of *unmasking of pre-existing connections*, as in the case of rapid expansion of the cortical sensory territory of one thalamocortical projection following experimental inactivation of a neighboring projection. The most likely mechanism of additional pyramidal cell recruitment appears to be one of *disinhibition*, probably by the premotor cortex, involving activation of sequential pairs of GABAergic neurons in the manner illustrated in Figure 6.2.

In this general context, it has also been shown that performance improvement in weight lifting is optimal when subjects *mentally rehearse* weight lifting during the days between performing the exercises.

Finally, Box 31.1 includes an experiment in which TMS has been used to assess the supposed usefulness of acupuncture in improving motor performance.

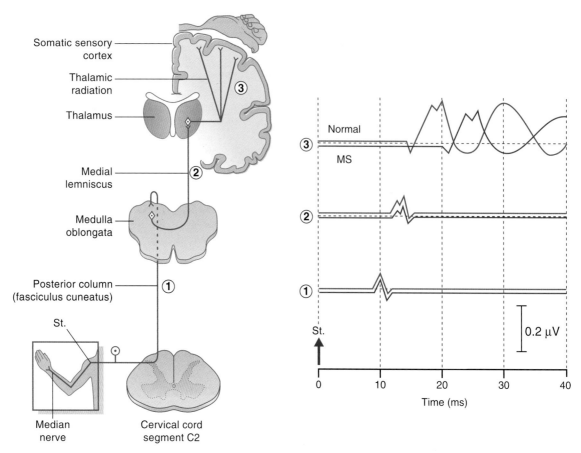

Figure 31.3 Short latency somatosensory evoked potentials derived from stimulation (St.) of the median nerve at the wrist. The pathway has four segments. **1** is purely PNS. **2** is PNS from brachial plexus to spinal cord and CNS within the cord. **3** and **4** are purely CNS. In the recordings from a patient with multiple sclerosis (MS), trace 1 is normal; trace 2 shows reduced amplitude of the negative (upward) and positive peaks within the posterior column; trace 3 shows slowing as well as reduced amplitude. (Adapted in part from Adams and Victor 1993.)

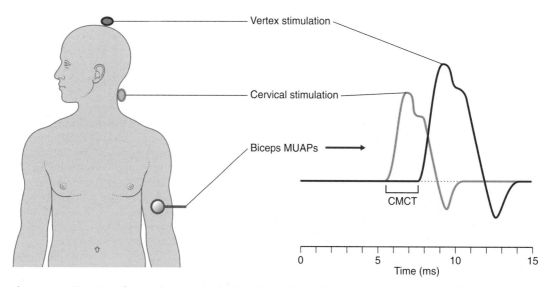

Figure 31.4 Laboratory estimation of central motor conduction time. The (*red*) coil over the vertex has delivered a 200 ms current to pyramidal tract neurons serving upper limb spinal motor neurons. A large compound motor action potential (CMAP) is elicited in the biceps. The (*green*) coil over the cervical spine has delivered a weaker pulse to cervical anterior nerve roots eliciting a smaller CMAP. The difference between the two latencies (stimulus–response intervals) represents the central motor conduction time (CMCT).

Figure 31.5 Five-finger exercise. As explained in the main text, Group A volunteers imagined performing a daily five-finger piano exercise for the right hand, whereas Group B actually did perform it. Transcranial magnetic stimulation (TMS) showed remarkable enlargement of the area of motor cortex activating the finger flexors and extensors in both groups. (Based on data in Pascual-Leone et al., 1995.)

Box 31.1 Acupuncture

'There is sufficient evidence of acupuncture's value to expand its use into conventional medicine and to encourage further studies of its physiology and clinical value.' (NIH Consensus Conference on Acupuncture, 1997, cited by Stux et al., 1997).

Sensation
For relief of pain, fine (0.25 mm) needles are inserted bilaterally through appropriate acupoints, coming to rest among superficial muscle fibers underlying the subcutaneous fat (Figure 31.1.1). The needle is then briefly spun to excite Types II and III sensory nerve fibers in its immediate neighborhood. A subjective sense of numbness or heaviness in the acupoint area is usually reported.

The accepted explanation of the rapid pain relief produced by this form of stimulation is release of

Figure Box 31.1.1 Standard positioning of acupuncture needle.

Box 31.1 *Continued*

enkephalin by (a) spinal antinociception via the segmental reflex mentioned in 'rubbing the sore spot' combined with (b) supraspinal antinociception via spinoreticular activation of the PAG–MRN–RST–Enk pathway shown in Figure 24.8. Pain relief is not achieved if the subject has received a prior injection of the opiate antagonist naloxone.

The term *acupuncture analgesia* refers to low-frequency (1 Hz) electrical stimulation of needles inserted at appropriate acupoints (electroacupuncture). The remarkable result is analgesia so complete as to permit open surgery in alert awake patients. Clearly the ascending reticular activating system is not paralyzed, unlike the case with general anesthesia. Animal experiments indicate that electroacupuncture, in addition to the above-mentioned effects, produces co-release of β-endorphin from the arcuate nucleus of the hypothalamus and ACTH from the adenohypophysis.

With availability of fMRI as a research tool, attention is being focused on the effects of acupuncture on higher-level sensory functions. Figure 31.1.2 is composite, reproducing the remarkable results of two quite separate experiments. In each volunteer, needling was performed *bilaterally,* one acupoint being traditional for relief of disorders of vision, the other for disorders of hearing. Areas of increased cortical blood flow closely resemble those associated with retinal/cochlear activation. Surprisingly, the volunteers did not report visual/auditory hallucinations. And an obvious question persists concerning the mysteriously specific anatomical pathways from the acupoints to the appropriate areas of cortex.

Movement
Movement disorders also have tradional therapeutic acupoints. One of these acupoints, on the lateral side of the proximal forearm, has been selected for low-

Figure Box 31.1.2 Bilateral needling of acupoint GB 37 generates increased blood flow in the visual cortex. Bilateral needling of acupoint GB 43 generates increased blood flow in the auditory cortex. (Adapted from Cho et al., 2000, with permission of Pabst.)

Box 31.1 *Continued*

☐	0.25–0.5
■	0.5–0.75
■	0.75–1.0
■	1.0–1.26
■	1.26–1.5
■	1.5–1.75
■	1.75–2.0

Figure Box 31.1.3 Surface EMG activity recorded over flexor carpi ulnaris muscle in response to TMS over and beyond the arm area of the left motor cortex. **A** marks an acupoint traditionally used to improve motor function, **B** marks the sham needling point (needling in the same manner 2 cm medial to A). Both points are well clear of ulnar nerve motor and sensory territories.
Numbers 0, 10, and 15, respectively, refer to baseline (no needling), 10 min with needle in place, and 15 min after needle removal. The table records voltage of MUAPs in response to TMS over equal areas of the frontal lobe at each time interval. (Based on Lo et al., 2005.)
(Assistance of Dr.Y.L. Lo, Department of Neurology, National Neuroscience Institute, Singapore is gratefully acknowledged.)

frequency (1 Hz) electroacupuncture in the experiment illustrated in Figure Box 31.1.3.

The upper three figures show expansion of the cortical area eliciting a twitch response in the EMG records related to acupoint needling; the lower three, related to sham needling, show no significant expansion.

REFERENCES

Chen K: Neuroanatomical basis of acupuncture treatment for some common illnesses, *Acupuncture in Medicine* 27:61–64, 2009.

Gruccu G, Aminoff MJ, Curio G, et al: Recommendations for the clinical use of somatosensory-evoked potentials, *Clin Neurophysiol* 1705–1719, 2008.

Lo YL, Cui SL: Acupuncture and the modulation of cortical excitability, *Neuroreport* 14:1229–1231, 2003.

Lo YL, Cui SL, Fook-Chong S: The effect of acupuncture on motor cortex excitability and plasticity, *Neurosci Lett* 384:385–389, 2005.

Olssen C-J, Jonnson B, Nyberg L: Learning by doing and learning by thinking: an fMRI study of combining motor and mental training, *Front Hum Neurosci* 2:5–12, 2008.

Pomeranz P, Berman B: Scientific basis of acupuncture. In Stux G, Berman B, Pomeranz B, editors: *Basics of acupuncture*, ed 5, Berlin, 2003, Springer, pp 52–86.

Stux G, Berman B, Pomeraz B: *Basics of acupuncture*, ed 5, Berlin, 1997, Springer-Verlag.

Tageshige C: Mechanisms of acupuncture analgesia produced by low frequency electrical stimulation of aupuncture points. In Stux G, Hammerschlag R, editors: *Clinical acupuncture: scientific basis*, Berlin, 2003, Springer, pp 29–50.

Yan B, Li K, Xu J, et al: Acupoint-specific fMRI patterns in human brain, *Neurosci Lett* 383:236–240, 2005.

Core Information

Sensory evoked potentials

Recordings of sensory evoked potentials are used to assess conduction rates and amplitudes in central sensory pathways that may be under suspicion on clinical grounds.

Potentials in the visual cortex are evoked by means of checkerboard pattern reversal, one eye being tested at a time. Conduction deficits caused by demyelination are usually expressed in the form of latency delays.

Potentials in the auditory cortex are evoked by click sounds. The montage normally shows seven successive waveforms generated by the seven cell groups involved in the pathway from cochlea to cortex. The auditory evoked potential technique is the most sensitive test available for detection of an aoustic neuroma.

Potentials in the somatosensory cortex are elicited by electrical pulses delivered to a peripheral nerve, e.g. median at wrist, peroneal at knee, with recording electrodes in place to detect waveforms in the brachial/lumbar plexus, posterior column of spinal cord, medial lemniscus and thalamocortical projection.

Different disorders impair conduction in different segments of the pathway from skin to cortex.

Motor evoked potentials

Transcranial magnetic stimulation (TMS) is used clinically to estimate conduction time in the pyramidal tract, in patients with motor weakness originating in the CNS. Surface EMG recordings of compound action potentials are taken from selected muscles while a magnetic coil delivers very brief currents over the scalp to excite the motor cortex and repeats the technique over the cervical and/or lumbar spine to excite anterior nerve roots innervating the selected muscle(s). The central motor conduction time is provided by subtraction of the peripheral nerve time segment from the total cortex-to-muscle time.

TMS is also used in neurophysiology laboratories to study activity changes in the motor cortex occurring in the course of training for motor skill or strength tasks.

REFERENCES

Adams RD, Victor M: *Principles of neurology*, ed 5, New York, 1993, McGraw-Hill.

Cho Z, Na C, Wong E, Lee S, Hong I: Investigation of acupuncture using fMRI. In Litscher G, Cho Z, editors: *Computer-controlled acupuncture*, Berlin, 2000, Pabst, pp 45–64.

Maccabee PJ, Amassian VE, Ziemann U, Wassermann E, Deletis V: Emerging applications in neuromagnetic stimulation. In Levin KH, Lüders HO, editors: *Comprehensive clinical neurology*, Philadelphia, 2000, Saunders, pp 325–347.

Misulis KE, Fakhoury T: *Spehlman's evoked potential primer*, ed 3, Boston, 2000, Butterworth-Heinemann.

Pascual-Leone A, Dang N, Cohen LG: Modulation of muscle responses evoked by transcranial magnetic stimulation during the acquisition of new motor skills, *J Neurophysiol* 74:1037–1045, 1995.

Tata MS, Ward LM: Spatial attention modulates activity in a posterior "where" pathway, *Neuropsychologia* 43:509–516, 2005.

Walsh P, Kane N, Butler S: The clinical role of evoked potentials, *J Neurol Neurosurg Psychiatry* 76:ii16–ii22, 2005.

STUDY GUIDELINES

1 Language functions, with their strikingly asymmetrical distribution in the majority of the population, are of great significance in the contexts of clinical diagnosis and speech rehabilitation.
2 Also asymmetrical as a rule are the functional emphases of the parietal lobes.
3 A first reading of relevant parts of Chapter 35 should follow, in order to integrate the clinical information with the regional distribution of the cerebral arteries.

The two cerebral hemispheres are *asymmetrical* in certain respects. Some of the asymmetries have to do with handedness, language, and complex motor activities; other, more subtle differences come under the general rubric of *cognitive style*. (Limbic asymmetries are described in Ch. 34.)

HANDEDNESS AND LANGUAGE

Handedness often determines the hemisphere that is dominant for motor control. Left hemisphere/right-hand dominance is the rule. Advances in ultrasound technology have made it possible for motor behavior in the fetus to be observed, and it has been noted that handedness is already established before birth on the basis of the preferred hand used for thumb sucking during fetal life.

The best indicator available for population estimates of handedness is the preferred hand for writing: this criterion indicates a left hemisphere dominance for motor control in about 90% of the population.

In 90% of subjects, the left hemisphere is dominant for language. In a further 7.5%, the right hemisphere is dominant in both sexes, and in the remaining 2.5%, the two hemispheres have an equal share. Although the left hemisphere is dominant in respect of both motor control and language, the two features are statistically independent: many left-handers have their language areas in the left hemisphere.

Language areas

Although several areas of the cortex, notably in the frontal lobe, are active during speech, two areas are specifically devoted to this function.

Broca's area (Figure 32.1)

The French pathologist Pierre Broca assigned a motor speech function to the inferior frontal gyrus of the left side in 1861. The principal area concerned occupies the opercular and triangular parts of the inferior frontal gyrus corresponding to areas 44 and 45 of Brodmann. Both areas are larger on the left side in people who are right handed. The main output of Broca's area is to cell columns in the face and tongue areas of the adjacent motor cortex.

Lesions involving Broca's area are associated with expressive aphasia (see Clinical Panel 32.1). Some workers believe that expressive aphasia requires that the lesion also includes the lower end of the precentral gyrus.

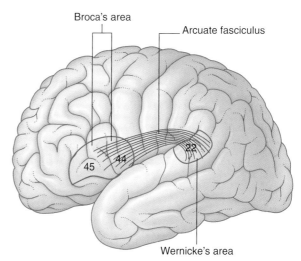

Figure 32.1 Broca's and Wernicke's language areas and the arcuate fasciculus.

Clinical Panel 32.1 The aphasias

Aphasia is a disturbance of language function caused by a lesion of the brain. The usual cause is a stroke produced by vascular occlusion in the anterior cortical territory of the left middle cerebral artery.

Motor (anterior) aphasia

Patients having a lesion that includes Broca's area suffer from motor aphasia. These patients have difficulty in expressing what they want to say. Speech is slow, labored, and characteristically 'telegraphic' in style. The important nouns and verbs are spoken but prepositions and conjunctions are omitted. The patient comprehends what other people are saying and is well aware of being unable to speak fluently. There is usually an associated agraphia (inability to express thoughts in writing).

   If the lesion involves a substantial amount of the cortical territory of the middle cerebral artery, there will be a motor weakness of the right lower face and right arm. Because the lips and tongue are affected on the right side, the patient will also have *dysarthria* (difficulty in speech articulation) in the form of slurring of certain syllables. In the example shown in Figure CP 32.1.1A, Broca's aphasia would be associated with right-sided weakness of the lower face but not of the arm, together with some dysarthria.

Sensory (posterior) aphasia

A lesion in Wernicke's area is accompanied by a deficit of auditory comprehension. If the lesion includes the angular gyrus, the ability to read will also be compromised. In addition to their difficulty in understanding the speech of others, these patients lose the ability to monitor their own conversation, and usually have difficulty in retrieving correct descriptive names. Speech fluency is normal but two kinds of abnormality occur in the use of nouns:

* Verbal paraphasia (use of words usually of allied meaning): instead of 'use a knife', 'use a fork'.
* Phonemic paraphasia (use of made-up but similar-sounding syllables): instead of 'knife and fork', 'bife and dork'.

   The most striking feature of Wernicke's aphasia is that, despite garbling to the point of being unintelligible (*jargon aphasia*), the patient may be quite unaware of making mistakes.

A

B

Figure CP 32.1.1 (A) Vascular lesion involving Broca's area. **(B)** Vascular lesion involving Wernicke's area.

   In the example shown in Figure CP 32.1.1B, Wernicke's aphasia would be associated with alexia (angular gyrus), ideomotor apraxia (supramarginal gyrus) and probably with a right upper quadrant visual deficit (lower fibers of left optic radiation in the temporal white matter).

Aprosodia

Lesions of the right hemisphere may affect speech in subtle ways. Lesions that include area 44 (corresponding to Broca's area on the left) tend to change the patient's speech to a dull monotone. On the other hand, lesions that involve area 22 (corresponding to Wernicke's area) may lead to listening errors, e.g. being unable to detect inflections of speech; the patient may not know whether a particular remark is intended as a statement or as a question.

Wernicke's area (Figure 32.1)

The German neurologist Karl Wernicke made extensive contributions to language processing in the late 19th century. He designated the posterior part of area 22 in the superior temporal gyrus of the left hemisphere as a sensory area concerned with understanding the spoken word. The upper surface of Wernicke's area is called the temporal plane (Figure 32.2). The volume of cerebral cortex in the temporal plane is larger on the left side in 60% of subjects. The horizontal part of the lateral fissure is longer in consequence – a feature readily identified on MRI scans. Lesions involving Wernicke's area in adults are associated with receptive aphasia (see Clinical Panel 32.1).

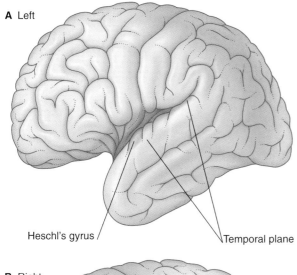

A Left

Heschl's gyrus   Temporal plane

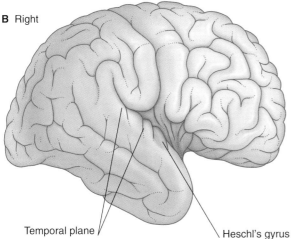

B Right

Temporal plane   Heschl's gyrus

Figure 32.2 Views of the opened lateral sulcus, showing the upper surface of the temporal lobes.

Wernicke's area is linked to Broca's area by association fibers of the arcuate fasciculus curving around the posterior end of the lateral fissure within the underlying white matter (Figure 32.1). The two areas are also linked through the insula.

It is difficult to assess the significance of the asymmetry of the temporal plane. The 60% incidence of left-sided relative enlargement does not match the 95% left hemisphere dominance for speech. Moreover, the *overall* length of the lateral sulcus is much the same on both sides. The *parietal plane* of that sulcus is longer on the right side because the right supramarginal gyrus is larger than the left one. This feature has been advanced as an explanation for the shorter temporal plane on the right.

Maldevelopment of the left temporal plane is a significant feature in cases of schizophrenia (Clinical Panel 32.4).

Right hemisphere contribution

During normal conversation there is some increase in blood flow in areas of the right hemisphere matching those of the left. These areas are believed to be concerned with melodic aspects of speech – the cadences, emphases, and nuances, collectively called *prosody*. Disturbances of the melodic function are called *aprosodias* (Clinical Panel 32.1).

Recovery of speech function – when it occurs – depends upon the age of the subject, and in adults upon the extent of the lesion. Occasional cases have been reported of recovery of near-normal speech in right-handed patients 7 years of age or less following complete removal of the left hemisphere as a treatment for intractable epilepsy. This can only be explained by language processing, including speech, being not fully lateralized at the time of operation. In adults, PET studies have shown increased activity in Broca's and Wernicke's equivalents on the right side following cerebrovascular accidents on the left. However, significant improvement is possible only if the left temporal plane is sufficiently viable to be able to process signals passed to it from the right side through the corpus callosum.

Angular gyrus

The angular gyrus (area 39) belongs descriptively to the inferior parietal lobule. The *left* angular gyrus receives a projection from the inferior part of area 19 (the lingual gyrus, shown in Figure 2.6), and itself projects to the temporal plane. It is commonly included as a part of Wernicke's area.

The angular gyrus seems to contain a neural lexicon (dictionary) of words, syllables, and numerical or other symbols, which can be retrieved by visual inputs – or even by visual imagery – and forwarded in the form of impulse trains to Wernicke's area within area 22. During reading, it is engaged in the conversion of written syllables ('graphemes') into the corresponding sound equivalents ('phonemes'). The angular gyrus is also active during listening to spoken words.

Listening to spoken words

Figure 32.3 contrasts regional increases in blood flow during PET scanning when a volunteer listens to words ('active listening') vs random tone sequences ('passive listening'). As expected, tone sequences activate the primary auditory cortex (bilaterally). Wernicke's area (left side) also becomes active, probably in screening out this non-verbal material from further processing. Area 9 in the frontal lobe is thought to be part of a supervisory, vigilance system.

During active listening to words, areas 21 (middle temporal lobe), 37 (posteroinferior temporal lobe), and 39 (angular gyrus) all participate in auditory word processing. Area 39 identifies phonemes. Areas 21 and 37 identify words in the sound sequence and tap into lexicons (dictionaries) stored in memory in a search for meaning – a process called *semantic retrieval*.

Activity in the left dorsolateral prefrontal cortex (DLPFC) expands to include area 46. Engagement of Broca's area is thought to signify 'subvocal articulation' of words heard (see Neuroanatomy of reading, later).

When listening to one's own voice, the areas of the temporal lobe identified above become active. An important function being served here is *meta-analysis* (*post hoc* analysis) of speech, whereby 'slips of the tongue' can be identified. Speech meta-analysis is singularly lacking in cases of receptive aphasia (Clinical Panel 32.1).

Modular organization of language

In alert subjects, electrical studies of the cortex exposed during neurosurgical procedures indicate the presence of a

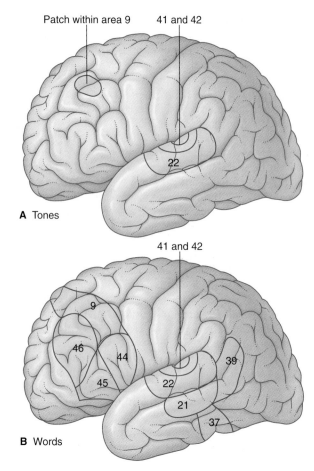

Figure 32.3 Regions of increased blood flow during listening **(A)** to tones, and **(B)** to words.

vast cortical mosaic for language. The mosaic of modules extends along the entire length of the frontoparietal operculum above the lateral sulcus and of the temporal operculum below the sulcus. The frontoparietal operculum is predominantly concerned with the motor functions of speaking and writing, and the temporal operculum with the sensory functions of hearing and reading.

It is well known that children have greater facility than adults in acquiring a second language. fMRI and other approaches have shown that the loci of second-language acquisition before the age of 7 years overlap extensively with those processing the native language. A second language learned in later years is non-overlapping with the first. One possibility is that in children, the syntactical systems for processing nouns, verbs, etc., are able to cope with two or more languages simultaneously.

It is of interest that following a small vascular lesion in an adult, *either* a late-acquired language *or* the native language may be lost, leaving the other relatively intact.

COGNITIVE STYLE

Hemispheric specializations in relation to information processing have been revealed by various forms of visual, auditory, and tactile tests. Results show that the left hemisphere is superior in processing information that is susceptible to *sequential analysis* of its parts, whereas the right is superior in respect of *shapes* and of *spatial relationships*. Accordingly, the left hemisphere is described as being *analytical* and the right as *holistic*. The right is also 'musical': there is a relative increase in blood flow in the right auditory association area when listening to music, versus a left-sided increase for words.

The analytical character of the left hemisphere may be owed to its unique capacity to perform the 'inner speech' that usually accompanies problem-solving.

Neuroanatomy of reading (Figure 32.4)

Glossary

- **Graphemes**. Written syllables.
- **Orthography** (*Gr.* 'correct writing'). Word and sentence construction.
- **Phonemes** (*Gr.* 'sounds'). The sounds of syllables. 'Cat' is a single syllable containing three phonemes, [k], [a], and [t].
- **Phonology**. The rules governing the sounds of words. Testing could include: 'How many of these words have two syllables?' or 'How many of these words rhyme with one another?'
- **Retrieval**. Matching words, phrases, and sentences with those previously entered into memory.
- **Semantics** (*Gr.* 'meaning'). Meaning of words and sentences.

Reading sequence

A *Carry out visual processing*
B *Perform orthographic processing*
C *Perform phonological assembly*
D *Perform semantic retrieval*
E *Execute motor plans*

   A *Visual processing* is performed bilaterally in areas 17, 18, and 19. It includes: analysis of letter shapes for their identification; distinguishing between letters in upper vs lower case, and between real letters and meaningless shapes ('false fonts'). Processed information in the right extrastriate cortex (areas 18 and 19) is transferred to the left side through the forceps major traversing the splenium of the corpus callosum – a point of clinical significance (see later).

   B *Orthographic processing* means discerning whether or not each letter string in a sentence represents a real or a pseudoword, e.g. 'word' vs 'wurd'. Medial area 19 (V4) is especially involved.

   C *Phonological processing* means the conversion of graphemes to phonemes. The angular gyrus (area 39) and middle temporal gyrus (area 21) participate.

   D *Semantic retrieval* means performance of a memory search, using both orthographical and phonological cues from the text to extract the meaning of words and sentences. The anterior part of Broca's area (area 45) becomes active at this advanced stage, together with area 37 in the posterior temporal lobe and area 40 (supramarginal gyrus) in the inferior parietal lobule.

   E *Execution of motor plans (phonological execution)* is the performance of 'inner speech' ('subvocal articulation'). Both parts of Broca's area become active, as do the adjacent parts of premotor and motor cortex,

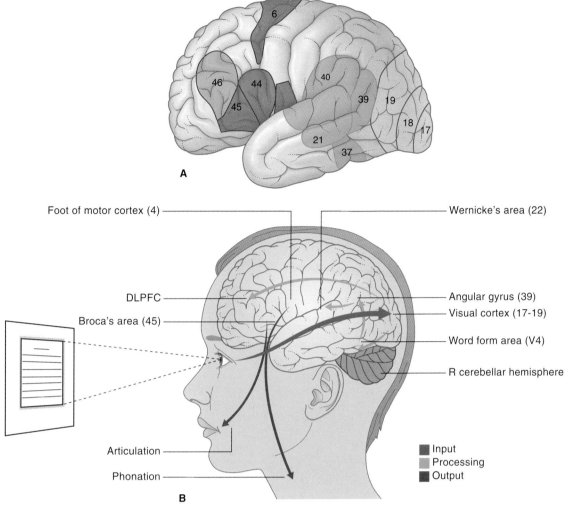

Figure 32.4 (A) Areas of increased cortical blood flow in the left hemisphere observed in PET scans during reading aloud. **(B)** Diagram representing input (*blue*), processing (*green*), and output (*red*) pathways active during reading aloud. DLPFC, dorsolateral prefrontal cortex.

the supplementary motor area (medial area 6), and the contralateral cerebellar hemisphere. The same four areas become much more active during reading aloud.

The left lateral prefrontal cortex, in and around area 46, is 'switched on' throughout A–E. Also active is part of area 32 in the left anterior cingulate cortex, which is involved in all cognitive activities requiring attention.

Developmental dyslexia is considered in Clinical Panel 32.2.

Schizophrenia, a psychiatric disorder involving the left hemisphere more than the right, is described in Chapter 34.

PARIETAL LOBE (Figure 32.5)

The parietal lobe – especially the *right* one – is of prime importance for appreciation of spatial relationships. There is also evidence that the parietal lobe – especially the *left* one – is concerned with initiation of movement.

Superior parietal lobule and the body schema

The term *body schema* refers to an awareness of the existence and spatial relationships of body parts, based on previous (stored) and current sensory experience. The reality of body schema has been established by the condition known as *hemineglect*, in which a patient with a lesion involving the superior parietal lobule ignores the contralateral side of the body.

Hemineglect is much more common following a right parietal lobe lesion than a left one. Under normal conditions, however, each parietal lobe exchanges information freely with its partner through the corpus callosum and the left and right hand are equally adept at distinguishing a key from a coin in a coat pocket without the aid of vision (*stereognosis*, Ch. 29).

Patients with a right hemisphere lesion involving the superior parietal lobule have difficulty in distinguishing between unseen objects of different shapes with the left hand. They have *astereognosis*. Patients with a comparable lesion

Clinical Panel 32.2 Developmental dyslexia

It is generally agreed that reading is a more skilled activity than speech, because it requires an exquisite level of integration of visual scanning and auditory (inner speech) comprehension. Reading is thought to activate two pathways in parallel: one passes via the angular gyrus to Wernicke's area and accesses a phonological representation of every syllable in a temporal lobe memory store; the other passes to the left dorsolateral prefrontal cortex and accesses a semantic (meaning) memory store for every word.

Developmental dyslexia is a specific and pronounced reading difficulty in children who are the match of their peers in other respects. The anomaly is widespread, affecting 10–15% of children and about half that number of adults. There is a 30% incidence in siblings of affected children and a similar incidence in one or other parent. There is a slightly higher incidence in boys, and in left-handed children of either gender.

A consistent finding in PET and fMRI studies during reading is diminished activity (compared to peers) in the left temporoparietal region (areas 22, 39 and 40).

Two commonly used classroom tests are: *rhyming*, e.g., in the alphabet, to identify the eight letters that rhyme with the letter B; and to pronounce *non-words (pseudowords)* within a word string, e.g. 'door', '*melse*', '*farm*', '*duve*', miss'. Both tests are used to detect *phonological impairment*, characterized by slow and inaccurate processing of the sound structure of language. The diagnostic label *phonological dyslexia* is usually used although other language-processing difficulties may also be present.

The performance of dyslexic children can often be improved by special training. Nevertheless, severe dyslexia tends to be associated with developmental deficiencies in one or more relevant parts of the brain, implicating as many as four different chromosomes.

- MRI scans tend to show a smaller than average left temporal plane. The cortex of the temporal plane (in dyslexic children dying from unrelated causes) may reveal evidence of incomplete migration of neurons from the ventricular zone to the temporal cortex during fetal life, with abnormally few neurons in laminae I–III, an excess in laminae IV–VI, and occasional clusters stranded in the subjacent white matter.
- The magnocells (M cells) of the ganglionic layer of the retina and lateral geniculate body are often smaller than normal, and their smaller axons conduct more slowly. One consequence is that the scanning movements used in reading, controlled by M cell inputs to the superior colliculus (Ch. 28), are so inefficient that written syllables tend to run together and individual letters may appear to be transposed.

- Magnocellular neurons of the medial geniculate body, projecting to the primary auditory cortex (Ch. 20), may also be smaller. The presumed effect is one of reduced detection of the frequency and amplitude of sounds, leading to below-normal perception of words that are read aloud.
- The right cerebellum tends to be smaller than average, and during PET scans to be less active during peformance of simple rapid motor tasks. Given that the cerebellovestibular system is responsible for keeping the eyes trained on visual targets, a cerebellar deficit could account for wobbly eye movements seen in about 1 in 10 dyslexics during reading. These children often try to stabilize their gaze by running an index finger below the line they are reading.
- Some dyslexic children are rather clumsy in executing fine movements such as buttoning a coat or tying a shoelace. The action tremor (intention tremor) characteristic of cerebellar disease is absent, and the label *dyspraxia* is used instead, to signify difficulty in controlling the rate and accuracy of fine learned movements in the absence of detectable loss of neuromuscular function. Here the fault appears to be at the interface between the processing and output pathways.
- A surprising finding is that the *insula* is inactive on certain language tasks on PET scans in dyslexics compared to controls. It has been postulated that the insula may be a station linking the supramarginal and angular gyri to Broca's area, and that a defect in this linkage may be significant in relation to the 'inner speech' that normally takes place during leisurely reading.

Commonly used classroom tests/indications on 5–7 year olds include:

Speech:
Slow, laborious reading with little or no expressive intonation
Vowel sounds, e.g. In the alphabet, to identify the eight letters that rhyme with the letter B.
Phoneme sounds, i.e. the sounds of normal word syllables; also ability to pronounce *non-words (pseudowords)* within a word string, e.g. 'door', '*melse*', 'farm', '*duve*', miss.
Syllable sequencing, e.g. a dyslexic child may say 'emeny' for 'enemy'

Writing:
Dyslexia tends to be accompanied by slow and poor-quality handwriting and spelling, e.g. letter transposition ('pelcin' for 'pencil'), reversal ('pad' for 'bad'), or inversion ('wad' for 'mad').

Clinical Panel 32.2 *Continued*

The assistance of Rena Lyons, Department of Speech and Language Therapy, NUI, Galway is gratefully acknowledged.

REFERENCES

Habib M: The neurological basis of developmental dyslexia, *Brain* 123:2373–2399, 2000.

Leonard CM, Eckert MA, et al: Anatomical risk factors for phonological dyslexia, *Cereb Cortex* 11:148–157, 2001.

Rumsey JM, Donohue BC, Brady DR, et al: An MRI study of planum temporale asymmetry in males with developmental dyslexia, *Arch Neurol* 54:1481–1489, 1997.

Temple E: Brain mechanisms in normal and dyslexic readers, *Curr Opin Neurobiol* 12:178–183, 2002.

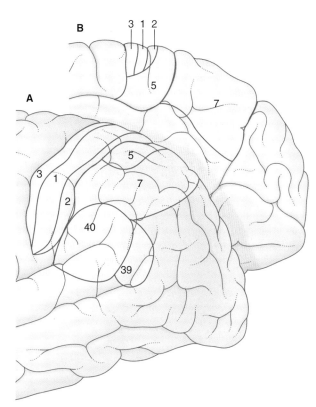

Figure 32.5 Brodmann's areas in the parietal lobe. **(A)** Lateral view; **(B)** medial view. 3/1/2, somesthetic cortex; 5, somesthetic association area; 7, posterior parietal cortex; 39, angular gyrus; 40, supramarginal gyrus.

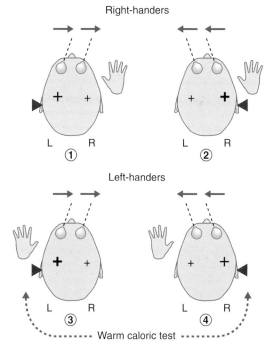

Figure 32.6 Diagrams illustrating hemispheric dominance in response to warm water irrigation of the outer ear canals of pronounced right-handers and left-handers. (The head was tilted back 20° to put the lateral semicircular canals in the horizontal position.) Arrows indicate the slow phase of caloric nystagmus. Note pronounced minor hemisphere response to ipsilateral caloric irrigation (2 and 3), and less marked major hemisphere response (1 and 4). (Based on diagrams in Dieterich et al., 2003.)

in the left hemisphere are able to make this distinction using the right hand but they have difficulty in announcing the *function* of a selected object. The left supramarginal gyrus participates in phonological retrieval, as already noted, and the deficit, although a semantic one, may be related to interference with the 'inner speech' that usually accompanies problem-solving.

Both deficits are forms of *tactile agnosia*. The right hemisphere deficit has become known as *apperceptive* tactile agnosia ('apperception', awareness of perception), and the left one as *associative* tactile agnosia (failure to identify functional associations).

Handedness and balance

In Chapter 18 we noted that the pathway from the vestibular nucleus to the parieto-insular vestibular cortex (PIVC) is mainly ipsilateral. Formal testing of static and dynamic vestibular functions, under fMRI monitoring, has revealed that maximal activation of the PIVC is produced in the *minor* hemisphere, as illustrated in Figure 32.6. The limited data available indicate a tight linkage between handedness and vestibular cortical activation, to the extent that the 'preferred' vestibular hemisphere, in view of its phylogenetic antiquity and early ontogenesis (e.g. presence of postural vestibular reflexes in the newborn), may *determine* handedness.

Parietal lobe and movement initiation

There are several sites for movement initiation in different behavioral contexts. The present context is the performance of learned movements of some complexity: examples would include turning a door knob, combing one's hair, blowing out a match, and clapping. It is logical to anticipate a starting point within the dominant hemisphere because they can all be performed in response to a verbal command (oral or written). This notion receives support from the observation that, if the corpus callosum has been severed surgically, the patient can perform a learned movement on command using the right hand, but not on attempting it with the left hand.

Failure to perform a learned movement on request is called *ideomotor apraxia*, or *limb apraxia*. It has been repeatedly observed immediately following vascular lesions at the sites listed and described in Figure 32.7. In that figure, a vascular stroke at site 2 injuring corticospinal fibers descending from the hand area of the motor cortex, would cause clumsiness of movement of both hands, whereas a similar lesion on the right side would only compromise movements of the left hand.

Ideomotor apraxia can be accounted for if the dominant parietal lobe is considered to contain a repertoire of learned movement programs which, on retrieval, elicit appropriate responses by the premotor cortex on one or both sides under directives from the prefrontal cortex. (The basal ganglia would also be involved, as described in Ch. 33.)

Ideomotor apraxia is a transient phenomenon. Because parietal blood flow increases almost equally on both sides during reaching movements, the right hemisphere seems to be able to assume a full role for the left arm when no longer overshadowed.

Clinical Panel 32.3 provides a brief account of parietal lobe dysfunction.

PREFRONTAL CORTEX

The prefrontal cortex has two-way connections with all parts of the neocortex except the primary motor and sensory areas; with its fellow through the genu of the corpus callosum; and with the mediodorsal nucleus of the thalamus. It is uniquely large in the human brain and is concerned with the highest brain functions, including abstract thinking, decision-making, anticipating the effects of particular courses of action, and social behavior.

The DLPFC, centered in and around area 9, is strongly active in both hemispheres during waking hours. It has been called the *supervisory attentional system*. It participates in all cognitive activities and is essential for conscious learning of all kinds. During conscious learning, it operates *working memory*, whereby memories appropriate to the task (work) in hand are retrieved and 'held in the mind'.

Figure 32.7 Association and commissural pathways serving motor responses to sensory cues. (Adapted from Kertesz and Ferro, 1984.) The premotor cortex is under higher control by the prefrontal cortex.

Lesions at site 1 effectively sever the anterior part of the corpus callosum and produce ipsilateral limb apraxia (left lesion, left limb). Lesions at either site 2 (superior longitudinal fasciculus) or site 3 (angular gyrus) may produce *bilateral* limb apraxia. In practice, a large lesion may render right-limb apraxia impossible to assess because of associated right hemiplegia or receptive aphasia.

The medial prefrontal cortex has auditory and verbal associations. The orbitofrontal cortex has been described as the *neocortical representative of the limbic system*, being richly connected to the amygdala, septal area, and the cortex of the temporal pole – three limbic structures described in Chapter 34.

In general terms, the left prefrontal cortex has an 'approach' bias, being engaged in all language-related activities, including the 'inner speech' that accompanies investigative activities. The right prefrontal cortex has a 'withdraw' bias, being particularly activated by fearful contexts, whether real or imagined.

Aspects of frontal lobe dysfunction are described in Clinical Panel 32.4.

Clinical Panel 32.3   Parietal lobe dysfunction

Anterior parietal cortex

Lesions of the somatic sensory cortex and somesthetic association area tend to occur together, causing cortical-type sensory loss and inaccurate reaching movements into contralateral visual hemispace (e.g. at mealtimes, the patient may tend to knock things over).

Supramarginal gyrus

Lesions affecting the supramarginal gyrus (area 40) are usually vascular (middle cerebral artery) and are usually concomitant with contralateral hemiplegia with or without hemianopia. However, the blood supply to the gyrus is sometimes selectively occluded, giving rise to a state known as *personal hemineglect*. The patient ignores the opposite side of the body unless attention is specifically drawn to it. A male patient will shave only the ipsilateral side of the face; a female patient will comb her hair only on the ipsilateral side. The patient will acknowledge a tactile stimulus to the contralateral side when tested alone; simultaneous testing of both sides will only be acknowledged ipsilaterally (*sensory extinction*).

Angular gyrus

Lesions of the anteroventral part of the angular gyrus (area 39, Figure 32.3.1) are notably associated with *spatial (extrapersonal) hemineglect*. The patient tends to ignore the contralateral visual hemispace, even if the visual pathways remain intact, and there is *visual extinction* (contralaterally) to simultaneous bilateral stimuli, e.g. when the clinician wiggles index fingers in both visual fields simultaneously.

Hemineglect is at least five times more frequent following lesions on the *right* side, irrespective of handedness.

An isolated vascular lesion of the posterior part of the left angular gyrus (very rare) produces *alexia*

Figure CP 32.3.1 Angular gyrus.

(complete inability to read) and *agraphia* (inability to write); letters on the page are suddenly without any meaning. If the temporal plane has survived, patients can still name words spelt aloud to them.

For *ideomotor apraxia*, see main text.

REFERENCES

Chokron S, Colliot P, Bartolomeo P, et al: Visual, proprioceptive and tactile performance in left neglect patients, *Neuropsychologia* 40:1965–1976, 2002.

Golay L, Schneider A, Ptak R: Cortical and subcortical anatomy of chronic spatial neglect following vascular damage, *Behav Brain Funct* 4:43–53, 2008.

Hanna-Pladdy B, Heilman KM, Foundas AL: Cortical and subcortical contributions to ideomotor apraxia, *Brain* 124:2513–2527, 2001.

Mort DJ, Malhotra P, Mannan SK, et al: The anatomy of visual neglect, *Brain* 126:1986–1987, 2003.

Clinical Panel 32.4 Frontal lobe dysfunction

Symptoms of *early* frontal lobe disease typically involve subtle changes in personality and social function rather than diminution of cognitive performance on objective tests. Lack of foresight (failure to anticipate the consequences of a course of action), distractibility (poor concentration), loss of willpower (*abulia*), and difficulty in 'switching cognitive sets' (e.g. inability to switch easily from one subject of conversation to another) are characteristic. These general symptoms are more often associated with bilateral disease with impending dementia than with a brain tumor. With increasing disease, especially if bilateral, the *gait* is affected. '*Marche à petit pas*' ('Walk with small steps') refers to a characteristic short, shuffling gait often associated with disequilibrium (tendency to fall), and 'freezing' (especially when turning). This syndrome may give rise to a mistaken suspicion of Parkinson's disease.

Large *dorsolateral lesions* are associated with slowing of mental processes of all kinds, leading to hypokinesia, apathy, and indifference to surrounding events. The picture resembles that of the 'withdrawn' type of schizophrenia, and it is of interest, that in 'withdrawn' schizophrenic patients, cortical blood flow may not show the anticipated increase in the dorsolateral region, in response to appropriate psychological tests.

Large *orbitofrontal* lesions are associated with hyperkinesia, and with increased instinctual drives in relation to food and sexual behavior. With disease more pronounced (or only) in the right orbitofrontal cortex, the 'fearful' side of the patient's nature may be lost, leading to puerile jocularity and compulsive laughter. Compulsive crying may be a clue to left-sided disease. A well-known cause of orbitofrontal disturbance is a meningioma arising in the groove occupied by the olfactory nerve; *anosmia* (loss of the sense of smell) may be discovered on testing, and optic atrophy may follow pressure on the optic nerve where it emerges from the optic canal. Hyperkinetic frontal lobe disorders have been treated in the past by means of *lobotomy* – a surgical procedure in which the white matter above the orbital cortex was severed through a temporal incision.

Gliomas within the frontal lobe may become large before any cognitive or physical defects appear. Eventually, a left-sided tumor may invade or compress Broca's area and cause motor aphasia. On either side, a progressive hemiparesis may supervene.

REFERENCES

Wheaton LA, Bohlhalter S, Nolte G, et al: Cortico-cortical networks in patients with ideomotor apraxia, *Neurosci Lett* 433:87–92, 2008.

Golay L, Schnider A, Ptak R: Cortical and subcortical anatomy of chronic spatial neglect following vascular damage, *Behav Brain Funct* 4:43–53, 2008.

Core Information

Hemispheric asymmetries mainly concern handedness, language, and cognitive style. Some 10% of people are left-handers. Language areas are left-sided in 90%, right-sided in 2.5%, and bilateral in 2.5%. Broca's motor speech area occupies the inferior frontal gyrus; lesions here give rise to motor aphasia with difficulty in writing. Wernicke's sensory speech area in the temporal plane is required for understanding the spoken word; lesions here result in receptive aphasia plus difficulty in reading if the angular gyrus is involved. The left hemisphere is usually superior in processing information susceptible to sequential analysis; the right hemisphere is superior for analysis of shapes and spatial relationships. The inferior parietal lobule is concerned with the body schema; lesions here may result in neglect of personal and (sometimes) extrapersonal space on the opposite side. Finally, the left parietal lobe may initiate complex motor programs; lesions here may be associated with ideomotor apraxia.

The prefrontal cortex is involved in the highest brain functions. The dorsolateral prefrontal cortex (DLPFC) contains a supervisory attentional system especially involved in conscious learning, where it operates working memory appropriate to the task at hand. The orbitofrontal cortex is a neocortical representative of the limbic system. The left prefrontal cortex has investigative, 'approach' characteristics, the right has 'withdraw' characteristics. General signs of frontal lobe disease include lack of foresight, distractibility, and difficulty in switching cognitive sets. The gait may take the form of short shuffling steps with instability and 'freezing'. DLPFC lesions lead to slowing of mental process, apathy, and indifference. Orbitofrontal lesions tend to produce a hyperkinetic state with increased instinctual drives and puerile behavior.

REFERENCES

Behrmann M, Geng JJ, Shomstein S: Parietal cortex and attention, *Curr Opin Neurobiol* 14:212–217, 2004.

Buchsbaum BR, Olsen RK, Koch PF, et al: Reading, hearing, and the planum temporale, *NeuroImage* 24:444–454, 2005.

Dieterich M, Bense S, Lutz S, et al: Dominance for vestibular cortical function in the non-dominant hemisphere, *Cereb Cortex* 13:994–1007, 2003.

Di Russo F, Aprile T, Spitoni G, Spinelli D: Impaired visual processing of contralesional stimuli in neglect patients: a visual-evoked potential study, *Brain* 131:842–854, 2008.

Farne A, Roy AC, Paulignan Y, et al: Visuo-motor control of the ipsilateral hand: evidence from right brain-damaged patients, *Neuropsychologia* 41:739–757, 2003.

Gross RG, Grossman M: Update on apraxia, *Curr Neurol Neurosci Rep* 8:490–496, 2008.

Kertesz A, Ferro JM: Lesion size and location in ideomotor apraxia, *Brain* 107:921–933, 1984.

Liotti M, Gay CT, Fox PT: Functional imaging and language, *J Clin Neurophysiol* 11:175–190, 1994.

Price CJ: The anatomy of language: contributions from functional imaging, *J Anat* 197:335–339, 2000.

Reed CL, Caselli RJ, Farah MJ: Tactile agnosia, *Brain* 119:875–888, 1996.

Thompson-Schill SL, Bedny M, Goldberg RF: The frontal lobes and the regulation of mental activity, *Curr Opin Neurobiol* 15:219–224, 2005.

STUDY GUIDELINES

The contribution of the basel ganglia to motor control systems is the subject of intensive research at basic and clinical levels.

In this account, the open-loop pathways linking different areas of the cerebral cortex through the basal ganglia are highlighted. Particular emphasis is put on the breaking and release mechanisms inherent in the arrangement of sequential sets of inhibitory neurons.

Pathological changes within the basal ganglia are associated with several kinds of motor disorders both in children and adults.

INTRODUCTION

The term *basal ganglia* is used to designate the areas of basal forebrain and midbrain known to be involved in the control of movement (Figure 33.1). It includes:

- The **striatum** (caudate nucleus, putamen – a part of the lentiform – and nucleus accumbens).
- The **pallidum** (globus pallidus – a part of the lentiform), which is comprised of a **lateral segment** and a **medial segment**. The medial segment has a midbrain extension known as the **reticular part (pars reticulata)** of the **substantia nigra**.
- The **subthalamic nucleus**.
- The pigmented, **compact part (pars compacta)** of **substantia nigra**.

BASIC CIRCUITS

It is possible to demonstrate at least four circuits which commence in the cerebral cortex, traverse the basal ganglia, and return to the cortex. The four comprise:

1 A *motor loop*, concerned with learned movements;
2 A *cognitive loop*, concerned with motor intentions;
3 A *limbic loop*, concerned with emotional aspects of movement;
4 An *oculomotor loop*, concerned with voluntary saccades.

Motor loop

The motor loop commences in the sensorimotor cortex and returns there via the striatum, thalamus, and SMA (supplementary motor area).

Figure 33.2 is derived from Figure 33.1A. It is a schematic coronal section including the posterior part of the striatum, depicting component parts of the motor loop. Two pathways are known. The 'direct' pathway traverses the corpus striatum and thalamus and involves five consecutive sets of neurons (Figure 33.2A). The 'indirect' pathway engages the subthalamic nucleus in addition and involves seven sets of neurons (Figure 33.2B). Separate from these pathways are two thalamic projections from the medial pallidum (**ansa lenticularis** and **lenticular fasciculus**) shown in Figure 33.3.

All projections from the cerebral cortex arise from pyramidal cells and are excitatory (glutaminergic). So, too, is the projection from thalamus to SMA. Those from striatum and from both segments of pallidum arise from medium-sized spiny neurons and are inhibitory. They are GABAergic, and also contain neuropeptides of uncertain function.

The *nigrostrial pathway* projects from the compact part of the substantia nigra to the striatum, where it makes two kinds of synapses upon the projection neurons there (Figure 33.4). Those upon 'direct' pathway neurons are facilitatory, by way of dopaminergic type 1 (D_1) receptors on the dendritic spines; those upon 'indirect' pathway neurons are inhibitory, by way of type 2 (D_2) receptors. Cholinergic internuncial neurons within the striatum are excitatory to projection neurons, and they are inhibited by dopamine.

A healthy substantia nigra is tonically active, favoring activity in the 'direct' pathway. Facilitation of this pathway is necessary for the SMA to become active before and during movement. SMA activity immediately prior to movement can be detected by means of recording electrodes attached to the scalp. This activity is known as the (electrical) *readiness potential*, and its manner of production is described in the caption to Figure 33.4. Impulses pass from SMA to the motor cortex, where a cerebello-thalamocortical projection selectively enhances pyramidal and corticoreticular neurons within milliseconds prior to discharge.

The putamen and globus pallidus are somatotopically organized, permitting selective facilitation of neurons relevant to (say) arm movements via the direct route, with simultaneous disfacilitation of unwanted (say) leg movements via the indirect route. For suppression of unwanted movements, the subthalamic nucleus (STN), acting upon the body map in the medial pallidal segment, is especially important, since we

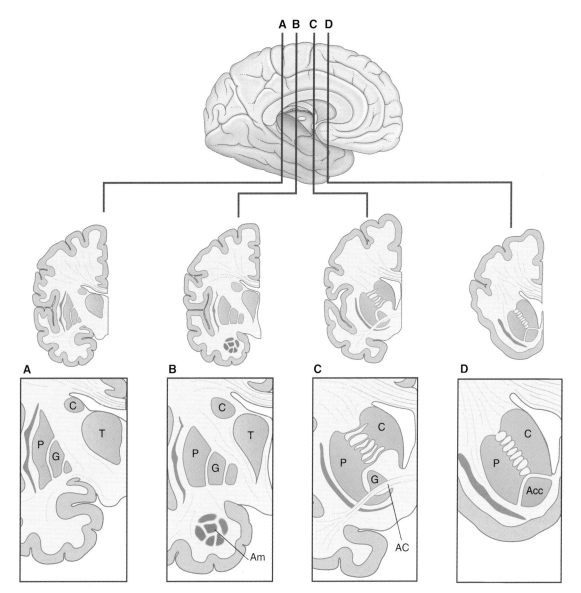

Figure 33.1 (A–D) Four coronal sections of the brain, viewed from behind. Ventral parts are enlarged below. Acc., nucleus accumbens; AC, anterior commissure; Am., amygdala; C, caudate nucleus; G, globus pallidus; P, putamen; T, thalamus.

know that destruction of STN results in uncontrollable flailing movements of one or more body parts on the opposite side (see later).

Progressive failure of dopamine production by the compact part of substantia nigra is the precipitating cause of *Parkinson's disease* (PD) (Clinical Panel 33.1).

What are the normal functions of the motor loop?

Although movements can be produced on the opposite side of the body by direct electrical stimulation of the healthy putamen, the basal ganglia do not normally initiate movements. Nevertheless, they are active during movements of all kinds, whether fast or slow. They seem to be involved in *scaling the strength* of muscle contractions and, in collaboration with SMA, in *organizing the requisite sequences* of

excitation of cell columns in the motor cortex. They come into action after the corticospinal tract has already been activated by 'premotor' areas including the cerebellum. Because patients with PD have so much difficulty in performing internally generated movement sequences, it is believed that the putamen provides a reservoir of learned motor programs which it is able to assemble in appropriate sequence for the movements decided upon, and to transmit the coded information to SMA.

Cognitive loop

The head of the caudate nucleus receives a large projection from the prefrontal cortex, and it participates in *motor learning*. PET scan studies have demonstrated increased contralateral blood flow through the head of the caudate when novel motor actions are performed with one hand. There is

Figure 33.2 Coronal section through the motor loop, based on Figure 33.1A. **(A)** The sequence of five sets of neurons involved in the 'direct' pathway from sensorimotor cortex to thalamus with final return to sensorimotor cortex via SMA. **(B)** The sequence of seven sets of neurons involved in the 'indirect' pathway.

The *red/pink* neurons are excitatory utilizing glutamate. The *black/gray* neurons are inhibitory utilizing γ-aminobutyric acid. The *brown*, nigrostriatal neuron utilizes dopamine which is excitatory via D_1 receptors on target striatal neurons and inhibitory via D_2 receptors on the same and other striatal neurons. CST/CRST, corticospinal, corticoreticular fibers; GPL, GPM, lateral and medial segments of globus pallidus; SMA, supplementary motor area; SNpc, compact part of substantia nigra; STN, subthalamic nucleus; VLN, ventral lateral nucleus of thalamus.

also increased activity in the anterior part of the contralateral putamen, globus pallidus and ventral anterior (VA) nucleus of the thalamus. The VA nucleus completes an 'open' cognitive loop through its projection to the premotor cortex, and a 'closed' loop through a return projection to the prefrontal cortex. The cortical connections of the caudate suggest that it participates in *planning ahead*, particularly with respect to complex motor intentions. When the novel motor task has been practiced to the level of automatic execution, the motor loop becomes active instead.

Limbic loop

Figure 33.5 depicts the *limbic* basal ganglia loop. This loop passes from inferior prefrontal cortex through **nucleus accumbens** (anterior end of the striatum, Figure 33.1D) and ventral pallidum, with return via the mediodorsal nucleus of thalamus to the inferior prefrontal cortex. (The nucleus accumbens, along with the nearby *olfactory tubercle* (not shown) are known as the *ventral striatum*.)

The limbic loop is likely to be involved in giving motor expression to emotions, e.g. through smiling or gesturing, or

adoption of aggressive or submissive postures. The loop is rich in dopaminergic nerve endings, and their decline may account for the mask-like facies and absence of spontaneous gesturing characteristic of Parkinson's disease, and for the *dementia* which may set in after several years.

Oculomotor loop

The oculomotor loop commences in the *frontal eye field* and *posterior parietal cortex* (area 7). It passes through the caudate nucleus and through the reticular part of the substantia nigra (SNpr). It returns via the ventral anterior nucleus of the thalamus to the frontal eye field and prefrontal cortex. SNpr sends an inhibitory GABAergic projection to the superior colliculus, where it synapses upon cells controlling automatic saccades (Ch. 23). These cells are also supplied directly from the frontal eye field.

While the eyes are fixated, SNpr is tonically active. Whenever a deliberate saccade is about to be made toward another object, the oculomotor loop is activated and the superior colliculus is *disinhibited*. The superior colliculus then discharges to reinforce the activity of the direct pathway.

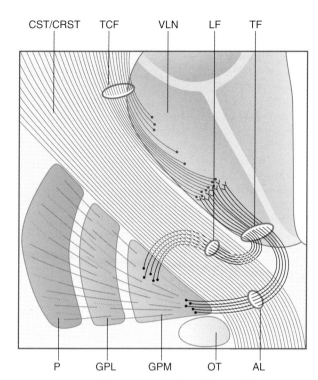

Figure 33.3 Part of the projection from the medial segment of globus pallidus (GPM) to the ventral lateral nucleus (VLN) of the thalamus sweeps around the base of the internal capsule as the **ansa lenticularis** (AL); the remainder traverses this region as the **lenticular fasciculus** (LF). The two parts come together as the **thalamic fasciculus** (TF) before entering the thalamus. CST/CRST, corticospinal and corticoreticular fibers; GPL, lateral segment of globus pallidus; OT, optic tract; P, putamen; TCF, thalamocortical fibers.

Figure 33.5 The limbic basal ganglia loop, right hemisphere. The medial dorsal nucleus of thalamus (MDN) is being released by means of disinhibition.

Figure 33.4 Activities in the striatal motor loops, prior to movement.

The SMA (supplementary motor area) is activated through the 'direct' pathway as follows. (1) Corticostriate fibers from the sensorimotor cortex activate those GABAergic spiny neurons in striatum having D_1 receptors tonically facilitated by nigrostriatal inputs. (2) The activated striatal neurons inhibit medial pallidal (GPM) neurons (3) with consequent *disinhibition* of ventral lateral nucleus (VLN) thalamocortical neurons (4) and activation of SMA (5), which both modifies ongoing corticostriate activity and initiates impulse trains along corticospinal (CST) and corticoreticular (CRST) fibers.

Activity along the 'indirect' pathway is relatively slight because of tonic dopaminergic inhibition of the relevant striatal neurons via D_2 receptors. However, the subthalamic nucleus (STN) is tonically activated by corticosubthalamic fibers, curtailing the inhibition of GPM. GPL, lateral segment of globus pallidus; SNpc, compact part of substantia nigra. (Cerebello-thalamocortical projection is not shown.)

Maximum speed (80 km/h) is achieved instantly, the eyeballs are flicked to the target, and SNpr resumes its vigilance.

In PD, *oculomotor hypokinesia* can be revealed by special tests. Saccades toward targets in the peripheral visual field tend to be slow, and sometimes inadequate. This hypokinesia can be explained on the basis of faulty disinhibition of the superior colliculus following associated neuronal degeneration within SNpr.

Other disorders involving the basic ganglia include several *hyperkinetic states* briefly described in Clinical Panel 33.2.

Clinical Panel 33.1 Hypokinesia: Parkinson's disease

Parkinson's disease (PD) affects about 1% of people over 65 years of age in all countries. The primary underlying pathology is degeneration of nigrostriatal neurons, resulting in diminished dopamine content within the striatum. *[¹⁸F]fluorodopa* is a mildly radioactive compound which, when injected intravenously, binds with dopamine receptors in the striatum. In symptomatic PD, a significant reduction of [¹⁸F]fluorodopa binding (and therefore of receptors) is revealed by means of PET scanning (Figure CP 33.1.1). One consequence is *increased* striatal activity, with a shift from the direct to the indirect motor pathway (Figure CP 33.1.2).

Nigrostriatal degeneration seems to take the form of a *dying back neuropathy*, because dopamine is lost from the striatum earlier than in the midbrain. The spiny striatal neurons also deteriorate, with reduction in the length of dendrites and the numbers of spines. It may be that the spiny neurons depend upon dopaminergic inputs for protection against potentially toxic effects of ongoing glutamate activity.

Some 60% of nigral neurons have been lost before the first symptoms appear. This delay is accounted for by (a) increased dopamine production by surviving neurons, and (b) increased production ('upregulation') of dopamine receptors in the target striatal neurons.

The following symptoms/signs are characteristic: tremor, bradykinesia, rigidity, and impairment of postural reflexes. Not all are expressed in every patient.

Tremor

Tremor, at 3–6 Hz (*hertz*, times per second) in one limb is the initial feature in two-thirds of patients with PD. The commonest sequence of limb involvement is from one upper limb to the ipsilateral lower limb within 1 year, followed by contralateral limb involvement within 3 years. Rhythmic tremor of lips and tongue, pronation–supination of the forearm, and flexion–extension of the fingers may be obvious. A 'pill-rolling' movement of the index and middle fingers against the thumb pad is characteristic. Typically, the tremor only involves muscle groups that are 'at rest' and vanishes during voluntary movement. A patient with an exclusively resting tremor has no difficulty in raising and draining a tumblerful of water. The term *resting tremors* is used to distinguish it from the *intention tremor* of cerebellar disease. Intention tremor is absent at rest (unless cerebellar dysfunction is severe) and is brought on by voluntary movement.

Tremor is associated with rhythmic bursting activity within all five cell groups of the direct motor loop (Figure 28.2A) and in anterior horn cells of the spinal cord. The contribution of disordered autogenic inhibition to both resting tremor and rigidity is described below.

A fine *action tremor* is often detectable in patients having pronounced resting tremor, and it is more pronounced on the side more affected by resting tremor. The action tremor is best seen in the fingers when the arms are fully outstretched, and it may be manifested by tremulous handwriting. Note particularly

Head of caudate nucleus   Putamen

A   B   Thalamus   Lateral ventricle

Figure CP 33.1.1 Diagram showing typical results of brain scans following intravenous injection of [¹⁸F]fluorodopa. Intensity of uptake is indicated as *red* (greatest), *yellow*, *green*, *blue* (least). **(A)** Control; **(B)** Parkinson's disease.

(Continued)

Clinical Panel 33.1 *Continued*

Left motor cortex

Corticostriate neuron

Precentral sulcus

SMA

⑦ (weak)

D₁ receptors (inactive)

① ⑥ (weak)

D₂ receptors (active)

VLN (inhibited)

⑤

STN (disinhibited)

④

②

Striatum

GPL (inhibited)

③

GPM

SNpc (degenerating)

CST/CRST (weak activity)

Figure CP 33.1.2 Consequences of degeneration of the pathway from the compact part of the substantia nigra (SNpc) to the striatum (S) in Parkinson's disease. The effects arise from loss of tonic facilitation of spiny striatal neurons bearing D₁ receptors, together with loss of tonic inhibition of those bearing D₂ receptors. The 'direct' pathway is disengaged, and the 'indirect' pathway is activated by default. (1) Corticostriate neurons from the sensorimotor cortex now strongly activate those GABAergic neurons (2) in the striatum that synapse upon others (3) in the lateral pallidal segment (GPL). The double effect is *disinhibition* of the subthalamic nucleus (STN). STN discharges strongly (4) onto the GABAergic neurons of the medial pallidal segment (GPM); these in turn discharge strongly (5) into the ventral lateral nucleus (VLN) of thalamus, resulting in reduced output along thalamocortical fibers (6) traveling to the supplementary motor area (SMA). Inputs (7) from SMA to corticospinal and corticoreticular fibers (CST/CRST) become progressively weaker, with pathetic consequences for initiation and execution of movements.

that in the *absence* of a resting tremor, a fine action tremor is indicative of *benign essential tremor* (see later).

Rigidity

Rigidity affects all of the somatic musculature simultaneously, but a predilection for flexors imposes

a stooped posture. Passive flexion and extension of the major joints evince resistance through the full range of movement. The term 'lead pipe rigidity' is used to distinguish this type of resistance from the 'clasp knife rigidity' of the spastic state that accompanies upper motor neuron lesions. The clinician may detect a subtle underlying tremor in the form of ratchety, 'cogwheel' sensation (tremor superimposed on rigidity).

Historically, rigidity has been abolished by section of dorsal nerve roots, thus proving its peripheral sensory origin. It can also be alleviated by a surgical lesion of the pallidum or of the VL nucleus of the thalamus. Because muscle spindle stretch reflexes are not exaggerated in PD, attention has focused on the Golgi tendon organ afferents responsible for autogenetic inhibition. As illustrated in Chapter 10, these afferents synapse upon inhibitory, 1b internuncials which, when activated by muscle contraction, dampen activity of motor neurons supplying the same muscle and any homonymous contributors to the same movement (e.g. impulses generated in biceps brachii tendon organs will depress both brachialis and biceps motor neurons). In PD patients, autogenetic inhibition is reduced, and it is also delayed to the extent that it becomes entrained with the pulses descending from the brain, with the effect of contributing to the tremor. It may also contribute to the rigidity, because in PD there is some degree of co-contraction of prime movers and antagonists.

Given that muscular contraction is required to activate tendon organs, why do patients display 'resting tremor', with supposedly inactive muscles? It transpires that, when the forearms (say) are resting on the lap or on the arms of a chair, the forearm/hand muscles are *not* fully at rest. If the limb is properly supported at elbow and wrist, the tremor disappears. The tremor also disappears during sleep.

Normally, both corticospinal and reticulospinal fibers are tonically facilitatory to 1b inhibitory internuncials. In PD, activation of the primary motor cortex by SMA is known to be both reduced and oscillatory, thus accounting for the pronounced effects in the forearm and hand. Impaired reticulospinal activity is more likely to be significant with respect to the lower limbs.

In addition to its massive projections into the pallidum, the putamen projects to another group of GABAergic neurons, namely the reticular part of the substantia nigra. The compact part of the substantia nigra also projects to the reticular part. The reticular part projects in turn to the brainstem locomotor center (Ch. 24). In PD, the overactive putamen would be expected to have the knock-on effect of inhibiting impulse traffic in the projections from the locomotor area to the pontine and medullary reticular reticulospinal tracts.

Difficulty in writing is a common early feature of PD. The individual written letters become small and irregular. Loss of writing skill is attributable to

Clinical Panel 33.1 *Continued*

co-contraction of wrist flexors and extensors, owing to a marked reduction of supraspinal activation of 1a internuncials synapsing on antagonist motor neurons.

Bradykinesia

Bradykinesia means slowness of movement. Patients report that routine activities, such as opening a door, require deliberate planning and consciously guided execution. Electromyographic studies of the limb musculature show a reduction of the 'initial agonist burst' of electrical charge accompanying the first contraction of relevant prime movers. Normally, the basal ganglionic contribution to movement comes on stream some milliseconds after the premotor cortex and cerebellum have raised the firing rate of motor-cortex neurons to threshold at a spinal lower motor neuron level. In PD, the boost to lower motor neuron activation is weak because of the weakened contribution from SMA.

Impairment of postural reflexes

Patients go off balance easily, and tend to fall stiffly ('like a telegraph pole') in response to a mild accidental push. The underlying fault is an impairment of anticipatory postural adjustments: normally, a push to the upper part of the body elicits immediate contraction of lower limb muscles appropriate for the maintenance of equilibrium.

Two other symptoms, *oculomotor hypokinesia* and *dementia*, are mentioned in the main text.

Misdiagnosis

PD has two principal kinds of presentation. In one, tremor is the predominant feature. In the other, akinesia and rigidity predominate. It is now known that more than one in five people initially diagnosed and treated as suffering from PD either do not have PD at all, or have a 'Parkinson plus' syndrome.

Benign essential tremor is more than twice as prevalent as PD and is often mistaken for it. It is characterized initially by a faint trembling, most noticeable when the arms are fully outstretched. Later, head-bobbing – not a feature of PD – and orthostatic (when upright) trunk tremor may appear, and a tremulous diaphragm may impart a vocal tremor. Benign essential tremor is sometimes called *familial tremor* because of autosomal dominant inheritance; it commonly becomes manifest during the fifth decade. When observed in the elderly, it may be called *senile tremor*.

The cause is unknown. Levodopa (L-dopa) (see below) is ineffective, whereas it relieves both kinds of tremor in Parkinson's disease.

Multisystem atrophy is a 'Parkinson plus' degenerative disorder of brainstem, basal ganglia, and central autonomic neurons. Patients present with one or more of the following:

- akinesia/rigidity with little or no tremor
- one or more signs of autonomic failure: postural hypotension, bladder/bowel dysfunction, impotence, dry eyes and mouth, pupillary abnormalities, impaired sweating
- bilateral pyramidal tract degeneration leading to pseudobulbar palsy (Ch. 18) and 'upper motor neuron signs' (Ch. 16) in the limbs
- poor ocular convergence.

L-dopa is of little value.

Clinical neurology texts describe other relevant disorders, e.g. *progressive supranuclear palsy* and *corticobasal degeneration*.

Treatment of Parkinson's disease
Drugs

The first line of treatment of PD is administration of L-dopa which can cross the blood–brain barrier and is metabolized to dopamine by surviving nigral neurons. Some 75% of patients benefit, with a reduction of symptoms by 50% or more. After several years of L-dopa therapy, many patients develop spontaneous choreiform movements (described in Clinical Panel 33.2) owing to excessive striatal response. After a year or more, the effectiveness of L-dopa declines with the progressive loss of nigral neurons, and dopamine agonist drugs are often used instead to stimulate striatal postsynaptic dopamine receptors.

Anticholinergic drugs reduce activity of the cholinergic internuncials in the striatum. They ameliorate tremor (of both kinds) in particular, but the required dosage is liable to produce one or more of the autonomic side effects listed in Clinical Panel 12.3.

Surgery

The optimal approach at present is to *paralyze* STN neurons by high-frequency (133 Hz) stimulation through implanted electrodes. The paralysis is caused by specific inactivation of Ca^{2+} and Na^+ voltage-dependent channels. This approach is being used in the STN to dramatic effect in patients with full-blown tremor, bradykinesia, and rigidity. All three are greatly ameliorated in most cases. Unilateral stimulation may be sufficient for bilateral relief, of rigidity in particular. The bilateral effect of *deep brain stimulation* has been accounted for (in monkey experiments) by paralysis of an excitatory projection from STN to the GABAergic reticular part of the substantia nigra which, as already mentioned, gives an inhibitory supply to the cross-connected right and left locomotor center. According to this interpretation, STN blockage *disinhibits* the locomotor center. It is also possible that deep brain stimulation generates a new type of discharge endowed with beneficial effects.

Clinical Panel 33.1 *Continued*

Other approaches are under intense investigation, including grafts of fetal substantia nigra, striatal infusion of growth factors, and gene therapy.

The assistance of Dr. Tim Counihan, Department of Medicine, University College Hospital, Galway is gratefully acknowledged.

REFERENCES

Axelrad JE, Louis ED, Honig LS, et al: Reduced Purkinje number in essential tremor, *Arch Neurol* 65:101–107, 2008.

Benabid AI: Deep brain stimulation of the subthalamic nucleus for the treatment of Parkinson's disease, *Lancet Neurol* 8:67–81, 2009.

Benarroch EE: Subthalamic nucleus and its connections, *Neurology* 70:1991–1995, 2008.

Braak H, Tredici KT: Nervous system pathology in sporadic Parkinson disease, *Neurology* 70:1916–1927, 2008.

Defazio G, et al: Pain as a nonmotor symptom of Parkinson disease, *Arch Neurol* 65:1191–1194, 2008.

Manto M: Tremorgenesis: a new conceptual scheme using reciprocally innervated circuits of neurons, *J Transl Med* 6:71–76, 2008.

Romanelli P, Esposito V, Schaal DW, Heit G: Somatotopy in the basal ganglia: experimental and clinical evidence for segregated sensorimotor channels, *Brain Res Rev* 48:112–128, 2005.

Schapira AHV: Etiology and pathogenesis of Parkinson Disease, *Neurol Clin* 27:583–603, 2009.

Timmermann L, Gross J, Dirks M, et al: The cerebral oscillatory network of parkinsonian resting tremor, *Brain* 126:199–212, 2003.

Clinical Panel 33.2 Other extrapyramidal disorders

Cerebral palsy

Cerebral palsy is an umbrella term covering a variety of motor disorders arising from damage to the brain during fetal life or in the perinatal period. The incidence is about 2 per 1000 live births in all countries.

The most frequent type of congenital motor disorder is *spastic diplegia*. During the early postnatal months, most affected children are usually 'floppy' (atonic), changing to a spastic state (of the lower limbs in particular) by the end of the first year. Remarkably, many children who are spastic at the age of 2 will be completely normal by the age of 5. Most of the remainder 'grow into their disability' and become more severely affected.

The ventricular system in spastic diplegia is dilated owing to maldevelopment of periventricular oligodendrocytes in the 6th to 8th month of gestation, notably those myelinating corticospinal fibers destined for lumbosacral segments of the spinal cord are affected. Intrauterine infection (Figure CP 33.2.1), ischemia, and metabolic disorders are etiological suspects.

Extrapyramidal or *dyskinetic* cerebral palsy is statistically correlated with perinatal asphyxia. In this condition, the striatum is particularly affected, perhaps

Figure CP 33.2.1 Horizontal MRI slice at the level of the corpus striatum from a 2-year-old girl suffering from severe choreoathetosis as a result of intrauterine damage to her basal ganglia by toxoplasmosis. The putamen on both sides has been partly replaced by cysts. (MRI kindly provided by Professor J. Paul Finn, Director, Magnetic Resonance Research, Department of Radiology, David Geffin School of Medicine, UCLA, California, USA.)

Clinical Panel 33.2 *Continued*

because it is normally highly active metabolically in establishing synaptic connections with the pallidum.

Choreoathetosis is characteristic. *Chorea* refers to momentary spontaneous twitching of muscle groups in a more or less random manner, interfering with voluntary movements. *Athetosis* refers to writhing movements which are continuous except during sleep and may be so severe as to prevent sitting or standing. Waxing and waning of muscle tone commonly cause the head to roll about. Both movements are regarded as escape phenomena resulting from damage to the striatum.

Huntington's chorea

Huntington's chorea is an autosomal (chromosome 4) dominant, inherited disease which occurs in 50% of the offspring of affected families. Onset of symptoms is usually delayed until the 40s. The clinical history is one of chronic, progressive chorea, often with athetoid movements superimposed. Sooner or later, a progressive dementia sets in.

Hemiballism

Hemiballism (or hemiballismus) tends to occur in the elderly. It is known to result from thrombosis of a small branch of the posterior cerebral artery supplying the STN. The condition is perhaps the most remarkable one in the whole of clinical neurology. It is marked by the abrupt onset of wild, flailing movements of the contralateral arm, sometimes of the leg as well. The appearances suggest that the thalamocortical pathway from VLN to SMA has become intensely overactive.

This question may well be asked: If vascular destruction of STN results in hemiballism, why does STN paralysis by high-frequency stimulation not have the same effect? Occasionally it does, requiring immediate withdrawal of the electrode. But, in general, the VLN–SMA pathway remains sufficiently inhibited by underactivity in the 'direct' pathway.

REFERENCE

Lin J: The cerebral palsies: a physiological approach, *J Neurol Neurosurg Psychiatry* 74:23–29, 2003.

Core Information

The basal ganglia are nuclear groups involved in movement control. They comprise the striatum (including nucleus accumbens), pallidum, subthalamic nucleus (STN), substantia nigra, and thalamic motor nuclei VL, VA, and MD. The pallidum has a lateral and a medial segment (GPL, GPM), the latter tapering into the midbrain as the reticular part of substantia nigra (SNpr). Four circuits commence in the cerebral cortex, pass through the basal ganglia, and return to the cortex. The compact part of substantia nigra (SNpc) stands aside of the circuits but influences them by way of the nigrostriatal pathway.

Cortical inputs to striatum and STN are excitatory. Striatal outputs are inhibitory to the pallidum; so, too are the pallidal outputs to STN and thalamus. STN is excitatory to GPM.

The 'direct' pathway, striatum → GPM, is facilitated by the normal tonic activity of nigrostriatal dopaminergic neurons. The 'indirect' pathway, striatum → GPL → GPM, is inhibited. In the *motor loop*, facilitation of the direct pathway is necessary for the SMA to become active before and during movement. SMA activity immediately prior to movement is detectable as the readiness potential, and is produced by silencing of GPM neurons with consequent liberation (disinhibition) of thalamocortical neurons to SMA, with follow-through to the motor cortex for initiation of movement.

Striatum and pallidum are somatotopically organized, permitting selective activation of body parts; STN is especially important for inhibition of unwanted movements.

The main function of the motor loop seems to be the appropriate sequencing of serial order actions for the execution of learned motor programs. In PD, the loss of nigrostriatal dopaminergic neurons causes the 'indirect' pathway to become dominant, with follow-through suppression of VL and reduced SMA activity, thus accounting for the characteristic bradykinesia. PD symptomatology also includes rigidity, tremor, and impairment of postural reflexes. Benign essential tremor and multisystem atrophy are too often misdiagnosed as PD.

The *cognitive loop* begins in the association cortex, and returns via VA nucleus of thalamus to the premotor and prefrontal cortex. It is actively engaged during motor learning, and also seems concerned with planning ahead for later movements.

The *limbic loop* begins in cingulate cortex and amygdala, passes through nucleus accumbens, and returns to SMA; it is probably involved in giving physical expression to the current emotional state.

The *oculomotor loop* disinhibits SNpr, thereby liberating the superior colliculus to execute a saccade.

Hyperkinetic states include many cases of cerebral palsy; also Huntington's chorea and hemiballism.

REFERENCES

Benarroch EE: Subthalamic nucleus and its connections, *Neurology* 70:1991–1995, 2008.

Brown P, Steiger MJ: Basal ganglia disorders. In Bronstein AM, Brandt T, Woollacott M, editors: *Clinical disorders of balance, posture and gait*, London, 2004, Arnold, pp 156–166.

Crossman AR: Functional anatomy of movement disorders, *J Anat* 196:519–525, 2000.

Haber SN, Calzavara R: The cortico-basal ganglia integrative network: the role of the thalamus, *Brain Res Bull* 78:69–74, 2008.

Kuban KCK, Leviton A: Cerebral palsy, *N Engl J Med* 333:88–195, 1994.

Meunier S, Pol S, Houeto JL, Vidailhet M: Abnormal reciprocal inhibition between antagonist muscles in Parkinson's disease, *Brain* 123:1017–1026, 2000.

STUDY GUIDELINES

Olfactory system
In most vertebrates the olfactory system is altogether more important than it is in humans. Clinically, its main interest is that damage to the olfactory pathway on one side is associated with anosmia on that side.

Limbic system
Cortical and subcortical limbic areas are prominent features of the brain in primitive mammals, where they are intimately concerned with mechanisms of attack and defense, procreation, and feeding. The principal effector elements of the limbic system are the hypothalamus and the reticular formation.
   The elements, pathways, and transmitters of the human limbic system provide the bedrock on which most of psychiatry and clinical psychology are built.

OLFACTORY SYSTEM

The olfactory system is remarkable in four respects:

1 The somas of the primary afferent neurons occupy a surface epithelium.
2 The axons of the primary afferents enter the cerebral cortex directly; second-order afferents are not interposed.
3 The primary afferent neurons undergo continuous turnover, being replaced from basal stem cells.
4 The pathway to the cortical centers in the frontal lobe is entirely ipsilateral.

   The olfactory system comprises the olfactory epithelium and olfactory nerves; the olfactory bulb and tract; and several areas of olfactory cortex.

Olfactory epithelium

The olfactory epithelium occupies the upper one-fifth of the lateral and septal walls of the nasal cavity. The epithelium contains three cell types (Figure 34.1):

Figure 34.1 Connections of olfactory epithelium (1) and olfactory bulb (2). The second glomerulus from the left is 'on line' (see text).

1 **Olfactory neurons**. These are bipolar neurons, each with a dendrite extending to the epithelial surface and an unmyelinated axon contributing to the olfactory nerve. The dendrites are capped by immotile cilia containing molecular receptor sites. The axons run upward through the cribriform ('sieve-like') plate of the ethmoid bone and enter the olfactory bulb. The axons (some 3 million on each side) are grouped into fila (bundles) by investing Schwann cells. The collective fila constitute the **olfactory nerve**.
2 **Sustentacular cells** are interspersed among the bipolar neurons.
3 **Basal stem cells** lie between the other two cell types. Olfactory bipolar neurons are unique in that they undergo a continuous cycle of growth, degeneration, and replacement. The basal cells transform into fresh bipolar neurons, which survive for about a month. Replacement declines over time, accounting for the general reduction in olfactory sensitivity with age.

Olfactory bulb (Figure 34.1)

The olfactory bulb consists of three-layered allocortex surrounding the commencement of the olfactory tract. The chief cortical neurons are some 50 000 **mitral cells**, which receive the olfactory nerve fibers and give rise to the olfactory tract.

Contact between olfactory fibers and mitral cell dendrites takes place in some 2000 **glomeruli**, which are sites of innumerable synapses and have a glial investment. Glomeruli which are 'on-line' (active) inhibit neighboring, 'off-line' glomeruli through the mediation of GABAergic **periglomerular cells** (cf. the horizontal cells of the retina). Mitral cell activity is also sharpened at a deeper level by **granule cells**, which are devoid of axons (cf. the amacrine cells of the retina). The granule cells receive excitatory dendrodendritic contacts from active mitral cells and they suppress neighboring mitral cells through inhibitory (GABA) dendrodendritic contacts.

Central connections

Mitral cell axons run centrally in the **olfactory tract** (Figure 34.2). The tract divides in front of the anterior perforated substance into **medial** and **lateral olfactory striae**.

The medial stria contains axons from the **anterior olfactory nucleus**, which consists of multipolar neurons scattered within the olfactory tract. Some of these axons travel to the septal area via the diagonal band (see later, under Limbic system). Others cross the midline in the anterior commissure and inhibit mitral cell activity in the contralateral bulb (by exciting granule cells there). The result is a relative enhancement of the more active bulb, providing a directional cue to the source of olfactory stimulation.

The lateral olfactory stria terminates in the **piriform lobe** of the anterior temporal cortex. The human piriform lobe includes the cortical part of the amygdala, the uncus, and the anterior end of the parahippocampal gyrus. The highest center for olfactory discrimination is the posterior part of the orbitofrontal cortex, which receives connections from the piriform lobe via the mediodorsal nucleus of the thalamus.

The medial forebrain bundle links the olfactory cortical areas with the hypothalamus and brainstem. These linkages trigger autonomic responses such as salivation and gastric contraction, and arousal responses through the reticular formation.

Points of clinical interest are mentioned in Clinical Panel 34.1.

LIMBIC SYSTEM

The limbic system comprises the limbic cortex (so-called *limbic lobe*) and related subcortical nuclei. The term 'limbic' (Broca, 1878) originally referred to a *limbus* or rim of cortex immediately adjacent to the corpus callosum and diencephalon. The limbic cortex is now taken to include the three-layered *allocortex* of the hippocampal formation and

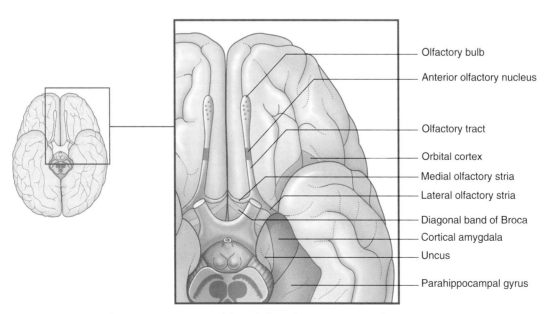

Olfactory bulb
Anterior olfactory nucleus
Olfactory tract
Orbital cortex
Medial olfactory stria
Lateral olfactory stria
Diagonal band of Broca
Cortical amygdala
Uncus
Parahippocampal gyrus

Figure 34.2 Brain viewed from below, showing cortical olfactory areas.

Clinical Panel 34.1 Olfactory disturbance

A routine test of olfactory function is to ask the patient to identify strong-smelling substances such as coffee and chocolate through each nostril in turn. Loss of smell, or **anosmia**, may not be detected by the patient without testing if it is unilateral. If it is bilateral, the complaint may be one of loss of taste because the flavor of foodstuffs depends on the olfactory qualities of volatile elements; in such cases, the four primary taste sensations (sweet, sour, salty, bitter) are

preserved. Unilateral anosmia may be caused by a *meningioma* compressing the olfactory bulb or tract, or by a head injury with fracture of the anterior cranial fossa. Anosmia may be a clue to a fracture, and should prompt tests for leakage of cerebrospinal fluid into the nasal cavity.

Olfactory auras are a typical prodromal feature of *uncinate epilepsy* (see Clinical Panel 34.3).

Figure 34.3 Medial view of cortical and subcortical limbic areas. MDN, mediodorsal nucleus of thalamus.

septal area, together with transitional *mesocortex* in the parahippocampal gyrus, cingulate gyrus, and insula. The principal subcortical component of the limbic system is the amygdala, which merges with the cortex on the medial side of the temporal pole. Closely related subcortical areas are the hypothalamus, reticular formation, and the nucleus accumbens. Cortical areas closely related to the limbic system are the orbitofrontal cortex and the temporal pole (Figure 34.3).

Figure 34.4 is a graphic reconstruction of mainly subcortical limbic areas.

Parahippocampal gyrus

The parahippocampal gyrus is a major junctional region between the cerebral neocortex and the allocortex of the hippocampal formation. Its anterior part is the **entorhinal cortex** (area 28 of Brodmann), which is six-layered but has certain peculiar features. The entorhinal cortex can be said to face in two directions. Its *neocortical face* exchanges massive numbers of afferent and efferent connections with all four association areas of the neocortex. Its *allocortical face* exchanges abundant connections with the hippocampal formation. In the broadest terms, the entorhinal cortex receives a constant stream of cognitive and sensory

information from the association areas, transmits it to the hippocampal formation for consolidation (see later), retrieves it in consolidated form, and returns it to the association areas where it is encoded in the form of memory traces. The fornix and its connections form a second, circuitous pathway from hippocampus to neocortex.

Hippocampal complex

The hippocampal complex (or hippocampal formation) comprises the **subiculum**, the **hippocampus proper**, and the **dentate gyrus** (Figure 34.5). All three are composed of temporal lobe allocortex which has tucked itself into an S-shaped scroll along the floor of the lateral ventricle. The band-like origin of the fornix from the subiculum and hippocampus is the **fimbria**. The hippocampus is also known as *Ammon's horn* (after an Egyptian deity with a ram's head). For research purposes, it is divided into four *cornu ammonis* (CA) zones (Fig. 34.6A).

The principal cells of the subiculum and hippocampus are **pyramidal cells**; those of the dentate gyrus are **granule cells**. The dendrites of both granule and pyramidal cells are studded with dendritic spines. The hippocampal complex is also rich in inhibitory (GABA) internuncial neurons.

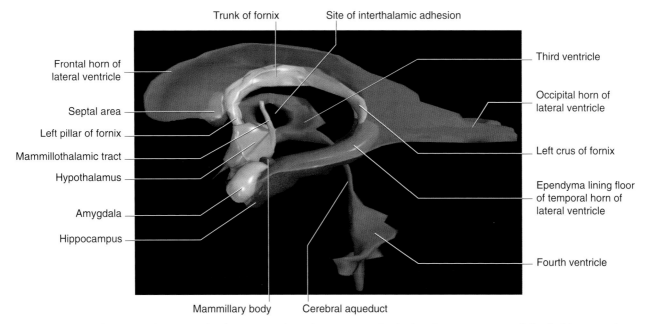

Trunk of fornix

Site of interthalamic adhesion

Frontal horn of
lateral ventricle

Septal area

Left pillar of fornix

Mammillothalamic tract

Hypothalamus

Amygdala

Hippocampus

Third ventricle

Occipital horn of
lateral ventricle

Left crus of fornix

Ependyma lining floor
of temporal horn of
lateral ventricle

Fourth ventricle

Mammillary body

Cerebral aqueduct

Figure 34.4 Three-dimensional computerized reconstruction of postmortem brain showing components of the limbic system in relation to the ventricular system. (Excerpt of figure from Kretschmann and Weinrich, 1998, with kind permission of the authors and the publisher.)

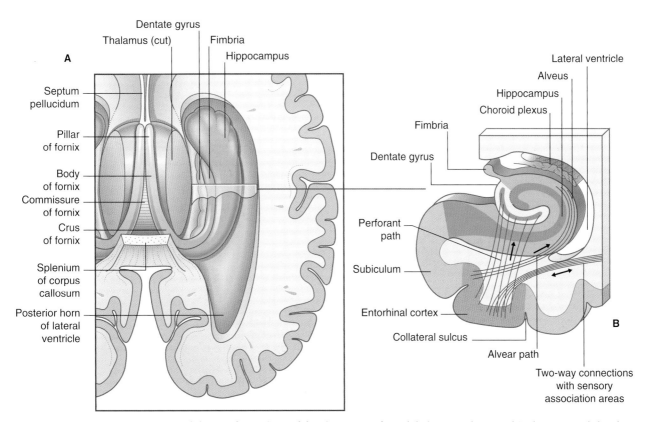

Dentate gyrus

Thalamus (cut)

Fimbria

Hippocampus

A

Septum
pellucidum

Pillar
of fornix

Body
of fornix

Commissure
of fornix

Crus
of fornix

Splenium
of corpus
callosum

Posterior horn
of lateral
ventricle

Lateral ventricle

Alveus

Hippocampus

Choroid plexus

Fimbria

Dentate gyrus

Perforant
path

Subiculum

Entorhinal cortex

Collateral sulcus

Alvear path

B

Two-way connections
with sensory
association areas

Figure 34.5 Hippocampal formation. **(A)** View from above. **(B)** Enlargement from (A) showing the entorhinal cortex and the three component parts of the hippocampal formation.

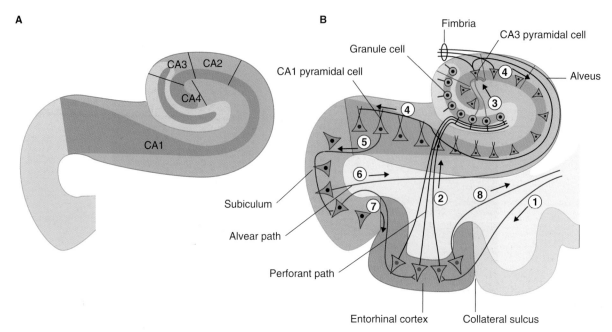

Figure 34.6 (A) The four sectors of Ammon's horn. **(B)** Input–output connections of the hippocampal formation.
1 Afferent from sensory association cortex.
2 Entorhinal cortex projecting perforant path fibers to dentate gyrus.
3 Dentate granule cell projecting to CA3.
4 CA3 principal neuron projecting into fimbria and CA1.
5 CA1 principal cell projecting to subiculum.
6 Subicular principal cell projecting into fimbria.
7 Subicular principal cell projecting into entorhinal cortex.
8 Entorhinal pyramidal cell projecting to sensory association cortex.

It should be mentioned that in general discussions related to memory, it is customary to use the term 'hippocampus' as synonymous with 'hippocampal complex'.

Connections

Afferents

The largest afferent connection of the hippocampal complex is the **perforant path**, which projects from the entorhinal cortex onto the dendrites of dentate granule cells (Figure 34.6B). The subiculum gives rise to a second, *alvear* path which contributes to a sheet of fibers on the ventricular surface of the hippocampus, the **alveus**.

The axons of the granule cells are called **mossy fibers**; they synapse upon pyramidal cells in the CA3 sector. The axons of the CA3 pyramidal cells project into the fimbria; before doing so they give off *Schaffer collaterals*, which run a recurrent course from CA3 to CA1. CA1 projects into the entorhinal cortex.

Auditory information enters the hippocampus from the association cortex of the superior and middle temporal gyri. The supramarginal gyrus (area 40) transmits coded information about personal space (the *body schema* described in Ch. 32) and extrapersonal (visual) space. From the occipitotemporal region on the inferior surface, information concerning object shape and color, and facial recognition, is projected to cortex called *perirhinal*, or *transrhinal*, immediately lateral to the entorhinal cortex. From here, it enters the hippocampus. A return projection from entorhinal to perirhinal cortex is linked to the temporal polar and prefrontal cortex.

In addition to the discrete afferent connections mentioned above, the hippocampus is diffusely innervated from several sources, mainly by way of the fornix:

- A dense *cholinergic* innervation, of particular significance in relation to memory, is received from the septal nucleus.
- A *noradrenergic* innervation is received from the cerulean nucleus.
- A *serotonergic* innervation enters from the raphe nuclei of the midbrain. The linkage between serotonin depletion and major depression is mentioned in Chapter 26.
- A *dopaminergic* innervation enters from the ventral tegmental area of the midbrain. The linkage between dopamine and schizophrenia is discussed in Clinical Panel 34.2.

Efferents

The largest efferent connection is a massive projection via the entorhinal cortex to the association areas of the neocortex. A second, forward projection is the **fornix** (Figure 34.5A). The fornix is a direct continuation of the **fimbria**, which receives axons from the subiculum and hippocampus proper. The **crus** of the fornix arches up beneath the corpus callosum, where it joins its fellow to form the **trunk** and links with its opposite number through a small **hippocampal commissure**. Anteriorly, the trunk divides into two **pillars**. Each pillar splits around the anterior commissure, sending *precommissural* fibers to the septal area and *postcommissural* fibers to the anterior hypothalamus, mammillary body, and medial

Clinical Panel 34.2 Schizophrenia

Schizophrenia occurs in about 1% of the population in all countries where the prevalence has been studied. It is a heritable illness with around a 10% risk of occurrence if a person's first-degree relative is affected, and as much as 50% risk of occurrence if both parents or an identical co-twin is affected. Although the onset of illness is typically in early adulthood, there is substantial evidence for neurodevelopmental disturbance in the illness, with increased rates of birth complications, early developmental insults, and childhood social, motor, and academic underperformance in those who later develop schizophrenia. Cognitive dysfunction is present in the illness, but relatively stable throughout life, unlike the progressive dementias.

MRI studies reveal enlargement of lateral ventricles and regionally specific atrophy predominantly affecting frontal and temporal parts of the cortex, the medial temporal lobe, and thalamus. There is a reduction or even a reversal of the usual left–right difference in the size of the temporal plane on the upper surface of the superior temporal gyrus. There is some progression of these neuroimaging abnormalities in the early years of the illness which then plateau. Postmortem studies indicate that the atrophy identified by imaging studies is related to loss of neuropil and reduced neuronal size rather than neuronal loss. No evidence of astrogliosis or of neurodegenerative disease pathology has been identified. Consistent with neurodevelopmental disturbance, underlying the illness are findings of aberrantly located neurons, for example in the entorhinal cortex and in white matter.

The clinical presentation is quite variable but the symptoms and behavioral changes can be categorized into two broad spectra – positive symptoms and negative symptoms.

- *Positive psychotic symptoms* include hallucinations, delusions, and disorganized thoughts and behavior. Hallucinations are typically auditory (the patient hears voices, which are commonly derogatory in nature and refer to the patient in the third person). Delusions often take a paranoid form, with a belief that the patient is being monitored or the subject of a conspiracy. Other typical delusions include a belief that one's thoughts and actions are being controlled by an outside agency and that thoughts are not private, but are somehow accessible by other people. Thought processes frequently become disorganized with the normal flow and logic of speech breaking down and in severe cases becoming incoherent. Disorganized behavior includes disinhibited, socially inappropriate behaviour or in some cases physical aggression in response to hallucinations or delusions.

Although positive symptoms cause great distress to patients and their families, they are much more responsive to antipsychotic medication treatment than the negative ones, which in the long term are more disabling.

- *Negative (deficit) psychotic symptoms* refer to an inability to engage in normal emotional and social interactions with people and frequently lead to impaired capacity to self-care. The patient lacks motivation, has little to say, and in conversation rambles from one inconsequential theme to another. There is a loss of emotional responsiveness (*flattening of affect*), including inability to experience pleasure (*anhedonia*). Personal hygiene and ability to live independently and manage affairs are often impaired. The negative symptoms appear to be associated with 'hypofrontality,' i.e. diminished prefrontal function. Functional imaging studies using fMRI and PET support this idea by demonstrating failure of the normal response of the dorsolateral prefrontal cortex to standard tests of cognitive function.

Medications used to treat psychotic disorders such as schizophrenia are called *antipsychotics, neuroleptics* or *major tranquillizers*. All such antipsychotic medications block dopamine D_2 receptors to some extent (e.g. haloperidol or olanzapine). In the normal brain, the D_2 receptors are on spiny (excitatory) stellate cells in the mesocortical projection territory of the ventral tegmental nucleus. D_2 receptors are inhibitory, for one or more of three possible reasons noted in Chapter 8. Interestingly, symptoms closely resembling the positive psychotic ones of schizophrenia may be induced by consuming excessive amounts of dopamine-stimulating drugs such as cocaine or amphetamine ('speed'). Amphetamine is known to increase the amount of dopamine in the forebrain extracellular space (Clinical Panel 34.5). In schizophrenia, dopaminergic overactivity seems not to be a matter of overproduction but of greater effectiveness through an increased number of postsynaptic dopamine receptors on the spiny stellate neurons. (The assistance of Professor Colm McDonald, Department of Psychiatry, NUI, Galway, Ireland is gratefully appreciated.)

REFERENCES

Harrison PJ, Weinberger DR: Schizophrenia genes, gene expression, and neuropathology: on the matter of their convergence, *Mol Psychiatry* 10:40–68, 2005.

Leonard BE: Drug treatment of schizophrenia and the psychoses. In *Fundamentals of psychopharmacology*, Chichester, 2003, Wiley, pp 255–294.

Picchioni MM, Murray RM: Schizophrenia, *BMJ* 335:91–95, 2007.

forebrain bundle. The mammillary body projects into the anterior nucleus of thalamus, which projects in turn to the cingulate cortex, completing the *Papez circuit* from cingulate cortex to hippocampus, with return to cingulate cortex via fornix, mammillary body, and anterior thalamic nucleus (Figure 34.7).

The term *medial temporal lobe* is clinically inclusive of the hippocampal complex, parahippocampal gyrus, and amygdala. The term is most often used in relation to seizures (Clinical Panel 34.3).

Memory function of the hippocampal complex

The evidence for a *mnemonic* (memory-related) function in the hippocampal formation is discussed at considerable length in psychology texts. Some insights are given below.

Glossary

- **Short-term memory**: Holding one or more items of new information briefly in mind (e.g. a new telephone number, while pressing the buttons).
- **Long-term (remote) memory**: Stored information capable of retrieval at appropriate moments. Two kinds of long-term memory are recognized: explicit and implicit.
  Explicit memory has to do with recollections of facts and events of all kinds that can be explicitly stated – or declared; hence the term *declarative memory*. The term *episodic memory* is also used, in the autobiographical sense of recollection of episodes involving personal experience. Yet another term, *semantic memory*, was devised in the context of memory for the meaning of written and spoken words,

but is now also used to include knowledge of facts and concepts.
  Implicit memory has to do with performance of learned motor procedures, e.g. riding a bicycle, assembling a jigsaw puzzle. The term *procedural memory* is commonly used.

- **Working memory**: Effortless brief simultaneous retrieval of several items from long-term memory stores for a task in hand, e.g. driving a car along a familiar route while making appropriate decisions based on previous experience.
- **Consolidation**: The process of storing new information in long-term memory. Novel factual information is relayed from the relevant sensory association areas to the hippocampal complex for encoding. Following a prolonged period of processing, the encoded information is relayed back to the same association areas and (with the exception of strongly autobiographical episodes) no longer depends on the hippocampal complex for retrieval.

Clinical and experimental observations

Bilateral damage or removal of the anterior part of the hippocampal formation is followed by *anterograde amnesia*, a term used to denote absence of conscious recall of newly acquired information for more than a few minutes. When asked to name a commonplace object, the subject will have no difficulty because access to long-term memories does not require the anterior hippocampus. However, when the same object is shown a few minutes later, the subject will not remember having seen it. There is loss of explicit/declarative memory.

Procedural (how-to-do) memory is preserved. If asked to assemble a jigsaw puzzle, the subject will do it in the normal way. When asked to repeat the exercise the next day, the subject will do it faster, although there will be no recollection of having seen the puzzle previously. *The hippocampus is not required for procedural memory.* We have previously noted that the basal ganglia are the storehouse of routine motor programs, and the cerebellum the storehouse of motor adaptations to novel conditions.

Long-term potentiation (LTP) is uniquely powerful in the dentate gyrus and hippocampus. It is regarded as vital for preservation (consolidation) of memory traces. Under experimental conditions, LTP is most easily demonstrated in the perforant path–dentate granule cell connections and in the Schaffer collateral–CA1 connections. A strong, brief (milliseconds) stimulus to the perforant path or Schaffer collaterals induces the target cells to show long-lasting (hours) sensitivity to a fresh stimulus. LTP is associated with a cascade of biochemical events in the target neurons, following activation of appropriate glutamate receptors, as described in Chapter 8 in the context of pain sensitization. Repetitive stimuli may cause cAMP to increase its normal rate of activation of protein kinases involved in phosphorylation of proteins that regulate gene transcription. The outcome is increased production of proteins (including enzymes) required for transmitter synthesis, and of other proteins for construction of additional channels and synaptic cytoskeletons.

LTP is described as an *associative* phenomenon, because the required expulsion of the magnesium plug from the NMDA receptor (Figure 34.8) is facilitated when the powerful depolarizing stimulus is coupled with a weaker

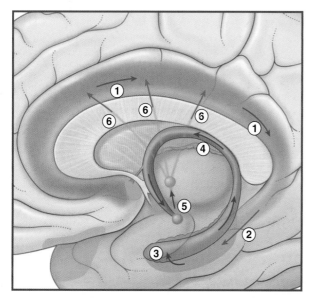

Figure 34.7 The Papez circuit.
1 Backward-projecting neurons in the cingulate gyrus.
2 Projection into the entorhinal cortex.
3 Projection into hippocampus.
4 Fornix.
5 Mammillothalamic tract.
6 Projections from anterior nucleus of thalamus to cingulate cortex.

Clinical Panel 34.3 Temporal lobe epilepsy

Complex focal (partial) seizures are synonymous with *temporal lobe epilepsy*. The initial event, or *aura*, may be a simple partial seizure whose electrical activity escapes into the temporal lobe. Many originate in a focus of runaway neural activity within the temporal lobe and spread over the general cortex within seconds to trigger a *secondarily generalized* tonic–clonic seizure (Figure CP 34.3.1) as mentioned in Chapter 30. Types of temporal lobe auras include well-formed visual or auditory hallucinations (scenes, sound sequences), a sense of familiarity with the surrounding scene ('*déjà vu*'), a sense of strangeness ('*jamais vu*') or a sense of

fear. Attacks originating in the uncus are ushered in by unpleasant olfactory or gustatory auras. Bizzare *psychic* auras can occur, where the patient has an 'out of body experience' in the form of a sensation of floating in the air and looking down at themselves and any others present.

Following accurate localization of the ictal (seizure) focus by means of recording electrodes inserted into the exposed temporal lobe, a tissue block including the focus may be removed, with abolition of seizures in four out of five cases. Histological examination of the surgical biopsy typically reveals *hippocampal sclerosis*: the picture is one of glial scarring, with extensive neuronal loss in CA2 and CA3 sectors. The granule cells of the dentate gyrus are relatively well preserved. Loss of inhibitory, GABA internuncials has been blamed in the past but these cells have recently been shown to persist. Instead, the granule cells appear to be *disinhibited*, because of loss of minute, inhibitory basket cells from among their dendrites.

Because 30% of sufferers from temporal lobe epilepsy have first-degree relatives similarly afflicted, often from childhood, a genetic influence must be significant. One possibility could be 'faulty wiring' of the hippocampus during mid-fetal life. Histological preparations show areas of congenital misplacement of hippocampal pyramidal cells, some lying on their sides or even in the subjacent white matter.

The sclerosis is regarded as a typical CNS healing process following extensive loss of neurons. The neuronal loss in turn seems to be inflicted by *glutamate toxicity* – a known effect of excessively high rates of discharge of pyramidal cells in any part of the cerebral cortex. Dentate granule cells are the main source of burst-firing, which is no surprise in view of their natural role in long-term potentiation and kindling (see main text).

REFERENCES

Emerson RG, Pedley TA: EEG and evoked potentials. In Bradley WG, Daroff RB, Finichel GM, Jankovic J, editors: *Neurology in clinical practice: principles of diagnosis and management*, Philadelphia, 2004, Elsevier, pp. 465–490.

Bernasconi N, Bernasconi A, Caramanos Z, et al: Mesial temporal damage in temporal lobe epilepsy: a volumetric MRI study of the hippocampus, amygdala and parahippocampal region, *Brain* 126:462–469, 2003.

Jay V, Becker LE: Surgical pathology of epilepsy, *Pediatr Pathol* 14:731–750, 2003.

Kempermann G: The neurogenic reserve rehypothesis: what is adult hippocampal neurogenesis good for? *Trends Neurosci* 89:1169–1176, 2008.

Niedergerger E, Kuhlein H, Geissler G: Update on the neuropathology of neuropathic pain, *Expert Rev Proteomics* 5:719–818, 2008.

Shin C: Mechanism of epilepsy, *Ann Rev Med* 45:379–389, 1994.

Willis WD, Westland KR: Pain system. In Paxinos G, Mai JK, editors: *The human nervous system*, ed 2, Amsterdam, 2004, Elsevier, pp 1125–1170.

Figure CP 34.3.1 Complex focal seizure. The ictal focus (*arrow*) occupies the middle–posterior junctional zone of the right temporal lobe (cf. electrode positions in Figure 30.2). Within a second the entire cortex exhibits a secondarily generalized seizure (to the right of the dashed line).

stimulus to the depolarized neuron from another source. *Norepinephrine* and *dopamine* are suitable associative candidates, one or both being released during elevation of the attentional or motivational state at the appropriate time.

Cholinergic activity in the hippocampus is also significant for learning. In human volunteers, central ACh blockade (by administration of scopolamine) severely impairs memory for lists of names or numbers, whereas a cholinesterase inhibitor (physostigmine) gives above-normal results.

Figure 34.8 Long-term potentiation.

Clinically, hippocampal cholinergic activity is severely reduced in Alzheimer's disease (AD), which is particularly associated with amnesia (see Clinical Panel 34.4).

Kindling ('lighting a fire') is a property unique to the hippocampal formation and amygdala, although its relationship to learning is not obvious. Kindling is the progressively increasing group response of neurons to a repetitive stimulus of uniform strength. In both humans and experimental animals, it can spread from mesocortex to neocortex and cause generalized convulsive seizures.

The contribution of the fornix projection to memory is uncertain. Indirect evidence has been adduced from *diencephalic amnesia*, a state of anterograde amnesia which may follow bilateral damage to the diencephalon. Such damage may interrupt the *Papez circuit* linking the fornix to the cingulate gyrus by way of the mammillary body and the anterior nucleus of the thalamus. Particularly impaired is relational memory (e.g. recollection of the sight and sound of a particular waterfall with the wind blowing spray over some fleeing viewers; recollection of the structure and the function of the (say) left vestibular labyrinth, along with inevitable symptoms and signs that follow sudden occlusion of the left labyrinthine artery.)

Left vs right hippocampal functions

In keeping with known hemispheric asymmetries, the left anterior hippocampus and dorsolateral prefrontal cortex (DLPFC) are engaged in encoding novel material involving language function. Also consistent is the finding that the right hippocampus and right inferior parietal lobe are engaged in spatial tasks such as driving a car (Figure 34.9). Blood flow in the DLPFC increases more on the left side during driving,

Figure 34.9 Navigation in a virtual environment. **(A)** Scene from a virtual town. Subjects navigated through the town using a keypad to stay clear of obstacles. PET scans taken during the virtual journey showed increased activation, **(B)** and **(C)**, within the right hippocampus and **(D)** and **(E)** within the right supramarginal gyrus. Orientation (L, R) of the MRIs is for a more general readership. (Kindly provided by Dr Eleanor Maguire, Wellcome Department of Cognitive Neurology, Institute of Neurology, University College, London, UK, and with permission from the Editor of *Current Opinion in Neurobiology*.)

presumably because of the 'inner speech' that occurs when exploring novel territory.

Anterior vs posterior hippocampal functions

The hippocampus is about 8 cm in length, and there is evidence for anteroposterior functional specialization with respect to novelty vs familiarity, e.g. when novel material is being read on a screen the left anterior hippocampus is especially active, but with development of familiarity with repeated exposure, activity shifts to the posterior part, suggesting that this region is involved in encoding material into long-term memory.

Long-term medial temporal lobe dependency

Autobiographical recollections typically are mainly visual, whereby we revisit scenes from the past, sometimes from childhood. Clinical studies indicate that medial temporal lobe damage impairs or even deletes such ego-centered (personal) memories whereas allocentered (impersonal), map-like recall of past scenes is preserved. On the other hand, damage to the visual association cortex has the opposite effect.

Prefrontal cortex and working memory

Volunteers have been examined under fMRI while preparing to give a motor response to one or more sensory cues. The mid-region of the prefrontal cortex (area 46) tends to be especially active. It is in a position to tap into memory stores in relevant sensory association areas and to organize motor responses including speech.

Insula

The anterior insula is a cortical center for pain (Box 34.1). The central region is continuous with the frontoparietal and temporal opercular cortex, and it seems to have a *language* rather than a limbic function. During language tasks, PET scans show activity there as well as in the opercular speech receptive and motor areas – but not in people with congenital dyslexia, where it remains silent (Ch. 32). The posterior insula is interconnected with the entorhinal cortex and the amygdala, and is therefore presumed to participate in emotional responses – perhaps in the context of pain evaluation.

Cingulate cortex and posterior parahippocampal gyrus

The cingulate cortex is part of the Papez circuit, receiving a projection from the anterior nucleus of the thalamus and becoming continuous with the parahippocampal gyrus behind the splenium of the corpus callosum.

The *anterior* cingulate cortex belongs to the *rostral limbic system*, which includes the amygdala, ventral striatum, orbitofrontal cortex, and anterior insular cortex.

Six functional areas can be discerned in the anterior cingulate cortex (Figure 34.10).

1 An *executive area* is connected directly with the DLPFC and with the supplementary motor area (SMA). The executive area becomes active prior to execution of willed movements, including voluntary saccades (Ch. 29) – and even prior to the SMA itself. The executive area is thought

Figure 34.10 Functional areas in the anterior cingulate cortex. SMA, supplementary motor area.

to have special significance, together with the DLPFC, in generating *appropriate motor plan selection* by the SMA.

2 A *pain perception area* receives afferents from the medial dorsal nucleus of the thalamus (Box 34.1).

3 An *emotional area* lies close to the pain perception area. When volunteers 'think happy' while undergoing PET scans, the anterior cingulate cortex 'lights up' and the amygdala 'switches off'. A reverse result occurs when volunteers 'think sad'. Anterior cingulectomy has often been performed in the past, yielding successful control of aggressive psychiatric disorders.

4 A *bladder control area* becomes increasingly active during bladder filling (Ch. 24).

5 A *vocalization area* becomes active, together with the DLPFC, during *decision-making* about appropriate sentence construction for speech activity. Electrical stimulation of this area causes jumbling of speech. *Stammering* in children is associated with *reduced* blood flow in the left anterior cingulate gyrus during speech. Blood flow there is also reduced in people suffering from *Tourette's syndrome*, which is characterized by brief, loud utterances of a single syllable or phrase, often offensive to the ear.

6 An *autonomic area*, below the rostrum of the corpus callosum, elicits autonomic and respiratory responses when stimulated electrically. This area is thought to participate in eliciting the visceral responses typical of emotional states.

The posterior cingulate gyrus (area 23 of Brodmann) merges with the posterior parahippocampal gyrus (area 36). This cortical complex is richly interconnected with visual, auditory, and tactile/spatial association areas. The complex evidently contains memory stores related to these functions because PET studies reveal increased activity there when scenes or experiences are conjured up in the mind. The complex is also engaged during reading (Ch. 32).

Amygdala

The **amygdala** (*Gr.* 'almond'; also called the *amygdaloid body* or *amygdaloid complex*) is a large group of nuclei above and in front of the temporal horn of the lateral ventricle and anterior to the tail of the caudate nucleus. *The amygdala is*

Box 34.1 Pain and the brain

The International Association for the Study of Pain has given the following definition: *Pain is an unpleasant sensory and emotional experience associated with actual or potential tissue damage or described in terms of such damage.*

This definition emphasizes the *affective* (emotional) component of pain. Its other component is *sensory-discriminative* ('Where and how much?').

Table Box 34.1.1 is a glossary of conventional terms used in relation to pain.

Table Box 34.1.1

Term	Meaning
Allodynia	Pain produced by normally innocuous stimuli. Examples: stroking sunburned skin; moving an inflamed joint.
Central pain-projecting neurons (CPPNs)	An inclusive conventional term denoting all posterior horn neurons projecting pain-encoded information to contralateral brainstem and thalamic nuclei. Pathways included are: *spinothalamic*, the lateral pain pathway to posterior nucleus of thalamus; *spinoreticulothalamic*, medial pain pathway to the medial and intralaminar nuclei of thalamus via brainstem reticular formation; *spinoamygdaloid*, to the amygdala via the reticular formation; and *spinotectal*, to the superior colliculus.
Central pain state	A state of chronic pain, resistant to therapy, sustained by hypersensivity of peripheral and/or central neural pathways.
Wind-up phenomenon	Sustained state of excitation of CPPNs induced by glutamate activation of NMDA receptors.
Fast pain	Stabbing pain perceived following activation of Aδ nociceptors.
Hyperalgesia	Hypersensitivity to stimulation of injured tissue, and of surrounding uninjured tissue. Causes include mechanical or thermal damage, bacterial/viral inflammation, small-fiber peripheral axonal neuropathy, radiculopathy (posterior nerve root injury).
Neurogenic inflammation	Inflammation caused by liberation of substance P (in particular) following antidromic depolarization of fine peripheral nerve fibers.
Neuropathic pain	Chronic stabbing or burning pain resulting from injury to peripheral nerves. Examples: postherpetic neuralgia; amputation neuroma.
Nociceptors	Peripheral receptors whose activation generates a sense of pain. These receptors occupy the plasma membrane of fine nerve endings and contain transduction channels that convert the requisite physical or chemical stimulus into trains of impulses decoded by the brain as a sense of pain.
Polymodal nociceptors	Peripheral nociceptors (notably in skin) responsive to noxious thermal, mechanical, or chemical stimulation.
Sensitization	Lowering the threshold of peripheral nociceptors by histamine (in particular) following peripheral release of peptides via the axon reflex.
Slow pain	Aching pain perceived following activation of C-fiber nociceptors.

Peripheral pain pathways

As already noted in Chapter 9, pain is served by finely myelinated (Aδ) and unmylinated (C) fibers belonging to unipolar spinal ganglion cells. These fibers are loosely known as 'pain fibers', although others of similar diameters are purely mechanoreceptors and others again elicit pain only when discharging at high frequency, notably mechanical nociceptors and thermoreceptors. The latter are referred to as *polymodal nociceptors* in the general context of pain.

From somatic tissues including skin, parietal pleura and parietal peritoneum, muscle, joint capsules, and bone, the distal processes of the ganglion cells travel in all of the spinal nerves. The proximal processes branch within the dorsal root entry zone and span five or more segments of the spinal cord within the posterolateral tract of Lissauer before terminating in laminae I, II and IV of the posterior gray horn. The corresponding fibers of the trigeminal nerve terminate in the spinal nucleus of that nerve.

From the viscera, the distal processes share perineural sheaths with postganglionic fibers of the sympathetic system. The proximal processes mingle with the somatic fibers within Lissauer's tract and terminate in the same region. As noted in Chapter 13, overlap of somatic and visceral afferent terminals on the dendrites

Box 34.1 *Continued*

of central pain-projecting neurons is thought to account for *referred pain* in visceral disorders such as myocardial infarction and acute appendicitis.

Sensitization of nociceptors
Injured tissue liberates molecules including bradykinin, prostaglandin, and leukotrienes, which lower the activation threshold of nociceptors. Injured C fibers also initiate axon reflexes (Ch. 11), whereby substance P ± CGRP (calcitonin gene-related peptide) is liberated into the adjacent tissue, causing histamine release from mast cells. Histamine receptors may develop on the nerve terminals and (as already noted in Ch. 8) produce arachidonic acid by hydrolysis of membrane phospholipids. The enzyme *cyclooxidase* converts arachidonic acid into a prostaglandin. (The main action of aspirin and other non-steroidal anti-inflammatory analgesics is to inactivate that enzyme, thereby reducing synthesis of prostaglandins.)

The net result is sustained activation of large numbers of C-fiber neurons and sensitization of mechanical nociceptors, manifested by *allodynia*, where even gentle stroking of the area may elicit pain; and by *hyperalgesia*, where moderately noxious stimuli are perceived as very painful.

As already noted in Chapter 13, *irritable bowel syndrome* is characterized by sensitization of nociceptive *interoceptors* in the bowel wall. That event also underlies the painful urinary bladder condition known as *interstitial cystitis.*

Sensitization of C-fiber neurons may include *gene transcription* (Ch. 8), whereby abnormal sodium channels are inserted into the cell membrane of the parent neurons in the posterior root ganglion. Spontaneous trains of impulses generated here are thought to account for occasional failure of quite high-level nerve blocks to abolish the pain.

Neuropathic pain
When a peripheral nerve is severed, and the proximal and distal stumps separated by developing scar tissue, trapped regenerating axons form thread-like balls, called *neuromas,* that are exqisitely sensitive to pressure. Repetitive activation may prolong the victim's sufferering by engendering a central pain state (see below). *Postherpetic neuralgia* is a neuropathic pain that may be a sequel to *herpes zoster* ('creeping girdle'), manifested by clusters of watery blisters, usually along the cutaneous territory of an intercostal nerve. The virus concerned may perpetuate the pain by precipitating the gene transcription mentioned above.

Central pain pathways
Central pain-projecting neurons are of two kinds, as described in Chapter 15: nociceptive-specific, with small peripheral sensory fields (about 1 cm^2), and wide dynamic range, with fields of 2 cm^2 or more; these are mechanical nociceptors encoding tactile stimuli by low-frequency impulses and noxious stimuli by high-frequency impulses.

The current consensus is that there exists a *lateral, sensory-discriminative pathway* and a *medial, affective pathway* in relation to pain (Figures Box 34.1.1 and 34.1.2).

Lateral pain pathway
For the trunk and limbs, the lateral pathway arises in the posterior gray horn of the spinal cord and projects as the lateral spinothalamic tract to the posterior part of the contralateral ventral posterior lateral nucleus of thalamus. For the head and neck, it commences in the spinal nucleus of the trigeminal nerve and occupies the trigeminothalamic projection to the contralateral posterior medial thalamic nucleus. The onward projection is mainly to the primary somatic sensory cortex (SI), partly to the upper bank of the lateral sulcus (SII). The arrangement is somatotopic, as can be seen on PET scanning when a noxious heat stimulus is applied to different parts of the body. Animal investigations demonstrate intensity responsive, nociceptive-specific neurons in SI, having appropriately small peripheral receptive fields, ideal candidates for encoding the 'Where and how much?' aspects of pain.

Onward projections to the posterior parietal cortex and SII are indicated in Figures Box 34.1.1 and 34.1.2.

Not surprisingly, the spinothalamic early warning system stimulates orientation of head and eyes toward the source of pain. As mentioned in Chapter 15, the *spinotectal tract* ascends alongside the spinothalamic and terminates in the superior colliculus. Its imprint is somatotopic and it elicits a *spinovisual reflex* to orient the eyes/head/trunk toward the area stimulated. In addition to activation of this phylogenetically ancient (reptilian) reflex, the 'Where?' visual channel (Ch. 29) is engaged by association fibers passing to the posterior parietal cortex from SI.

Nociceptive neurons in SII are less numerous, and many also receive visual inputs. They are linked to the insula, which also receives direct inputs from the thalamus. Insular stimulation may elicit autonomic responses such as a rapid pulse rate, vasoconstriction, and sweating. Surprisingly, pre-existing lesions of the insula may abolish the aversive quality of painful stimuli while preserving the location and intensity aspects. The condition is known as *asymbolia for pain.*

Medial pain pathway
The medial pathway is polysynaptic, via spinoreticular and trigeminoreticular tracts to the contralateral medial dorsal thalamic nucleus (among others), with onward projection to the anterior cingulate cortex. That this area is concerned with the affective component of pain experience is strongly supported by the effect of

(Continued)

Box 34.1 Continued

A

Somatic sensory cortex

B

Anterior cingulate cortex

C

Secondary somatic sensory area

Lateral ventricle

D

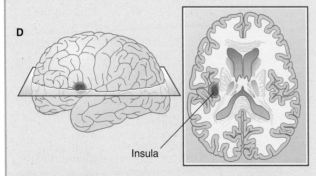

Insula

Figure Box 34.1.1 Areas showing increased metabolic activity following application of noxious heat to the right forearm.

surgical undercutting (cingulotomy) or removal (cingulectomy) as a treatment for chronic pain. Patients report that the intensity of their pain is unchanged but that it has lost its aggressive nature. Precisely the same result follows morphine injection – presumably because the anterior cingulate has the greatest number of opiate receptors in the cerebral cortex.

Following cingulotomy, edema of the bladder control area frequently causes temporary urinary incontinence. More importantly, more than half of all patients show permanent 'flatness of affect', i.e. low experience of either elation or depression.

An unexpected stab of pain from any source is likely to generate an immediate sense of fear. This is attributable to activation of *spinomesencephalic* fibers projecting to the midbrain reticular formation, with onward projection to the amygdala, a nucleus particularly associated with the sense of fear (see main text). Some of the fibers are believed to ascend in or alongside the posterolateral tract of Lissauer; they may account for the persistence of pain perception in some patients following the cordotomy procedure.

Central pain states
Central pain states are almost always generated by *wind-up* of the CPPNs of the spinothalamic and spinoreticular pathways. One or more of three mechanisms may be responsible:

- Repetitive activation of NMDA glutamate receptors by posterior nerve root inputs, over a period of weeks or months, tends to induce a state of long-term potentiation of CPPNs.
- The threshold of CPPNs may be lowered further by gene transcription whereby additional glutamate receptors are inserted into their dendrites.
- The term 'paradoxical' seems appropriate for the third mechanism. Reference was made in Chapter 24 to *supraspinal antinociception*, whereby serotonergic neurons projecting from the medullary magnus raphe nucleus (MRN) to the posterior gray horn may *inhibit* CPPNs by activating internuncial enkephalinergic neurons. Evidence from animal experiments now indicates that while either of the first two mechanisms may initiate a central pain state, its maintenance requires that non-serotonergic neurons in or near MRN *facilitate* CPPNs by a direct excitatory transmitter of uncertain nature. Following limb amputation, an ultimate expression of wind-up is *phantom limb pain*, where, following limb amputation, severe pain may be experienced in the distal part of the missing limb.

As mentioned in Chapter 27, the central pain state known as *thalamic syndrome* may develop following a vascular lesion in the white matter close to the ventroposterior nucleus of the thalamus. Explanation of

Box 34.1 *Continued*

Figure Box 34.1.2 Pain pathways. *Note:* Violet signifies having emotional significance.
The amygdala is in fact anterior to the plane of section in the diagram and areas 5 and 7 are posterior to it.
1. Peripheral nociceptive neurons project to posterior gray horn.
2. 'Fast' CPPNs project direct to contralateral posterolateral thalamus and
3. relay to somatic sensory cortex (SI).
4. Association fibers connect SI to posterior parietal cortex both for 'Where' and 'How much' tactile analysis, and to provide a 'Where?' visual alert.
5. Posterior parietal cortex projects to SII for tactile-visual integration. Onward relay to the insular cortex, supplemented by some direct thalamic inputs there, may elicit autonomic and emotional responses.
6. 'Slow' CPPNs relay via the reticular formation to the medial thalamus, with forward projection to the prefrontal cortex (not shown here) for overall evaluation.
7. Upward projection to the cingulate cortex normally generates an aversive (*L.* 'turn away') emotional evaluation.
8. Some CPPNs excite reticular neurons projecting to the amygdala, where they are likely to generate a sense of fear.

the bouts of severe contralateral pain sensation may lie in elimination of the normal inhibitory feedback to the posterior thalamus from the surrounding thalamic reticular nucleus.

REFERENCES

Benarroch EE: Descending monoaminergic pain modulation, *Neurology* 71:217–221, 2008.
Brooks J, Tracey I: From nociception to pain perception: imaging the spinal and supraspinal pathways, *J Anat* 207:19–33, 2005.

Froth M, Mauguiere M: Dual representation of pain in the operculo-insular cortex in humans, *Brain* 126:438–450, 2003.
Gatchel RJ: *Clinical essentials of pain management*, Washington, 2005, American Association.
Vanegas H, Schaible H-G: Descending control of persistent pain: inhibitory or facilitatory? *Brain Res Rev* 46:295–309, 2004.
Villanueva L, Nathan PW: Multiple pain pathways. In *Progress in pain research and management*, vol 16, Seattle, 2000, IASP Press, pp 371–386.
Willis WD, Westlund KR: Pain system. In Paxinos G, Mai JK, editors: *The human nervous system*, ed 2, Amsterdam, 2004, Elsevier, pp 1125–1170.

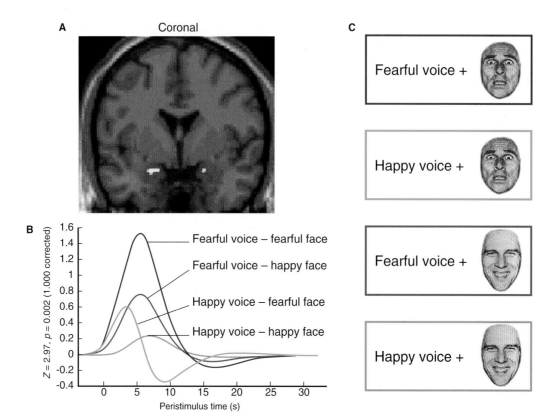

Figure 34.11 Cross-modal emotional responses. **(A)** Coronal structural MRI image showing a superimposed fMRI map of bilateral activation of the amygdala in a volunteer observing a fearful face accompanied by a fearful voice (see C). At the opposite end of the spectrum, amygdalar activity was below normal level in the presence of a happy face and voice. **(B)** The associated graph shows experimental condition-specific fMRI responses in the amygdala. (Kindly provided by Professor R.J. Dolan, Wellcome Department of Cognitive Neurology, Institute of Neurology, University College, London, UK.)

Table 34.1 Afferents to lateral nucleus of amygdala

Nature	Subcortical source	Cortical source
Tactile	Ventral posterior nucleus of thalamus	Parietal lobe
Auditory	Medial geniculate body	Superior temporal gyrus
Visual	Lateral geniculate body*	Occipital cortex
Olfactory	—	Piriform lobe
Mnemonic	—	Hippocampus/entorhinal cortex
Cardiac	Hypothalamus	Insula
Nociceptive	Midbrain reticular formation	—
Cognitive	—	Orbital cortex
Attention-related	Cerulean nucleus	Basal nucleus of Meynert

Afferents from LGB to amygdala have yet to be clearly identified.

primarily associated with the emotion of fear, as illustrated by the effect of looking at an angry or fearful face (Figure 34.11). Current clinical and basic science ambition is to gain diagnostic and therapeutic insights into the role of the amygdala with regard to various *phobias* and *anxiety states* prevalent in both the young and the adult population. The connections of the amygdala (inasmuch as these are understood) are consistent with the present perception of a 'bottleneck' position in the perception and expression of fear.

Afferent pathways

Within the amygdala, nuclear groups receiving afferents are predominantly laterally placed and are usually referred to collectively as the **lateral nucleus**. In Table 34.1 and related Figures, the afferents are segregated into subcortical and cortical.

Subcortical access, depicted in Figure 34.12, is thought to be especially important in infancy and childhood, at a time

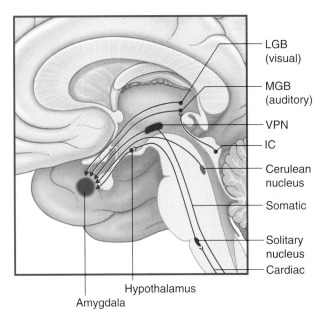

Figure 34.12 Subcortical afferents to lateral nucleus of amygdala. IC, inferior colliculus; LGB, MGB, lateral, medial geniculate body; VPN, ventral posterior nucleus of thalamus.

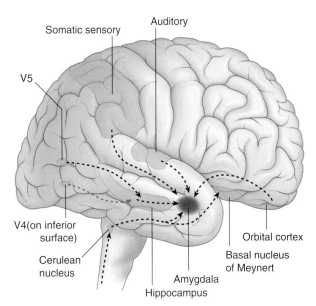

Figure 34.13 Cortical afferents to lateral nucleus of amygdala. V4, object/face recognition area; V5, motion detection area.

when the amygdala is developing faster than the hippocampus and is capable of acquiring fearful memory traces without hippocampal participation. Such memories cannot be *consciously* recalled at any later time despite generating physical responses of an 'escape' nature. The general-sense and special-sense pathways listed and depicted are sufficiently comprehensive to account for the acquisition of almost any specific 'unexplained' phobia (e.g. enclosed spaces, smoke, heights, dogs, faces).

As indicated in Figure 34.13, all sensory association areas of the cortex have direct access to the lateral nucleus of the amygdala. These areas are also linked to the prefrontal cortex through long association fiber bundles, rendering all conscious sensations subject to cognitive evaluation.

Activity of the visual association cortex is especially important in connection with phobias and anxiety states. Area V4 at the inferior surface of anterior area 19 is a link in the object/face recognition pathway. V5, at the lateral surface of anterior area 19, is a link in the movement detection pathway. Both are connected to the amygdala via the hippocampus, where fearful visual memories may be recalled by the current visual scene. The visual association cortex is also important in that fearful visual images conjured in the mind independently of current sensation may activate the amygdala. This capability has resonance in relation to *post-traumatic stress disorder*, where a seemingly innocent scene may cause the afflicted individual to 'relive' a horrific visual experience, up to 20 years or more after the event. In the multimodal anterior region of the superior temporal gyrus, where sound and vision coalesce, a door banged shut may induce a 'virtual reality' re-enactment of a horrific encounter, e.g. of a haunting war experience.

The orbital prefrontal cortex of the right side, with its bias toward 'withdrawal' rather than 'approach' (Ch. 32), is commonly active (in PET scans) along with the right amygdala in fearful situations, e.g. when a specific phobia is presented

to a susceptible subject. On the one hand, this offers the 'downside' potential to 'feed on one's fear'. On the other hand, expert social/psychological conditioning may eventually suffice to reduce the 'negative drive' of the orbital cortex. When conditioning is combined with use of anxiolytic drugs, specific phobias may be abolished completely.

The insula is omitted from Figure 34.13 but, as noted earlier, its posterior part also has direct access to the amygdala, probably related to the emotional evaluation of pain.

Finally, the basal nucleus of Meynert is listed. The cholinergic projection from this nucleus is thought to be of significance in facilitating cortical cell columns in the context of situations having negative emotional valence. Meynert activity appears to be heightened in association with *anxiety*, generating a raised level of autonomic activity involving the amygdala (and/or the adjacent bed nucleus of the stria terminalis, mentioned below).

Efferent pathways (Table 34.2)

Easily identified in the postmortem brain is the **stria terminalis** (Figure 34.14), which, upon emerging from the central nucleus of the amygdala, follows the curve of the caudate nucleus and accompanies the thalamostriate vein along the *sulcus terminalis* between thalamus and caudate nucleus. The stria sends fibers to the septal area and hypothalamus before entering the medial forebrain bundle and (downstream) the central tegmental tract. Some fibers of the stria terminate in a *bed nucleus*, above the anterior commissure. The bed nucleus is regarded by some workers as part of the 'extended amygdala'; it may be more active than the amygdala proper, on PET scans, in anxiety states.

A second efferent projection, the **ventral amygdalofugal pathway**, passes medially to synapse within the nucleus accumbens (Figure 34.15). This connection is considered in the context of schizophrenia (Clinical Panel 34.4).

Notes on the efferent target connections

Periaqueductal gray matter (PAG). A source of *supraspinal antinociception* was described in Chapter 24, namely the opioid-containing axons from the hypothalamus which disinhibit the excitatory projection from the PAG to the serotonergic cells of origin of the raphespinal tract. The excitatory cells of the *dorsal* PAG are directly stimulated by axon terminals entering from the amygdala via the medial forebrain bundle.

In laboratory animals, stimulation of the *ventral* PAG causes *freezing*, where a fixed, flexed posture is adopted. The ventral PAG contains neurons projecting to the cells of origin of the medullary reticulospinal tract. This tract activates flexor motor neurons during the walking cycle, and intense activation may cause a frightened person to 'go weak at the knees' and perhaps fall down.

Cerulean nucleus. Facilitation of excitatory cortical neurons by the noradrenergic projection from this pontine nucleus is to be expected.

Medullary adrenergic neurons. As noted in Chapter 24, these neurons are a component of the baroreflex pathway sustaining the blood pressure against gravitational force. Sudden stimulation by the direct projection from the amygdala may send the heart dullthudding and cause a major elevation of systemic blood pressure.

Hypothalamus. Fibers of the stria terminalis synapse upon two sets of hypothalamic neurons. The first, located in the

Table 34.2 Efferents from central nucleus of amygdala

Target nucleus/pathway	Function/effect
Periaqueductal gray matter (to medulla/raphespinal tract)	Antinociception
Periaqueductal gray matter (to medullary reticulospinal tract)	Freezing
Cerulean nucleus	Arousal
Norepinephrine medullary neurons (projection to lateral gray horn)	Tachycardia/hypertension
Hypothalamus/dorsal nucleus of vagus (to heart)	Bradycardia/fainting
Hypothalamus (liberation of corticotropin-releasing hormone)	Stress hormone secretion
Parabrachial nucleus (to medullary respiratory nuclei)	Hyperventilation

Figure 34.14 Efferents from central nucleus of amygdala via stria terminalis. The only postsynaptic pathways shown are autonomic. The periaqueductal gray matter (PAG) projects to magnus raphe neurons (MRN), giving rise to the raphespinal tract. ACTH, adrenocorticotropic hormone; BNST, bed nucleus of stria terminalis. CN, nucleus ceruleus; MRN, magnus raphe nucleus; PBN, parabrachial nucleus; RF, reticular formation; X, dorsal nucleus of vagus.

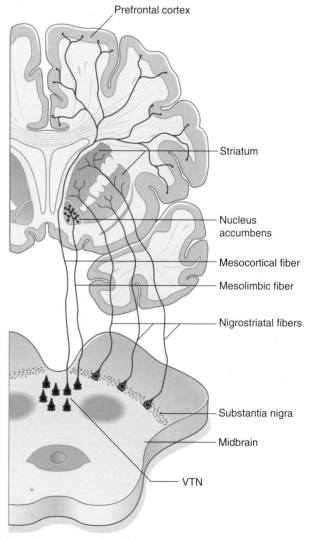

Figure 34.15 Coronal section at the level of the nucleus accumbens highlighting distribution of dopaminergic fibers arising in the ventral tegmental nuclei (VTN) of the midbrain.

Clinical Panel 34.4 Alzheimer's disease (AD)

Dementia is defined as a severe loss of cognitive function without impairment of consciousness. AD is the commonest cause of dementia, afflicting 5% of people in their seventh decade and 20% of people in their ninth. AD patients fill 20% of all beds in psychiatric institutions.

MRI brain scans usually reveal severe atrophy of the cerebral cortex, with widening of the sulci and enlargement of the ventricular system. As seen in Figure CP 34.4.1, the medial temporal lobe (hippocampal complex and entorhinal cortex) are most severely affected. The primary sensory and motor areas, and the upper regions of the prefrontal cortex, are relatively well preserved.

Postmortem histological studies of the cerebral cortex reveal:

- Extensive loss of pyramidal neurons throughout the brain.
- *Amyloid plaques* and *neurofibrillary tangles*, notably in the hippocampus and amygdala. The plaques begin in the walls of small blood vessels and have been explained in terms of an enzyme defect resulting in abnormal, *beta-amyloid* protein production. The tangles are made up of clumps of microtubules associated with an abnormal variant of a microtubule-associated *tau* protein. The tangles are progressively replaced by amyloid.

- Loss of up to 50% of the cholinergic neurons from the basal nucleus of Meynert and from the septal area, together with their extensive projections through the cerebral isocortex and mesocortex. Indeed, degenerating ACh terminals seem to contribute to the neurofibrillary tangles in the temporal lobe.

Hypometabolism can be shown on PET scans arranged to detect glucose utilization. This is attributable in part to loss of pyramidal cells, and in part to loss of cholinergic innervation of the pyramidal cells remaining. Healthy pyramidal neurons have excitatory ACh receptors in their cell membranes.

Although the pattern of degeneration varies from case to case, its general trend is to commence in the medial temporal lobe and to travel upward and forward. The following clinical features are explained in that sequence:

- *Dwindling hippocampal function.* Anterograde amnesia leads to *forgetfulness*, e.g. recounting a personal event within minutes of telling it (loss of present-time episodic memory); difficulty in finding one's way around familiar streets, or alarming misjudgments while driving an automobile (hippocampal activity is required to sustain parietal

Figure CP 34.4.1 Coronal MRI slices. **(A)** Normal control. **(B)** Alzheimer's patient. (Images supplied by Professor Clifford R. Jack, Jr., and the Alzheimer's Disease Research Center at the Mayo Clinic.)
Colors added: *green* = hippocampus; *red* = entorhinal cortex.

Clinical Panel 34.4 *Continued*

lobe *spatial sense*); *attentional deficit*, whose earliest manifestation is an inability to switch attention from one thing to another.

- *Dwindling occipitotemporal function.* Damage to area 37 leads to an inability to read and write. Damage to the temporal polar region leads to distressing failure to recognize the faces of family and friends. Involvement of the supramarginal and angular gyri leads to an inability to write.
- *Dwindling frontal lobe function.* Usually within 3 years of onset, the patient is 'spaced out', staring at walls and seemingly unaware of what is going on in the room. This 'vacant' state lasts for up to 5 or 6 years antemortem.

An unusual variant, known as *early-onset AD*, shows clear evidence of an autosomal dominant trait. The illness appears during the fourth or fifth decade. Chromosomal analyses have revealed a specific mutation in the gene coding for amyloid precursor protein on the long arm of chromosome 21. This mutation is also found in Down's syndrome, where sufferers surviving into middle age usually develop AD.

REFERENCES

Duara R, Loewenstein DA, Potter E, et al: Medial lobe temporal atrophy on MRI scans and the diagnosis of Alzheimer disease, *Neurology* 71:1986–1992, 2008.

Gendron TF, Petrucelli L: The role of tau in neurodegeration, *Mol Neurodegener* 4:13–51, 2009.

Whitwell JL, Jack CR Jr: Neuroimaging in dementia, *Neurol Clin* 25:843–857, 2007.

anterolateral region, sends axons into the dorsal longitudinal fasciculus to synapse in cells of origin of the vagal supply to the heart. The well-known condition, referred to by psychiatrists as *blood trauma phobia* (fainting at the sight of blood at the scene of an accident), is characterized by initial sympathetic excitation followed by vagus-induced bradycardia causing the individual to collapse (faint).

The second set of neurons secrete corticotropin-releasing hormone (CRH) into the adenohypophysis via the hypophyseal portal system, with consequent release of adrenocorticotropin (ACTH). Curiously, these CRH neurons send collateral branches into the central nucleus of the amygdala, with positive feedback enhancement of its activity.

Parabrachial nucleus. In individuals subject to *panic attacks*, hyperventilation, together with a sense of fear, may be triggered by what may appear to be relatively trivial environmental challenges. Normally, the respiratory alkalosis produced by washout of carbon dioxide reduces the respiratory rate causing the blood pH to return to normal, whereas susceptible individuals continue to hyperventilate. Because selective serotonin reuptake inhibitors (SSRIs) are highly successful in treatment, the prevailing view is that the normal inhibitory role of serotonergic terminals within the nucleus accumbens (see below) has become deficient. However, overactivity of the cerulean nucleus has also been implicated because the drug yohimbine can induce a panic attack, apparently through norepinephrine release.

Limbic striatal loop. This circuit is depicted in Chapter 33, passing from the prefrontal cortex through the nucleus accumbens and medial dorsal nucleus of thalamus, with return to the prefrontal cortex. However, the central nucleus of the amygdala participates in this circuit through an excitatory projection to the nucleus accumbens. In the right hemisphere, this projection is likely to facilitate a withdrawal response; in the left, it may facilitate an approach response.

Bilateral ablation of the amygdala has been carried out in humans for treatment of *rage attacks*, characterized by irritability, building up over several hours or days to a state of dangerous aggressiveness. This controversial operation has been successful in eliminating such attacks. In monkeys, bilateral ablation leads to placidity, together with a tendency to explore objects orally and to exhibit hypersexuality (*Klüver–Bucy syndrome*). A comparable syndrome has occasionally been observed in humans.

At the other end of the spectrum, PET studies of incarcerated murderers have revealed that the amygdala of the majority remains 'silent' even when gruesome scenes are presented on screen.

Nucleus accumbens

The full name is *nucleus accumbens septi pellucidi*, 'the nucleus leaning against the septum pellucidum'. More accurately, the nucleus abuts septal nuclei located in the base of the septum. Figures 34.15 and 34.18C show this relationship. The accumbens is one of many deep-seated brain areas where electrodes have been inserted on a therapeutic trial basis, notably in the hope of providing pain relief. Stimulation of the accumbens induces an intense sense of well-being (*hedonia*), comparable to that experienced by intake of drugs of addiction such as heroin (see Clinical Panel 34.5). This 'high' feeling is attributed to flooding of the nucleus, and of the medial prefrontal cortex, by synaptic and volume release of dopamine from the neurons projecting from the ventral tegmental area. Normally, dopamine is released in small amounts and quickly retrieved from the extracellular space by a specific dopamine reuptake transporter.

Septal area

The septal area comprises the **septal nuclei**, merging with the cortex directly in front of the anterior commissure, together with a small extension into the septum pellucidum (Figure 34.16).

Afferents to the septal nuclei are received from:

- the amygdala, via the *diagonal band* (of Broca), a slender connection passing alongside the anterior perforated substance;

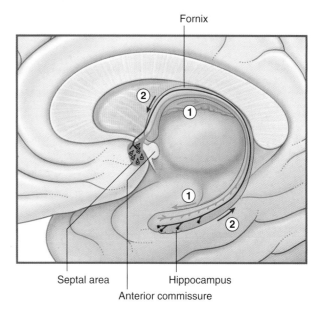

Figure 34.16 Connections of the septal area. MDN, mediodorsal nucleus of thalamus.

Figure 34.17 Septohippocampal pathway (1) with return projection from hippocampus (2).

- the olfactory tract, via the medial olfactory stria;
- the hippocampus, via the fornix; and
- brainstem monoaminergic neurons, via the medial forebrain bundle.

The two chief *efferent* projections are the:

- **stria medullaris**, a glutamatergic strand running along the junction of side wall and roof of the third ventricle to synapse upon cholinergic neurons in the **habenular nucleus**. The habenular nuclei of the two sides are connected through the **habenular commissure** located close to the root of the pineal gland, as shown earlier, in Figure 17.20. The habenular nucleus sends the cholinergic **habenulo-interpeduncular tract (fasciculus retroflexus)** to synapse in the **interpeduncular nucleus** of the reticular formation in the midbrain (Figure 17.19). The interpeduncular nucleus is believed to participate in the sleep–wake cycle together with the cholinergic neurons beside the cerulean nucleus, identified earlier (Figure 24.3).
- **septohippocampal pathway**, running to the hippocampus by way of the fornix (Figure 34.17). It is responsible for generating the slow-wave *hippocampal theta rhythm* detectable in EEG recordings from the temporal lobe. Glutamatergic neurons in this pathway are pacemakers determining the *rate* of theta rhythm; cholinergic neurons determine the *size* of the theta waves. Theta rhythm is produced by synchronous discharge of groups of hippocampal pyramidal cells, and is significant in the development of biochemical alterations within pyramidal glutamate receptors during the long-term potentiation involved in laying down episodic memory traces. The strength of theta rhythm is greatly reduced in AD, reflecting the substantial loss of both cholinergic neurons and episodic memory formation and retrieval in this disease.

Electrical stimulation of the human septal area produces sexual sensations akin to orgasm. In animals, an electrolytic lesion may evince signs of extreme displeasure (so-called 'septal rage'). This surprising response may be due to destruction of a possible inhibitory projection from septal area to amygdala.

Basal forebrain

The basal forebrain extends from the bifurcation of the olfactory tract as far back as the infundibulum, and from the midline to the amygdala (Figure 34.18). In the floor of the basal forebrain is the **anterior perforated substance**, pierced by anteromedial central branches arising from the arterial circle of Willis (Ch. 5). Here the cerebral cortex is replaced by scattered nuclear groups, of which the largest is the **magnocellular basal nucleus** of Meynert.

The *cholinergic neurons of the basal forebrain* have their somas mainly in the septal nuclei and basal nucleus of Meynert (Figure 34.19). The basal nucleus projects to all parts of the cerebral neocortex, which also contains scattered intrinsic cholinergic neurons.

The septal and basal nuclei, and small numbers contained in the diagonal band of Broca, are often referred to as the *basal forebrain nuclei*.

In the neocortex, the cholinergic supply from Meynert's nucleus is tonically active in the waking state, contributing to the 'awake' pattern on EEG recordings. All areas of the neocortex are richly supplied. Tonic liberation of ACh activates muscarinic receptors on cortical neurons, causing a reduction of potassium conductance, making them more responsive to other excitatory inputs. The cholinergic supply promotes long-term potentiation and training-induced synaptic strengthening of neocortical pyramidal cells.

Clinical Panel 34.5 Drugs of dependency

Experimental evidence from the injection of drugs of abuse has yielded the following results (Figures CP 34.5.1 and 34.5.2):

- Cocaine binds with the dopamine reuptake transporter, blocking reuptake of the normal secretion with consequent dopamine accumulation in the extracellular space.
- Amphetamine and methamphetamine are potent dopamine-releasing agents and also tend to block the reincorporation of dopamine into synaptic vesicles. These two drugs are also significantly active within the terminal dopaminergic network in the prefrontal cortex.
- Cannabinoids activate specific, excitatory, cannabinoid receptors on dopamine nerve endings.
- Nicotine attaches to specific excitatory receptors in the plasma membrane of parent somas in the midbrain.

- Opioids such as morphine and dihydromorphine (heroin) activate specific *inhibitory* receptors located in the plasma membrane of GABAergic internuncial neurons within the nucleus. These neurons normally exert a tonic braking action on the projection cells of the ventral tegmental nuclei. Opioid-induced hyperpolarization of the internuncials leads to functional disinhibition of the projection cells, with consequent increased activity of both mesolimbic and mesocortical neurons.
- Ethanol also interferes with normal GABAergic activity. It binds to postsynaptic GABA membrane receptors throughout the brain without activating them; again, the target neurons become more excitable.

Serotonergic and noradrenergic neurons projecting to limbic system and hypothalamus have also been implicated in connection with drug dependency, notably in expressing some of the effects of abrupt drug withdrawal.

Figure CP 34.5.1 Mesolimbic neuron supplying nucleus accumbens, showing sites of action of some drugs of dependency.

Figure CP 34.5.2 Intense activation (*red*) of D_3 receptors (D_2 variants) in the nucleus accumbens of a cocaine addict. (From Staley and Mash, 1996, with permission.)

REFERENCE

Heimer L, Van Hoesen GW, Trimble M, Zalm S: Anatomy of the basal forebrain. In *The anatomy of psychiatry*, Amsterdam, 2008, Elsevier, pp 27–67.

Staley JK, Mash DC: Adaptive increase in D_3 dopamine receptors in the brain reward circuits of human cocaine fatalities, *J Neurosci* 16:610–616, 1996.

Figure 34.18 Coronal sections of the basal forebrain in the planes indicated. Am, amygdala; Acc, nucleus accumbens; AC, anterior commissure; BLA, basolateral amygdala; BN, basal nucleus of Meynert; Cl, claustrum; CMA, corticomedial amygdala; CN, caudate nucleus; DB, diagonal band of Broca; IC, internal capsule; In, infundibulum; LV, lateral ventricle; OC, optic chiasm; ON, optic nerve; OT, optic tract; Pal, pallidum; Put, putamen; SN, septal nucleus; SP, septum pellucidum; Th, thalamus; VP, ventral pallidum.

The general psychic slow-down often observed in patients following a stroke may be accounted for by interruption of cholinergic fiber bundles in the subcortical white matter caused by arterial occlusion within the territory of the anterior or middle cerebral artery. The result may be virtual cholinergic denervation of the cortex both at and posterior to the site of the lesion.

Neurogenesis in the adult brain

The term *neurogenesis* signifies the development of neurons from stem cell precursors. It is now well established that neurogenesis within the brain continues into adult life and, at a much lower rate, into old age. In the brains of laboratory animals including monkeys, and in biopsies taken from human brains during neurosurgery, mitotic neuronal stem cells have been detected in two regions:

- In the subventricular zone, i.e. the zone immediately deep to the ependymal lining of the lateral ventricles. This is the original source of the stem cells of the olfactory bulb referred to earlier. In the adult, the stem cells of the subventricular zone generate cells that are incorporated into the gray matter of the frontal, parietal, and temporal lobes; however, whether they are destined to become neurons or neuroglia is uncertain.
- Within the hippocampal formation, in the zone immediately deep to the granule cell layer of the dentate gyrus. In all species examined, including humans, these stem cells when followed in cell cultures, exhibit branching and acquire electrical activity. Serial histological studies in rats prove that they become mature, integrated granule cells.

In adult rats, the numbers of mitotic stem cells may increase dramatically in response to appropriate sensory stimulation.

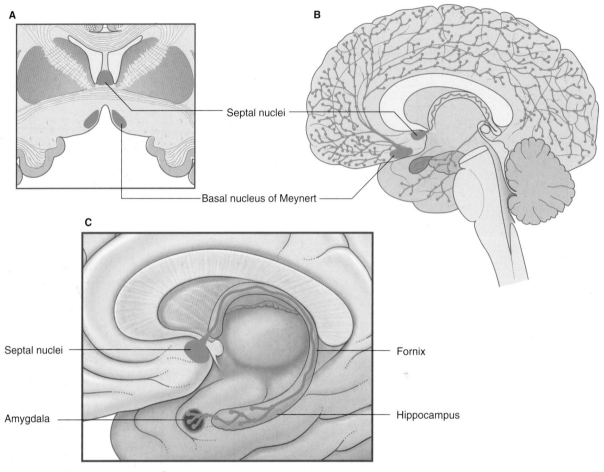

Figure 34.19 Cholinergic innervation of the cerebral cortex from the basal forebrain nuclei. **(A)** Section at level indicated in **(B)**. **(B)** Cortical innervation. **(C)** Septohippocampal pathway via the fornix. The amygdala is also supplied via this route.

For example, the numbers in the olfactory bulb increase five-fold in the presence of an odor-rich environment; in the dentate subgranular zone, a sharp increase is observed in the presence of learning opportunities provided by tread-wheels and mazes. These observations lend credence to the belief that continuing to exercise body and mind is beneficial to humans entering their retirement years.

There is evidence from animal experiments that existing pharmacological therapies for neurodegenerative and neuropsychiatric disorders exert beneficial neurotrophic effects. A high level of serotonin in the extracellular fluid of the dentate gyrus stimulates the proliferation of neurons there, notably following administration of serotonin reuptake or monoamine oxidase inhibitors.

Core Information

Olfactory system

The olfactory system comprises the olfactory epithelium in the nose, the olfactory nerves, olfactory bulb and olfactory tract, and several patches of olfactory cortex. The epithelium comprises bipolar olfactory neurons, supporting cells, and basal cells which renew the bipolar neurons at a diminishing rate throughout life. Central processes of the bipolar neurons form the olfactory nerves, which penetrate the cribriform plate of the ethmoid bone and synapse upon mitral cells in the bulb. Mitral cell axons form the olfactory tract, which has several low-level terminations in the anterior temporal lobe. Olfactory discrimination is a function of the orbitofrontal cortex, which is reached by way of the mediodorsal nucleus of the thalamus.

Limbic system

The limbic system comprises the limbic cortex and related subcortical nuclei. The limbic cortex includes the hippocampal formation, septal area, parahippocampal gyrus, and cingulate gyrus. The principal subcortical nucleus is the amygdala. Closely related are the orbitofrontal cortex, temporal pole, hypothalamus and reticular formation, and the nucleus accumbens.

The anterior part of the parahippocampal gyrus is the *entorhinal cortex*, which receives cognitive and sensory information from the cortical association areas, transmits it to the hippocampal formation for consolidation, and returns it to the association areas where it is encoded in the form of memory traces.

The hippocampal formation comprises the subiculum, hippocampus proper, and dentate gyrus. Sectors of the hippocampus are called cornu ammonis (CA) 1–4.

The perforant path projects from the entorhinal cortex on to the dendrites of dentate granule cells. Granule cell axons synapse on CA3 pyramidal cells which give Schaffer collaterals to CA1. CA1 back-projects to the entorhinal cortex, which is heavily linked to the association areas.

The fornix is a direct continuation of the fimbria, which receives axons from the subiculum and hippocampus. The crus of the fornix joins its fellow to form the trunk. Anteriorly the pillar of the fornix divides into precommissural fibers entering the septal area and postcommissural fibers entering anterior hypothalamus, mammillary bodies, and medial forebrain bundle.

Bilateral damage to or removal of the hippocampal formation is followed by anterograde amnesia, with loss of declarative memory. Procedural memory is preserved. Long-term potentiation of granule and pyramidal cells is regarded as a key factor in the consolidation of memories.

The insula has functions in relation to pain and to language. The anterior cingulate cortex has functions in relation to motor response selection, emotional tone, bladder control, vocalization, and autonomic control. The posterior cingulate responds to the emotional tone of what is seen or felt.

The amygdala, above and in front of the temporal horn of the lateral ventricle, is the principal brain nucleus associated with the perception of fear. Its afferent, lateral nucleus receives inputs from olfactory, visual, auditory, tactile, visceral, cognitive, and mnemonic sources. The central, efferent nucleus sends fibers via the stria terminalis to the hypothalamus, activating corticotropin release and vagus-mediated bradycardia, and to the brainstem activating dorsal and ventral periaqueductal gray matter and influencing respiratory rate and autonomic activity. The amygdalofugal pathway from the central nucleus facilitates defensive/evasive activity via the limbic striatal loop.

The nucleus accumbens is a clinically important component of the mesolimbic system in the context of drug dependency, based upon its abundance of dopaminergic nerve terminals derived from ventral tegmental nuclei. Dopamine levels in the extracellular space in nucleus accumbens and medial prefrontal cortex are raised by cocaine and amphetamines, which interfere with local dopamine recycling, and by cannabinoids, which activate specific terminal receptors. Nicotine activates specific receptors in the parent tegmental neurons. Opioids and ethanol interfere with the normal braking action of GABA tegmental internuncials.

The septal area comprises two main nuclear groups. One sends a set of glutamatergic fibers in the stria medullaris thalami to the habenular nucleus, which in turn sends the cholinergic fasciculus retroflexus to the interpeduncular nucleus, which participates in the sleep–wake cycle. The other forms the septohippocampal pathway to synapse upon hippocampal pyramidal cells. Glutamatergic and cholinergic elements govern the rate and strength, respectively, of hippocampal theta rhythm which facilitates formation of episodic memories.

The basal forebrain is the gray matter in and around the anterior perforated substance. It includes the cholinergic, nucleus basalis of Meynert, which projects to all parts of the neocortex, and the cholinergic, septal nucleus projecting to the hippocampus. Both lose about half of their neurons in Alzheimer's disease, and the neocortical distribution is vulnerable to stroke.

REFERENCES

Adolphs R: Fear, faces, and the human amygdale, *Curr Opin Neurobiol* 18:166–172, 2008.

Bayley PJ, Gold JJ, Hopkins RO, Squire L: The neuroanatomy of remote memory, *Neuron* 46:799–810, 2005.

Becerra L, Borsook D: Signal valence in the nucleus accumbens to pain onset and offset, *Eur J Pain* 12:866–869, 2008.

Benaroch EE: Descending monoaminergic pain modulation, *Neurology* 72:217–221, 2008.

Bruen PD, McGeown WJ, Shanks MF, Veneri A: Neuroanatomical correlates of neuropsychiatric symptoms in Alzheimer's disease, *Brain* 131:2455–2463, 2008.

Derntl B, Habel U, Windischberger C, et al: General and specific responsiveness of the amygdala during explicit motion recognition in females and males, *BMC Eurosci* 10:91–115, 2009.

Diederich NJ, Goetz CG: The placebo treatments in neurosciences, *Neurology* 71:677–684, 2008.

Doetch F, Hen R: Young and excitable: the function of new neurons in the adult mammalian brain, *Curr Opin Neurobiol* 15:121–128, 2005.

Dolan RJ, Paulesu E, Fletcher P: Human memory systems. In Frackowiak RSJ, Friston KJ, Frith CD, Dolan RJ, editors: *Human brain function*, London, 1997, Academic Press, pp 367–404.

Duvernoy HM: *The human hippocampas*, ed 2, with drawings by J.L. Vannson. Berlin, 1998, Springer.

Friedman JH, Dubinsky R: The placebo effect, *Neurology* 71:25–26, 2008.

Hansson E: Could chronic pain and spread of pain sensation be induced and maintained by glial activation? *Acta Physiol* 187:321–327, 2006.

Henriksen G, Willch I: Imaging of opioid receptors in the central nervous system, *Brain* 131:1171–1196, 2008.

Johansen-Berg H, Gutman DA, Behrens TJ, et al: Anatomical connectivity of the subgenual cingulate region targeted with deep brain stimulation for treatment-resistant depression, *Cereb Cortex* 18:1374–1383, 2008.

Kemperrmann G, Wiskott L, Gage FH: Functional significance of adult neurogenesis, *Curr Opin Neurobiol* 14:186–191, 2004.

Kim E, Shirvalkar P, Herrera DG: Regulation of neurogenesis in the aging vertebrate brain: role of oxidative stress and neuroactive trophic factors, *Clin Neurosci Res* 2:285–343, 2003.

Kretschmann H-J, Weinrich W: *Neurofunctional systems: 3D reconstructions with correlated neuroimaging: text and CD-ROM*, New York, 1998, Thieme.

Leonard BE: *Fundamentals of psychopharmacology*, ed 3, Chichester, 2003, Wiley.

Liddell BL, Brown KJ, Kemp AH, et al: A direct brainstem-amgdala-cortical 'alarm' system for subliminal signals of fear, *NeuroImage* 24:235–243, 2005.

Liss B, Roeper J: Individual dopamine midbrain neurons: functional diversity and flexibility in health and disease, *Brain Res Rev* 58:314–321, 2008.

Moscovitch M, Rosenbaum RS, Gilboa A, et al: Functional neuroanatomy of remote episodic, semantic and spatial memory, *J Anat* 207:35–66, 2005.

Passingham D, Sakai K: The prefrontal cortex and working memory: physiology and brain imaging, *Curr Opin Neurobiol* 14:163–168, 2004.

Perry RJ, Hodges JR: Attention and executive deficits in Alzheimer's disease, *Brain* 122:383–404, 1999.

Phelps EA: Human emotion and memory: interactions of the amygdala and hippocampal complex, *Curr Opin Neurobiol* 14:198–202, 2004.

Phelps EA: The human amygdala and the control of fear. In Tait MJ, Sadoun S, Bell A, Bass A, editors: *Water movements in the brain: role of aquaporins, Trends Neurosci* 31:37–43, 2008.

Richardson MP, Strange B, Dolan RJ: Encoding of emotional memories depends on the amygdala and hippocampus and their interactions, *Nat Neurosci* 7:278–285, 2000.

Schott G: Pain. In Clarke C, Howard R, Rossor M, Shorvon S, editors: *Neurology: A Queen Square Textbook*, London, 2009, Wiley-Blackwell, pp 847–870.

Selden NR, Gitleman DR, Salammon-Murayama N, Parrish T, Mesulam M-M: Trajectories of cholinergic pathways within the cerebral hemispheres of the human brain, *Brain* 121:2249–2257, 1998.

Staley JK, Mash DC: Adaptive increase in D_3 dopamine receptors in the brain reward circuits of human cocaine fatalities, *J Neurosci* 16:610–616, 1996.

Van der Werf YD, Scheltens P, Lindeboom J, et al: Disorders of memory, executive functioning and attention following infarction in the thalamus: a study of 22 cases with localised lesions, *Neuropsychologia* 41:1330–1344, 2003.

Whelan PJ, Phelps EA: *The human amygdala*, New York, 2009, Guilford Press.

Cerebrovascular disease

STUDY GUIDELINES

1 This final chapter touches upon a large range of neurological symptoms and signs, because it deals with vascular damage to every part of the brain. The great majority of the symptoms and signs have been already been mentioned, individually, in other contexts.
2 The Clinical Panels may convey the impression that clinical diagnosis is rather straightforward. However, following vascular insults, patients are seldom alert and cooperative.
3 An objective of this chapter is to demonstrate the value of understanding the regional as well as the systems anatomy of the brain, because cerebrovascular accidents cause injury to regions, with consequent effects on multiple systems.
4 The increasing range of diagnostic aids does not shrink the need for clinical acumen. The more accurate the tentative diagnosis, the more likely the most appropriate technology will be selected for further elucidation.
5 Perhaps refresh the blood supply (Ch. 5).

INTRODUCTION

Cerebrovascular disease is the third leading cause of death in adults, being superseded only by heart disease and cancer. The most frequent expression of cerebrovascular disease is that of a *stroke*, which is defined as a focal neurological deficit of vascular origin which lasts for more than 24 hours if the patient survives. The most frequent example is a hemiplegia caused by a vascular lesion of the internal capsule. However, it will be seen that many varieties of stroke symptomatologies are recognized, based upon place and size.

The chief underlying disorders are atherosclerosis within the large arteries supplying the brain, heart disease, hypertension, and 'leaky' perforating arteries.

- Atherosclerosis signifies fatty deposits in the intimal lining of the internal carotid and vertebrobasilar system – most notably in the internal carotid trunk or in one of the vertebral arteries. The deposits pose a dual threat: in situ enlargement may cause progressive occlusion of a main artery; and breakaway deposits may form emboli (plugs) blocking distal branches within the brain. However, gradual occlusion is often redeemed by routing of blood through alternative channels. For example, an internal carotid artery (ICA) may be progressively occluded over a period of 10 years or more without apparent brain damage; the contralateral ICA utilizes the circle of Willis to perfuse both pairs of anterior and middle cerebral arteries; and it is not unusual in such cases for external carotid blood to assist, by retrograde flow from the facial artery through the ophthalmic artery on the affected side. Similarly, occlusion of the stem of one of the three cerebral arteries may be compensated for through small (<0.5 mm) anastomotic arteries in the depths of cortical sulci, perfused by the other two cerebrals. The number of such small arteries varies greatly between individuals. The crescent-shaped anastomotic region is known as the *border zone* (Figure 35.1). On the other hand, all arteries penetrating the brain substance are end arteries, i.e. their communications with neighboring penetrating arteries are too fine to save brain tissue in the event of blockage.
- Many cerebral emboli originate as blood clots in the left side of the heart, in association with coronary or valvular disease.
- Hypertension is obviously associated with cerebral hemorrhage, which may be so massive as to rupture into the ventricular system and cause death within minutes or hours.
- Less obvious are *lacunae* ('small pools') up to 2 cm in diameter, in the white matter adjacent to one or more perforating end-arteries. The souce is now believed to be a 'leakiness' of the vascular endothelium (blood–brain barrier) permitting extravasation of plasma into the perivascular space. The fundamental cause is not understood: there is only a marginal association with hypertension and none with atherosclerosis or stenosis. Lacunar strokes are the most likely to recur, and such recurrence has a high association with a state of *multi-infarct dementia*. An *infarct* is an area of brain destruction produced by vascular occlusion, hemorrhage or extravasation.

Cerebral infarcts become swollen after a few days because of osmotic activity. Some become large enough to produce

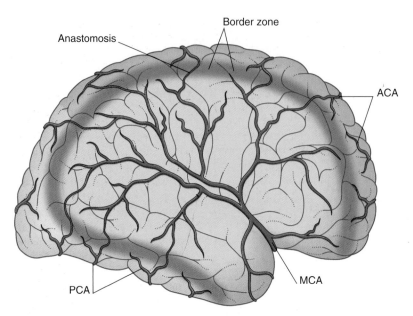

Figure 35.1 Border zone of anastomotic overlap between the middle cerebral artery (MCA) and the anterior and posterior cerebral arteries (ACA, PCA).

distance effects by causing subfalcal or tentorial herniation of the brain in the manner of a tumor (Ch. 4).

It is usually easy to distinguish the symptoms/signs of vascular disease from those of a tumor. A vascular stroke takes up to 24 hours to evolve, whereas the time frame for tumors is usually several months or more. However, hemorrhage into a tumor may cause it to expand suddenly and to mimic the effects of a stroke. Very often, the hemorrhage is into a metastatic tumor, notably from lung, breast, or prostate; in fact, a stroke may be the first manifestation of a cancer in one of those organs.

Some 10% of vascular strokes are caused by rupture of a 'berry' aneurysm into the brain. As explained later, berry aneurysms usually bleed directly into the subarachnoid space because they originate in or near the circle of Willis, but some arise at an arterial bifurcation point within the brain. A ruptured aneurysm is always a prime suspect when a stroke comes 'out of the blue' in someone less than 40 years old.

ANTERIOR CIRCULATION OF THE BRAIN

Clinicians refer to the ICA and its branches as the *anterior circulation* of the brain, and the vertebrobasilar system (including the posterior cerebral arteries) as the *posterior circulation*. The anterior and posterior circulations are connected by the posterior communicating arteries (Figure 35.2).

About 75% of cerebrovascular accidents (CVAs) originate in the anterior circulation.

Internal capsule

The following details supplement the account of the arterial supply of the internal capsule in Chapter 5.

The blood supply of the internal capsule is shown in Figure 35.3. The three sources of supply are the **anterior choroidal**, a direct branch of the internal carotid; the **medial striate**, a branch of the anterior cerebral, and **lateral striate (lenticulostriate)** branches of the middle cerebral artery.

The contents of the internal capsule are shown in Figure 35.4. The anterior choroidal branch of the internal carotid artery supplies the lower part of the posterior limb and the retrolentiform part of the internal capsule, and the inferolateral part of the lateral geniculate body. Some of its branches (not shown) supply a variable amount of the temporal lobe of the brain and the choroid plexus of the inferior horn of the lateral ventricle.

The medial striate branch of the anterior cerebral artery (recurrent artery of Heubner) supplies the lower part of the anterior limb and genu of the internal capsule.

The lateral striate arteries penetrate the lentiform nucleus and give multiple branches to the anterior limb, genu, and posterior limb of the internal capsule.

POSTERIOR CIRCULATION OF THE BRAIN

Additional information is confined to the stem branches of the posterior cerebral artery shown in Figure 35.5.

TRANSIENT ISCHEMIC ATTACKS

Transient ischemic attacks (TIAs) are episodes of vascular insufficiency that cause temporary loss of brain function, with total recovery within 24 hours. Most TIAs last for less than half an hour, with no residual signs at the time of clinical examination. Diagnosis is therefore usually based upon reported symptoms alone.

Figure 35.2 Circle of Willis and its branches. This is an magnetic resonance (MR) angiogram based on the principle that flowing blood generates a different signal to that of stationary tissue, without injection of a contrast agent. Conventional angiograms, e.g. those in Chapter 5, require arterial perfusion with a contrast agent. The vessels shown here are contained within a single thick MR 'slice'. Some, e.g. the calcarine branch of the posterior cerebral artery, could be followed further in adjacent slices. ACA, anterior cerebral artery; ICA, internal carotid artery; MCA, middle cerebral artery; PCA, posterior cerebral artery. (From a series kindly provided by Professor J. Paul Finn, Director, Magnetic Resonance Research, Department of Radiology, David Geffen School of Medicine at UCLA, California, USA.)

Most attacks follow lodgment of fibrin clots or detached atheromatous tissue at an arterial branch point, with subsequent dissolution.

- Transient symptoms originating in the anterior circulation include: motor weakness (a 'heavy feeling') in an arm or leg, hemisensory deficit (a 'numb feeling'), dysphasia, and monocular blindness from occlusion of the central artery of the retina.
- Transient symptoms originating in the posterior circulation include: vertigo, diplopia, ataxia, and amnesia.

Recognition of TIAs involving the anterior circulation is important because they serve notice of impending major illness. Without treatment, one patient in four will die from a heart attack within 5 years, and one in six will suffer a stroke.

CLINICAL ANATOMY OF VASCULAR OCCLUSIONS

In the Clinical Panels, the term *occlusion* encompasses all causes of regional arterial failure other than aneurysms. Symptoms of occlusions within the anterior circulation are summarized in Clinical Panels 35.1–35.4, within the posterior circulation in Clinical Panel 35.5, specifically within the terrirory of the posterior cerebral artery in Clinical Panel 35.6. Subarachnoid hemmorrhage is considered in Clinical Panel 35.7.

It should be emphasized that the majority of strokes originate in the territory of the middle cerebral artery.

Finally, recovery of motor function after a stroke is discussed in Clinical Panel 35.8.

Clinical Panel 35.8 *Continued*

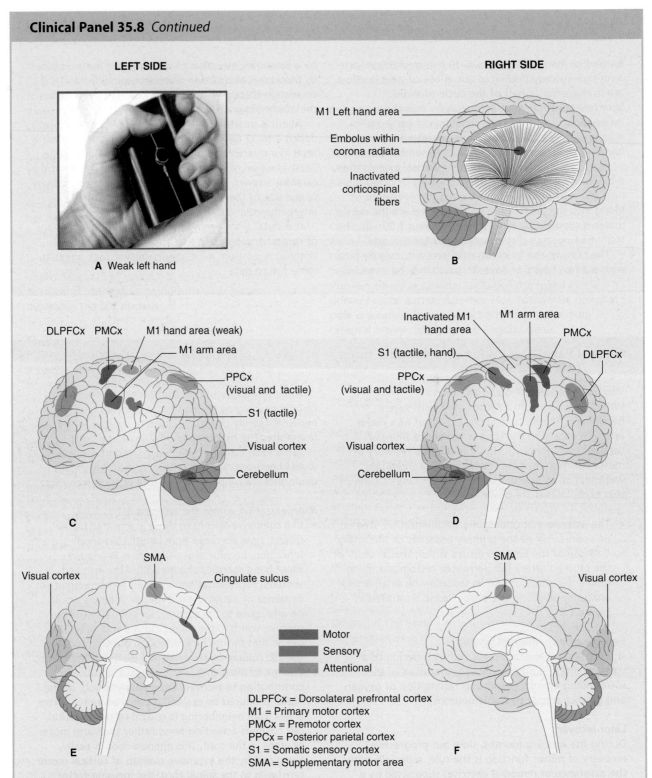

LEFT SIDE

RIGHT SIDE

A Weak left hand

M1 Left hand area

Embolus within corona radiata

Inactivated corticospinal fibers

B

DLPFCx PMCx M1 hand area (weak)

M1 arm area

PPCx (visual and tactile)

S1 (tactile)

Visual cortex

Cerebellum

C

Inactivated M1 hand area   M1 arm area

PMCx

DLPFCx

S1 (tactile, hand)

PPCx (visual and tactile)

Visual cortex

Cerebellum

D

Visual cortex   SMA

Cingulate sulcus

E

SMA

Visual cortex

F

Motor
Sensory
Attentional

DLPFCx = Dorsolateral prefrontal cortex
M1 = Primary motor cortex
PMCx = Premotor cortex
PPCx = Posterior parietal cortex
S1 = Somatic sensory cortex
SMA = Supplementary motor area

Figure CP 35.8.1 Areas of cortical activity revealed by fMRI during recovery from stroke caused by an embolus within the white matter containing the right corticospinal tract.
(A) The 'manipulandum' used by Ward et al. to register the squeezing power of the affected hand.
(B) Depiction of embolic compromise of the right corticospinal tract.
(C) Lateral view of areas of increased cortical activity in the left (contralesional) cortex of cerebrum and cerebellum.
(D) Corresponding view of the right (lesional) side.
(E) Medial view of the left side.
(F) Medial view of the right side.
(Assistance of Dr. Nick Ward, Honorary Consultant Neurologist, National Hospital for Neurology and Neurosurgery, Queen Square, London is gratefully acknowledged.)

Clinical Panel 35.8 *Continued*

Contributions originating outside the affected M1

- Active secondary motor areas contributing to the contralesional (left) corticospinal tract include premotor cortex, SMA (supplementary motor area) and anterior cingulate cortex, and the arm/shoulder area of the left M1 (Figure CP 35.8.1). All three are active during the recovery period. fMRI monitoring indicates that, in those patients with greatest damage to the corticospinal tract, there is greatest reliance on secondary motor areas to generate some motor output. Their recruitment is often bilateral, presumably because of bilateral hand representations.

  Opinions differ concerning the contribution of the *hand* area of the left M1 to motor recovery, although some contribution would be expected in view of its 10% contribution to the left lateral corticospinal tract.

- The cerebellum and motor thalamus (ventrolateral nucleus) are also active bilaterally throughout and share the progressive reduction of activity during later stages. Cerebellar activity during *motor learning* was touched upon in Chapter 23, whereby an 'efference copy' of pyramidal tract activity is sent to the cerebellar cortex via red nucleus and inferior olivary nucleus, representing intended movements. Sensory feedback during movement enables the cerebellum to detect any discrepancy between intention and execution, leading to adjustment of the cerebellar discharge via thalamus to motor cortex. As accuracy improves, cerebellar corrective activity declines.

Sensory system contributions

Visual and tactile areas of the cortex show above-normal activation during the recovery period; so too does the dorsolateral prefrontal cortex. These activities suggest a heightened level of sensory attention, with the objective of optimizing task performance.

Collectively, fMRI observations reveal the recruitment of alternative pathways capable of activating the anterior horn cells that have been functionally deprived by the stroke.

REFERENCES

Brozici M, van der Zwan A, Hillen B: Anatomy and functionality of leptomeningeal anastomoses: a review, *Stroke* 34:2750–2758, 2003.

Cramer SC: Repairing the human brain after stroke: I. Mechanisms of spontaneous recovery, *Ann Neurol* 63:272–287, 2008; II. Restorative therapies, *Ann Neurol* 63:549–560, 2008.

Giles MF, Rothwell PM: Transient ischaemic attack: clinical revelance, risk prediction and urgency of secondary prevention, *Curr Opin Neurol* 22:46–53, 2009.

Henry JL, Lalloo C, Yashpal K: Central poststroke pain: an abstruce outcome, *Pain Res Manage* 13:41–49, 2008.

Losseff L, Browne M, Grieve J: Stroke and cerebrovascular disease. In Clarke C, Howard R, Rossor M, Shorvon S, editors: *Queen Square Textbook of Neurology*, London, 2009, Wiley-Blackwell, pp 109–154.

Schaechter JD: Motor rehabilitation and brain plasticity after hemiparetic stroke, *Progr Neurobiol* 73:61–72, 2004.

Ward NS, Brown MM, Thompson AJ, Frockowiak RSJ: Neural correlates of motor recovery after stroke, *Brain* 126:2476–2496, 2003.

Ward NS, Cohen LG: Mechanisms underlying recovery of motor function after stroke, *Arch Neurol* 61:1844–1848, 2004.

Core Information

Etiology of cerebrovascular accidents

The three chief underlying disorders are atherosclerosis of the internal carotid artery or vertebrobasilar system, thrombi issuing from the left side of the heart, and hypertension. Hypertension may lead either to sudden hemorrhage into the white matter or to production of small lacunae there. Hemorrhage into a tumor may mimic the effects of a vascular stroke. Some 10% of vascular strokes are caused by rupture of a 'berry' aneurysm.

Arterial supply of internal capsule

The anterior choroidal artery supplies the posterior limb and the retrolentiform portion. The medial striate artery supplies the anterior limb and genu. Lateral striate branches supply anterior limb, genu, and posterior limb.

Transient ischemic attacks

Transient ischemic attacks (TIAs) are episodes of vascular insufficiency causing temporary loss of brain function with complete recovery within 24 hours. Anterior circulation TIAs may cause motor and/or sensory deficit and/or dysphasia, sometimes monocular blindness. Posterior circulation TIAs may cause vertigo, diplopia, ataxia, or amnesia.

Arterial occlusion within the anterior circulation

Anterior choroidal artery syndrome results from occlusion of the anterior choroidal artery. The complete syndrome comprises contralateral hemiparesis with upper limb ataxia ('ataxic hemiparesis'), hemihypesthesia and hemianopia.

Clinical effects of anterior, middle and posterior cerebral artery branch occlusion are summarized in Tables 35.1–35.4.

The effects of middle cerebral artery occlusion are shown in *Table 35.2*.

Small lacunar infarcts are commonly associated with chronic hypertension. Typical examples are in Table 35.3.

Cerebral hemorrhage most often spreads from the putamen into the internal capsule; contralateral severe, flaccid hemiplegia results. Sufficient recovery may eventually permit stick-supported spastic ambulation.

Clinical effects of vertebrobasilar arterial occlusion have been summarized in the main text.

Aneurysms

Subarachnoid hemorrhage follows spontaneous rupture of a berry aneurysm at the base of the brain. A typical sequence of clinical effects, in those who survive, is sudden, blinding headache followed by collapse into unconsciousness and development of neck rigidity. About a quarter of cases develop a neurological deficit within 2 weeks.

Table 35.1 Clinical effects of anterior cerebral artery branch occlusion

Branch	Clinical effects
Orbital/frontopolar	Apathy with some memory loss
Medial striate	Paresis of face and arm
Callosomarginal	Paresis and hypesthesia of face and arm ± abulia ± mutism ± inability to reach across
Pericallosal	Ideomotor apraxia (anterior lesion), tactile anomia (posterior lesion)

Table 35.3 Clinical effects of three common lacunar infarcts

Location	Clinical effects
Genu of internal capsule	Dysarthria-clumsy hand syndrome ± dysphagia
Posterior limb of internal capsule	Pure motor hemiparesis
Ventral posterior nucleus of thalamus	Pure sensory syndrome ± sensory ataxia

Table 35.2 Clinical effects of middle cerebral artery occlusion

Segment	Clinical effects
Left temporal	Wernicke aphasia
Either stem	Hemiplegia, hemihypesthesia, hemianopia
Left stem	Same + global aphasia
Right stem	Same + sensory neglect
Either upper division	Paresis and hypesthesia of face and arm, dysarthria
Left upper division	Same + Broca's aphasia
Right upper division	Same + hemineglect or expressive aprosodia
Either lower division	Hemianopia ± agitated state
Left lower division	Same ± Wernicke's aphasia, alexia, ideomotor apraxia
Branches	
Orbitofrontal	Prefrontal syndrome
Left precentral	Broca's aphasia
Right precentral	Motor aprosodia
Central	Loss of motor ± sensory function in face and arm
Inferior parietal	Hemineglect
Either angular	Hemianopia
Left angular	Alexia
Right temporal	Receptive aprosodia

Table 35.4 Clinical effects of posterior cerebral artery occlusion

Stem	Clinical effects
Either	Homonymous hemianopia
Left	Alexia in visible field
Both	Cortical blindness ± amnesia
Branch	
Midbrain	Ipsilateral third nerve palsy + contralateral hemiplegia
Thalamus	Contralateral numbness ± hemianopia ± thalamic syndrome
Subthalamic nucleus	Contralateral ballism
Corpus callosum	Alexia in contralateral visual field

REFERENCES

De Ruck J, de Groote L, Van Maele G: The classic lacunar syndromes: clinical and neuroimaging correlates, *Eur J Neurol* 15:681–684, 2008.

Lee JS, Han M-K, Kim SH, Kwon H-K, Kim JH: Fiber tracking by diffusion tensor imaging in corticospinal tract stroke: topographical correlation with clinical symptoms, *Neuroimage* 26:771–776, 2005.

Losseff N, Brown M, Grieve J: Stroke and cerebrovascular diseases. In Clarke C, Howard R, Rossor M, Shorvon S, editors: *Neurology: A Queen Square Textbook*, London, 2009, Wiley-Blackwell, pp 109–194.

Wardlaw JM: What causes lacunar stroke? *J Neurol Neurosurg Psychiatry* 76:617–619, 2005.

Glossary

ABBREVIATIONS: Chapter containing main reference. Fr. Signifies French origin; Gr. signifies Greek origin; L. signifies Latin origin.

Abducens L. 'leading away'. Abducens nerve stimulates lateral rectus muscle to abduct the direction of gaze (Ch. 23).

Absence seizures Childhood seizures associated with frequent brief spells of unconsciousness ('absence') (Ch. 30).

Absolute refractory period Time interval following generation of an action potential, during which the membrane is refractory to a second stimulus (Ch. 7).

Abulia Gr. 'lack of will'. Loss of willpower associated with prefrontal cortical disorders (Ch. 32).

Accommodation Focusing light by allowing the lens to become more convex (Ch. 23).

Action potential A brief fluctuation in membrane potential caused by rapid opening and closure of voltage-gated ion channels (Ch. 7).

Action tremor See *Intention tremor*.

Active zone Site of release of neurotransmitter through the presynaptic membrane (Ch. 6).

Adaptation Attenuation of response to a sustained sensory stimulus (Ch. 11).

Adrenaline Synonym for epinephrine (Ch. 13).

Adrenoceptor Sympathetic junctional receptor (Ch. 13).

Affective disorder A disorder of mood, e.g. major depression (Ch. 26).

Afferent L. 'carrying toward'. Strictly, applies to nerve impulses traveling toward CNS along sensory fibers; is loosely applied within CNS, e.g. afferent connections of the cerebellum (Ch. 2). See also *Centripetal*.

Agnosia Gr. 'without knowledge'. Inability to interpret sensory information (Ch. 29).

Agraphia Gr. 'without writing'. Inability to express oneself in writing, owing to a central lesion (Ch. 32).

Akinesia Gr. 'without movement'. Refers to immobility often seen in Parkinson's disease (Ch. 33).

Alexia Gr. 'without reading'. Inability to read (Ch. 32).

Allocortex Gr. 'other cortex'. Phylogenically old, three-layered cortex in the temporal lobe (Ch. 29).

Allodynia Pain produced by normally innocuous stimulation (Ch. 34).

Alpha (α) motor neuron The motor neuron that innervates extrafusal fibers of skeletal muscle (Ch. 10).

Alveus Gr. 'trough'. Refers to the thin layer of white matter on the surface of the hippocampus (Ch. 29).

Alzheimer's disease A form of dementia (Ch. 34).

Amino acid transmitters Glutamate, γ-aminobutyric acid, glycine (Ch. 8).

Amnesia Loss of memory (Ch. 34).

Amygdala Gr. 'almond'. Nucleus at the tip of the inferior horn of the lateral ventricle (Ch. 2).

Amyotrophic lateral sclerosis See *Motor neuron disease* (Ch. 16).

Analgesia Gr. 'without pain'. Absence of perception of a noxious stimulus (Ch. 15).

Aneurysm Gr. 'widening'. Localized dilation of an artery (Ch. 35).

Angiogram Image of blood vessels obtained by intraarterial injection of radiopaque fluid (Ch. 5).

Anomia Gr. 'without names'. Inability to name common objects (Ch. 32).

Anopsia Gr. 'without vision' (Ch. 28).

Anterior circulation The territory of the internal carotid artery and its branches (Chs 5, 35).

Anterograde amnesia Inability to lay down new memories (Ch. 34).

Anterograde transport Axonal transport from soma to nerve terminals (Ch. 6).

Antidromic Gr. 'running against'. Usually refers to nerve impulses that, traveling proximally along one branch of a Y-shaped sensory nerve fiber, arrive at the junction and travel distally along the other branch (Ch. 11).

Aphasia Gr. 'without speech', e.g. motor aphasia, sensory aphasia (Ch. 32).

Apperceptive tactile agnosia Right parietal lobe form of tactile agnosia (Ch. 32).

Apraxia Gr. 'without movement'. Inability to carry out voluntary movements in the absence of paralysis (Ch. 32).

Aprosodia Disturbance of the melodic interpretation of speech (Ch. 32).

Arachnoid Gr. 'spider-like'. Refers to the web-like delicacy of the arachnoid mater (Ch. 4).

Archi- (arche-) Gr. 'beginning'. Refers to oldest areas, e.g. archicerebellum (Ch. 25).

Area postrema L. 'back end area'. Refers to the posterior tip of the fourth ventricle (Ch. 17).

Arnold–Chiari malformation Maldevelopment of the posterior cranial fossa (Ch. 14).

Ascending reticular activating system (ARAS) A polysynaptic chain of reticular formation neurons involved in maintaining the conscious state (Ch. 24).

Assistance reflex During voluntary movement, positive feedback from actively stretched neuromuscular spindles assists the movement (Ch. 16). Cf. *Resistance reflex*.

Association cortex Area of cortex receiving afferents from one or more primary sensory areas (Ch. 29).

Associative agnosia Left parietal lobe style of tactile agnosia (Ch. 32).

Astereognosis Gr. 'without knowledge of solid'. Refers to inability to identify common objects by touch alone (Ch. 29).

Astrocyte The 'star-like' neuroglial cell (Ch. 5).

Asymbolia for pain Abolition of the aversive quality of painful stimuli while preserving the location and intensity aspects (Ch. 34).

Ataxia Gr. 'without order'. Describes the uncoordinated movements associated with posterior column (Ch. 15) or cerebellar (Ch. 25) disease.

Atherosclerosis Arterial degenerative disorder associated with fatty subintimal plaques capable of detachment with consequent embolism within the arterial territory (Ch. 35).

Athetosis Gr. 'without stability'. Describes the continuous writhing movements sometimes associated with damage to the basal ganglia (Ch. 34).

Autogenetic inhibition Negative feedback from Golgi tendon organs causing a muscle to relax (Ch. 10).

Autonomic Self-regulating (Ch. 13).

Autoreceptor A presynaptic receptor acted on by the transmitter released at the same nerve ending (Chs 8, 13).

Autoregulation The capacity of a tissue to regulate its own blood supply (Ch. 5).

Axolemma Gr. 'husk' covering the central part or 'axis' of a nerve fiber (Ch. 6).

Axon reflex Activation of the reflex arc producing the triple response in the skin (Ch. 11).

Axoplasm Gr. 'substance' (i.e. cytoplasm) of the axon (Ch. 6).

Axoplasmic transport Orthograde or retrograde transport of materials within an axon (Ch. 6).

Babinski sign Reflex fanning of the toes with extension of the great toe, following a scraping stimulus to the lateral part of the sole; sign of corticospinal tract disorder (Ch. 16).

Ballism Gr. 'throwing', with reference to the flailing movements that follow damage to the subthalamic nucleus (Ch. 33).

Baroreceptor Gr. 'weight' receptor. Refers to the blood pressure receptors of the carotid sinus and aortic arch (Ch. 24).

Baroreceptor reflex (Baroreflex) Reflex increase of sympathetic vascular tone in response to a fall in intracranial blood pressure, e.g. on assuming the upright position (Ch. 24).

Barosympathetic reflex Reflex reduction of sympathetic tone in response to a rise of arterial blood pressure (Ch. 24).

Barovagal reflex Reflex reduction of heart rate in response to a rise of arterial blood pressure (Ch. 24).

Bell's palsy Peripheral facial nerve paralysis caused by swelling of the nerve followed by its compression against the wall of the bony facial nerve canal (Ch. 22).

Benign essential tremor A tremulous disorder commonly erroneously attributed to Parkinson's disease (Ch. 33).

Benign rolandic epilepsy Childhood disorder having an ictal focus of origin in front of or behind the fissure of Rolando (central sulcus) (Ch. 30).

Berry aneurysm Blister-like aneurysm on or near the circle of Willis (Ch. 35).

Binocular visual field The visual field common to both eyes (Ch. 28).

Bipolar recording EEG montage using varying pairs of electrodes (Ch. 30). Cf. *Referential recording*.

Bitemporal hemianopia Lateral visual field defects resulting from pressure on crossover optic nerve fibers in the midregion of the optic chiasm, usually by a pituitary adenoma (Ch. 28).

Blind sight Patients with cortical blindness may perceive movement in the peripheral field without being able to see anything there (Ch. 29).

Blinking-to-light reflex Reflex blinking in response to a flash of bright light (Ch. 22).

Blinking-to-noise reflex Acousticofacial reflex causing the orbicularis oculi to twitch in response to a loud sound (Ch. 22).

Blood trauma phobia Fainting at the sight of blood at the scene of an accident (Ch. 34).

Body schema Consciousness of the relative position of body parts (Ch. 32).

Border zone Crescentic arteriolar anastomotic zone on the surface of the cerebral cortex (Ch. 35).

Bradykinesia Gr. 'slow movement' characteristic of Parkinson's disease (Ch. 33).

Brain Intracranial CNS.

Brain attack Stroke (Ch. 35).

Brain-derived neurotrophic factor (BDNF) A 'nourishing' factor that promotes survival and normal functioning of cortical neurons (Ch. 6).

Brainstem Comprises midbrain, pons and medulla oblongata (Ch. 3). In the embryo, also includes the diencephalon (Ch. 1).

Brainstem auditory evoked potentials Potentials evoked in the temporal cortex following click excitation of the cochlea (Ch. 31).

Broca aphasia Aphasia caused by damage to the motor speech area (Ch. 32).

Broca's area Pars triangularis (area 44) and pars anterior (area 45) of the frontal operculum, involved in generating speech (Ch. 32).

Brown–Sequard syndrome The constellation of signs that follows hemisection of the spinal cord (Ch. 16).

Bulbar L. 'bulb' of the brain. A discredited term usually meaning medulla oblongata.

Calcar avis L. 'spur of a bird'. Refers to the elevation produced by the calcarine sulcus in the medial wall of the atrium of the lateral ventricle (Ch. 2).

Glossary

Myelocele A form of spina bifida associated with an open neural tube (Ch. 14).

Myelogram Image of the spinal subarachnoid space produced by injection of a radiopaque substance into the lumbar cistern (Ch. 4).

Myoneural junction Gr. Motor end plate (Ch. 10).

Myotatic reflex Gr. 'muscle touching'. Tendon reflex (Ch. 10).

Narcolepsy Gr. 'sleep seizure'. Sleep disorder characterized by daytime distorted REM sleep attacks (Ch. 30).

Near response Passive thickening of the lens, miosis, and convergence, combined for close-up viewing (Ch. 23).

Needle electrode An EMG recording electrode in the lumen of a fine needle (Ch. 12).

Neglect Neglect of contralateral personal or extrapersonal space, associated with inferior parietal lobe disease (Ch. 32).

Neo- Gr. 'new', e.g. neocerebellum (Ch. 25), neocortex (Ch. 27).

Nervi erigentes L. 'erectile nerves'. Parasympathetic nerve fibers responsible for penile erection (Ch. 13).

Neurite Gr. process of a neuron, whether axon or dendrite (Ch. 6).

Neuroblast Gr. 'nerve germ'. Refers to embryonic neuron (Ch. 1).

Neuroeffector junctions Autonomic nerve endings within target tissues (Ch. 13).

Neurofibril L. Refers to matted neurofilaments seen by light microscopy (Ch. 6).

Neurofibrillary tangles Tangles of neurofibrils, most numerous in Alzheimer's disease (Ch. 34).

Neurofilament L. The fine filaments seen in neurons by electron microscopy (Ch. 6).

Neurogenic inflammation Inflammation caused by liberation of substance P (in particular) following antidromic depolarization of fine peripheral nerve fibers (Chs 11, 34).

Neurohumoral reflex Reflex with neural afferent limb and hormonal efferent limb, e.g. the milk ejection reflex (Ch. 26).

Neurolemma Gr. 'nerve sheath', comprising chains of Schwann cells (Ch. 9).

Neuron Gr. 'nerve'. Refers to the complete nerve cell (Ch. 6).

Neuropathic pain Chronic stabbing or burning pain resulting from injury to peripheral nerves (Ch. 34).

Neuropathy Pathology in one or more peripheral nerves (Ch. 12).

Neurotoxicity Refers to damage inflicted on target neurons by excess glutamate (Ch. 29).

Neurotransmitter A chemical liberated at a nerve terminal that activates postsynaptic and/or presynaptic receptors (Chs 6, 8).

Nicotinic receptor Acetylcholinergic receptor historically activated by nicotine (Chs 8, 13).

Nigrostriatal pathway Dopaminergic projection from substantia nigra to the striatum; especially relevant to Parkinson's disease (Ch. 33).

Nociceptive L. 'taking injury'. Responsive to noxious stimulation (Ch. 11).

Nociceptors Peripheral receptors whose activation generates a sense of pain (Ch. 34).

Non-conscious proprioception Sensory signals arising within the body that are not perceived, e.g. spinocerebellar tracts (Ch. 15).

Noradrenergic Neurons using norepinephrine (noradrenaline) as transmitter, e.g. postganglionic sympathetic (Ch. 13), cerulean nucleus (Ch. 17).

Norepinephrine (Also called noradrenaline) Hormone released by the adrenal medulla (Ch. 13); also a brainstem neurotransmitter (Ch. 17).

NREM sleep Non-rapid eye movement sleep (Stages 1–4); also called *slow-wave sleep* (Ch. 30).

Nuclear lesion Lesion of a motor nucleus in the brainstem.

Nucleus L. 'nut'. Refers either to the trophic center of a cell, or to a group of neurons within the CNS (Ch. 6).

Nystagmus Gr. 'nodding'. Refers to involuntary oscillation of the eyes (Ch. 19).

Occupational deafness Deafness brought on by noise in the workplace (Ch. 20).

Ocular dominance columns Cell columns in the primary visual cortex activated by geniculostriate neurons (Ch. 29).

Oculomotor hypokinesia Inadequate saccades associated with Parkinson's disease (Ch. 33).

Oculomotor L. 'eye-moving'. Refers to the oculomotor nerve (Ch. 23).

Olfactory aura Epileptic aura accompanied by illusion of an odor (Ch. 34).

Oligodendrocyte Gr. 'few tree cell'. A myelin-forming neuroglial cell with few processes (Ch. 6).

Operculum L. 'cover'. Refers to any of the three opercula covering the insula (Ch. 2).

Ophthalmoplegia Gr. 'eye stroke'. Signifies paralysis of extrinsic ocular muscles (Ch. 23).

Organ of Corti The spiral organ of hearing (Ch. 20).

Orthodromic Impulse conduction in a centrifugal direction.

Orthograde transneuronal degeneration Neuronal degeneration in a proximodistal direction (Ch. 9).

Orthograde transport Proximodistal axoplasmic transport (Ch. 6).

Orthography Processing of letter shapes by the visual cortex (Ch. 32).

Oscillation Spontaneous burst-firing of large groups of thalamic reticular neuron; thought to be responsible for occurrence of sleep spindles (Ch. 27).

Osteophytes Bony excrescences associated with spondylosis (Ch. 14).

Otitis media Middle ear disease (Ch. 20).

Otosclerosis Ear disease associated with ankylosis of the footplate of stapes (Ch. 20).

Ototoxic Term referring to drugs causing sensorineural deafness (Ch. 20).

Pachymeninx Gr. 'thick membrane'. The dura mater (Ch. 4).

Paleo- Gr. 'old', e.g. paleocerebellum (mainly the anterior lobe, Ch. 25), paleocortex (olfactory, Ch. 29), paleostriatum (globus pallidus, Ch. 33).

Pallidotomy Surgical lesion of globus pallidus, a treatment for Parkinson's disease (Ch. 33).

Pallidum L. 'pale'. Refers to globus pallidus (Chs 2, 33).

Pallium Gr. 'cloak'. The cerebral cortex.

Papez circuit An 'emotional' circuit of the limbic system first described by Papez (Ch. 34).

Papilledema Swelling of the optic papilla, usually in association with raised intracranial pressure (Ch. 4).

Para- Gr. 'beside'.

Paradoxical sleep Dreamy light sleep accompanied by EEG voltage patterns resembling those of the awake state (Chs 24, 30). See *REM sleep*.

Paralysis agitans See *Parkinson's disease*.

Paralysis Gr. 'disablement'. Loss of voluntary movement.

Paraplegia Gr. 'paralysis'. Refers to paralysis of both lower limbs (Ch. 16).

Paresis Gr. 'weakness'. Incomplete paralysis.

Paresthesia Gr. 'side feeling'. A sense of numbness or tingling.

Parkinson's disease Disorder of the basal ganglia associated with one or more characteristic features (Ch. 33).

Partial seizure See *Focal seizure*.

Passive stiffness Resistance of ankle dorsiflexors to slow passive plantar flexion in patients with long-standing hemiparesis; probably caused by collagen accumulation within these muscles (Ch. 16).

Pattern generators Patterned activities involving cranial or spinal nerves (Chs 16, 24).

Peduncle L. 'little foot'. Refers to stem, e.g. cerebral peduncle (Ch. 2).

Peri- Gr. 'around'.

Peroneal nerve entrapment Compression of the common peroneal nerve at the neck of the fibula (Ch. 12).

PET Positron emission tomography (Ch. 29).

PGO pathway Pathway from pontine reticular formation via lateral geniculate body to occipital cortex, responsible for rapid eye movements during light sleep (Ch. 30).

Phase cancellation A recording event (not a physiologic one) during compound sensory nerve action potential measurements, where positive and negative phases of adjacent waveforms tend to cancel each other out (Ch. 12).

Phasic motor neurons Motor neurons innervating squads of fast, glycolytic muscle fibers (Ch. 10).

Phoneme A syllable of sound corresponding to a grapheme (Ch. 32).

Phonemic paraphrasia In Wernicke aphasia, the use of incorrect but similar-sounding words (Ch. 32).

Phonology The sounds of words (Ch. 32).

Pia mater Gr. 'soft cover'. The innermost layer of the meninges (Ch. 4).

Pineal L. 'pine cone'. Pineal gland is part of the epithalamus (Ch. 27).

Plasticity Capacity of neurons to adapt to a changed environment (Ch. 29).

Plexopathy Neuropathy within one or more of the limb plexuses (Ch. 12).

Plexus L. 'interwoven'. Interwoven nerves or blood vessels.

Polymodal afferent Afferent neuron receptive to more than one sensory modality, e.g. touch and pain (Ch. 11).

Polymodal association cortex Association cortex processing signals in more than one sensory modality (Ch. 29).

Polymodal nociceptors Peripheral nociceptors (notably in skin) responsive to noxious thermal, mechanical, or chemical stimulation (Ch. 34).

Polyphasic MUAPs Compound motor unit action potentials having an abnormally large number of positive and negative phases, signifying *reinnervation* of motor end plates vacated by earlier degeneration of their nerve supply, followed by takeover by neighboring healthy axons (Ch. 12).

Pons L. 'bridge'. Part of brainstem in the interval between midbrain and medulla oblongata (Ch. 2).

Position sense Perception of the position of body parts (Ch. 15).

Positron emission tomography (PET) Imaging technique identifying radioactive atoms that emit positrons (Ch. 29).

Posterior circulation The vertebrobasal arterial system including the posterior cerebral arteries (Chs 5, 35).

Posterior columns The gracile and cuneate fasciculi (Ch. 3)

Postherpetic neuralgia Neuropathic pain sequel to *herpes zoster* inflammation (Ch. 34).

Postjunctional receptors Receptors in the plasma membranes of autonomic target tissues (Ch. 13).

Postsynaptic inhibition Inhibition of a target neuron (Ch. 6).

Posttraumatic stress disorder A disorder where a seemingly innocent sight may precipitate vivid recollection of a horrific experience (Ch. 34).

Postural fixation Fixation of axial musculature prior to voluntary movement of a limb (Ch. 25).

Postural hypotension Fall of arterial blood pressure on assuming the upright posture (Ch. 16).

Posture The position adopted between movements (Ch. 16).

Prejunctional receptors Receptors in the plasma membrane of postganglionic nerve terminals (Ch. 13).

Pressure coning Displacement of the cerebellar tonsils into the foramen magnum with compression of the medulla oblongata (Ch. 6).

Presynaptic inhibition Inhibition of conduction along the axon terminal of a target neuron (Ch. 6).

Priapism Persistent involuntary erection of the penis (Ch. 13).

Primary myopathy Degenerative change originating in muscle fibers, e.g. in muscular dystrophies (Ch. 12).

Primary neuropathy Neuropathy originating in peripheral nerve fibers; cf. *Secondary neuropathy* (Ch. 12).

Primary tonic–clonic seizures Seizures that are generalized from the start (Ch. 30).

Procedural memory 'How to do' memory (Ch. 33).

Progressive bulbar palsy Rapidly lethal medullary variant of progressive muscular atrophy (Ch. 16).

Projection L. 'forward throw'. Target of a neuronal pathway, e.g. spinothalamic tract projecting to the thalamus (Ch. 15).

Prolapsed intervertebral disk Herniation of the nucleus pulposus into the vertebral canal with consequent pressure on spinal nerve roots (Ch. 14).

Proprioception Gr. 'self perception'. Conscious or non-conscious reception, by the brain, of information from muscles, tendons, and joints (Ch. 15).

Propriospinal tract Fibers of internuncial neurons passing from one segment of the spinal cord to another (Ch. 15).

Pros- Gr. 'before', e.g. prosencephalon, the embryonic forebrain (Ch. 1).

Prosody Tonal variations during speech having emotional attributes (Ch. 32).

Prosopagnosia Gr. 'face-no-knowledge'. Inability to recognize faces (Ch. 29).

Pseudobulbar palsy Term given to the clinical picture arising from compromise of the corticonuclear supply to motor cranial nuclei in pons and medulla oblongata (Ch. 18).

Psychogenic impotence Impotence probably caused by excessive sympathetic activity (Ch. 13).

Psychosis Mental disorder involving a distorted sense of reality, e.g. schizophrenia (Ch. 32).

Ptosis Gr. 'falling'. Drooping of the upper eyelid (Ch. 23).

Pulvinar L. 'cushion'. Refers to posterior bulge of thalamus above the midbrain (Ch. 3).

Pure motor syndrome Syndrome associated with a lacuna in the posterior limb of the internal capsule (Ch. 35).

Pure sensory syndrome Syndrome associated with a lesion of the ventral posterior nucleus of the thalamus (Ch. 35).

Putamen L. 'shell'. Refers to outer part of lentiform nucleus (Ch. 2).

Quadrantic hemianopia Blindness in one quadrant of the visual field (Ch. 28).

Quadriplegia L., Gr. 'four-stroke'. Paralysis of all four limbs (Ch. 16).

Radiculopathy (L. *radix*, 'root'). Nerve root pathology (Ch. 12).

Rage attack Irritability increasing to a state of dangerous aggressiveness, attributed to hyperactivity of the amygdala (Ch. 34).

Raphe Gr. 'seam'. Refers to the midline. Greek genitive case is used in nucleus raphes magnus (Ch. 17).

Raynaud phenomenon Painful blanching of the fingers in cold weather (Ch. 13).

Receptor A term with two distinct meanings: (a) sensory receptors, e.g. photoreceptors, neuromuscular spindles, transduce sensory stimuli; (b) molecular receptors on or within cells are protein molecules acted on by messenger molecules, e.g. hormones, neurotransmitters.

Receptor blocker A drug that can occupy a membrane receptor without activating it (Ch. 13).

Receptor potential The membrane potential at peripheral sensory nerve endings at which action potentials are generated (Ch. 7).

Referential recording Montage following EEG recording where electrode pairs have one recording site in common, e.g. the auricle or mastoid area, (Ch. 30). Cf. *Bipolar recording.*

Referred pain Perception of pain at a site distant from the locus of nociceptive activity (Ch. 13).

Reflex reversal Term used to signify the 'change of sign' accompanying a switch from reflex resistance to reflex assistance (Ch. 16).

Reflexive impotence Impotence caused by damage to reflex arcs (Ch. 13).

Relative refractory period Time interval after firing one action potential, during which a greater-than-normal negative current is required to generating another (Ch. 7).

REM sleep Rapid eye movement sleep (Chs 24, 30).

Renshaw cells Neurons in the medial part of the anterior horn exerting tonic inhibition on alpha motor neurons (Ch. 16).

Resistance reflex Resistance to passive movement, notably at the knee joint, produced by passive stretching of neuromuscular spindles (Ch. 16). Cf. *Assistance reflex.*

Resting tremor Tremor at rest; characteristic of Parkinson's disease (Ch. 33).

Reticular L. 'net-like', e.g. reticular formation (Ch. 24).

Retrieval Calling up items from memory stores (Chs 32, 34)

Retrograde amnesia Amnesia for past events (Ch. 34).

Retrograde transport Transport of materials from axon terminals to soma (Ch. 6).

Rhinencephalon Gr. 'nose brain'. Refers to olfactory areas (Ch. 29).

Rhombencephalon Gr. 'rhomboid-brain' containing the rhomboid fourth ventricle. Embryologically, the hindbrain vesicle (Ch. 1).

Rolandic epilepsy See *Benign rolandic epilepsy.*

Rostral limbic system The anterior cingulate cortex and related areas (Ch. 34).

Rostrum L. 'beak'. Rostrum of corpus callosum extends from genu to lamina terminalis (Ch. 2).

Rubro- L. 'red'. Refers to projections from red nucleus.

Saccade Scanning movement of the eyes (Ch. 23).

Saltatory conduction Gr. 'jumping'. Mode of impulse conduction along myelinated fibers (Ch. 6).

Satellite L. 'attendant', e.g. the satellite cells in spinal ganglia.

Schizophrenia Gr. 'split mind'. Psychiatric state with variable manifestations (Ch. 32).

Scotoma Blind spot (Ch. 28).

Second messenger In the context of the transmitter activating a G-protein–coupled membrane receptor is the first messenger, the second messenger (e.g. cyclic AMP) is the responding molecule that initiates biochemical events in the cytoplasm and/or nucleus (Ch. 8).

Secondary neuropathy Neuropathy of motor nerve fibers brought about by collapse of myelin sheaths secondary to anterior horn disease (Ch. 12).

Secondary tonic–clonic convulsion Convulsion characteristic of temporal lobe epilepsy (Ch. 34).

Segmental antinociception Relief of pain at segmental level, e.g. by 'rubbing the sore spot' (Ch. 24).

Seizure Epileptic attack (Ch. 30).

Semantic Having to do with meaning (Ch. 32).

Semantic retrieval Retrieving the meaning of a word from memory stores (Ch. 32).

Senile tremor Benign essential tremor, often mistaken for a sign of Parkinson's disease (Ch. 33).

Sensitization Lowering the threshold of peripheral nociceptors (by histamine in particular) following peripheral release of peptides via the axon reflex (Ch. 34).

Sensorineural deafness Deafness caused by disease of the cochlea or of the cochlear nerve (Ch. 20).

Sensory competition An explanation for cortical sensory plasticity (Ch. 29).

Sensory modality A distinct mode of sensation, e.g. touch vs pain (Ch. 11).

Sensory unit A cutaneous nerve fiber together with all of its sensory terminals (Ch. 11).

Septal rage A rage attack thought to originate in the septal nuclei (Ch. 34).

Septum pellucidum L. 'transparent partition' separating the frontal horns of the lateral ventricles (Ch. 2).

Sign An objective indicator of a disorder, e.g. Babinski sign (Ch. 16).

Sleep paralysis A state of complete awareness accompanied by complete paralysis, at beginning and/or end of an attack of narcolepsy.

Slow pain Aching pain perceived following activation of C-fiber nociceptors (Ch. 34).

Slow receptor See *Metabotropic receptor*.

Slow-wave sleep Stages 3 and 4 of sleep, characterized by slow, delta waves (Ch. 30).

Sodium pump Membrane ion channel capable of simultaneously extruding Na^+ ions while importing K^+ ions (Ch. 7).

Sole plate An accumulation of nuclei, mitochondria, and ribosomes in the sarcoplasm at the myoneural junction (Ch. 10).

Soma Gr. The cell body of a neuron (Ch. 6).

Somatic Gr. 'body-related'. Implies body wall as distinct from viscera.

Somatosensory evoked potentials Waveforms recorded at surface landmarks en route from the point of stimulation of a peripheral nerve to the contralateral somatic sensory cortex (Ch. 31).

Somatotopic Containing a body map.

Somesthetic Somatic sensory, e.g. somesthetic cortex (Ch. 29).

Sound attenuation Dampening of sound by contraction of stapedius or tensor tympani (Ch. 20).

Sound field The peripheral field of sound perception by one ear (Ch. 20).

Spastic State of increased muscle tone induced by an upper motor neuron lesion (Ch. 16).

Spastic diplegia A form of cerebral palsy involving corticospinal fibers destined for lower-limb motor neurons (Ch. 33).

Spatial sense Perception of the position of objects in relation to one another (Ch. 29).

Speech meta-analysis Post hoc analysis if one's own speech (Ch. 32).

Sphincter–detrusor dyssynergia Failure of the urethral sphincter to relax at the onset of micturition; a feature of spinal cord injury (Ch. 16).

Spike Action potential (Ch. 7).

Spina bifida Varying degrees of failure of the embryonic neural arches to unite in the posterior midline (Ch. 14).

Spinal anesthesia Anesthesia induced by injection of local anesthetic into the lumbar cistern (Ch. 4).

Spinal lemniscus Conjoint anterior and lateral spinothalamic tracts (Ch. 15).

Spinal tap (lumbar puncture) Needle puncture of the lumbar cistern to obtain a sample of cerebrospinal fluid (Ch. 4).

Splanchnic Gr. 'visceral'.

Splenium L. 'pad'. Refers to posterior end of corpus callosum (Ch. 2).

Startle response Generalized muscle twitch in response to sudden loud noise (Ch. 20).

Static labyrinth The utricle and saccule (Ch. 19).

Static posturography Study of postural responses on an unstable platform (Ch. 25). Cf. *Dynamic posturography*.

Stellate L. 'star-like', e.g. stellate ganglion (Ch. 13).

Stereoanesthesia Inability to identify an unseen object held in the hand, as a consequence of cortical-type sensory loss (Ch. 29).

Stereopsis Three-dimensional vision (Ch. 29).

Stimulus-induced analgesia Analgesia induced by electrical stimulation of the periaqueductal gray matter (Ch. 24).

Strabismus Gr. 'squinting' (Ch. 23).

Stress incontinence Incontinence brought about by weakness of the pelvic floor (Ch. 13).

Stria L. 'narrow band', e.g. stria terminalis originating in the amygdala (Ch. 2).

Striatum L. 'furrowed'. Refers to caudate nucleus and putamen taken together (Ch. 2).

Stroke A disorder of brain function following a cerebrovascular accident that does not disappear within 24 h (Ch. 35).

Subfalcal herniation Displacement of brain tissue beneath the falx cerebri (Ch. 6).

Subiculum L. 'little layer'. Refers to transitional zone between six-layered parahippocampal gyrus and three-layered hippocampus (Ch. 34).

Substantia L. 'substance', e.g. substantia gelatinosa of the spinal gray matter (Ch. 15), and substantia nigra of the midbrain (Ch. 17).

Sulcus L. 'groove'.

Supervisory attentional system Attention center within the dorsolateral prefrontal cortex (Ch. 32).

Supraspinal antinociception Pain suppression by pathways descending to the posterior horn gray matter from the brainstem (Ch. 24).

Sympathetic Gr. 'with feeling', i.e. responsive to emotional state.

Symptom Clues about a disorder derived from the patient's account.

Synapse Gr. 'contact'. Refers to sites of contact between neurons (Ch. 6).

Syndrome Gr. 'running together'. A characteristic group of symptoms and signs.

Syringomyelia Gr. 'marrow tube'. Refers to central cavitation of the spinal cord (Ch. 15).

T channels Voltage-gated calcium channels causing transient (momentary) bursts of thalamic reticular neuronal activity during slow-wave sleep (Chs 27, 30).

Tactile agnosia Inability to identify common objects by touch alone (Ch. 32).

Tactile menisci Merkel cell–neurite complexes.

Tandem Romberg sign A toe-the-line test for presence of ataxia (Ch. 15).

Tapetum L. 'carpet'. Refers to sheet of callosal fibers above the lateral ventricles (Ch. 2).

Tarsal tunnel syndrome Compression of the tibial nerve within the tarsal tunnel (Ch. 12).

Tectum L. 'roof' of midbrain, comprising the four colliculi.

Tegmentum L. 'covering'. Refers to intermediate region of midbrain and pons (Ch. 17).

Tela choroidea L. 'membranous web', consisting of vascular pia-ependyma (Ch. 2).

Telencephalon Gr. 'endbrain', comprising the embryonic cerebral hemispheres (Ch. 1).

Teloglia Gr. 'distant'. Modified Schwann cells surrounding axons in encapsulated nerve endings (Ch. 11).

Temporal dispersion Elongation of the compound sensory nerve action potential over time (Ch. 12).

Temporal lobe epilepsy Temporal plane. Upper surface of temporal area (Ch. 32).

TENS Transcutaneous electrical nerve stimulation (Ch. 24).

Tentorium L. 'tent', e.g. tentorium cerebelli (Ch. 4).

Tetanus Gr. 'taut'. Spasmodic state of musculature, especially those of the face and lower jaw following infection with *Clostridium tetani* (Ch. 6).

Tetraplegia Gr. 'four-paralysis'. Synonymous with quadriplegia.

Thalamic syndrome Syndrome including contralateral intractable pain, following occlusion of the thalamogeniculate artery (Ch. 35).

Thalamus Gr./L. 'meeting place'.

Thermosensitive neurons Peripheral sensory neurons having sensory receptors activated by heat (Ch. 11).

Theta rhythm Slow-wave temporal lobe rhythm associated with the septohippocampal cholinergic pathway (Ch. 34).

Threshold The membrane voltage level at which action potentials are generated.

Thrombus L. 'clot' (of blood, Ch. 35).

TIA Transient ischemic attack (Ch. 35).

Tinnitus A ringing, booming, or buzzing sound heard in one or both ears (Ch. 20).

Todd paralysis A jacksonian seizure followed by weakness or paralysis of the affected limb(s) for a period of hours or days.

Tonic motor neuron Motor neuron innervating a squad of slow, oxidative–glycolytic muscle fibers (Ch. 10).

Tourette syndrome Involuntary exclamations associated with anterior cingulate cortex dysfunction (Ch. 34).

Tracking Smooth visual pursuit of a moving object (Ch. 23).

Tract L. tractus, 'district'. A group of CNS axons having the same origin and destination.

Transcranial electrical stimulation Recording central motor conduction time by means of transcranial magnetic stimulation of the motor cortex (Ch. 31).

Transduction L. 'leading across'. Refers to conversion of sensory stimuli into trains of nerve impulses.

Transient ischemic attack (TIA) Episode of vascular insufficiency causing focal loss of brain function, with total recovery within 24 h (Ch. 35).

Transneuronal atrophy Atrophic neuronal degeneration passing from one neuron to another, in either an orthograde or a retrograde manner (Ch. 9).

Trapezoid L. 'diamond-shaped'. Collection of second-order auditory fibers in the pons (Ch. 20).

Tremor Involuntary trembling of one or more body parts; may accompany cerebellar (Ch. 25) or basal ganglionic disease (Ch. 33).

Trigeminal L. 'triplet'. Refers to the ophthalmic, maxillary, and mandibular divisions of the trigeminal nerve (Ch. 21).

Trigger point A point or zone in the membrane of the initial segment of the axon where the generator potential arises (Ch. 7).

Triple response The line–flare–wheal response to a sharp stroke to the skin, involving an axon reflex (Ch. 11).

Trochlear L. 'pulley'. Transferred epithet: tendon of superior oblique muscle passes through a fascial pulley, and the name is applied to the nerve of supply (trochlear) (Ch. 23).

Trophic Gr. 'nourishing' (Ch. 9).

Tropic Gr. 'turning'. Chemotropic substances attract ('turn') axonal growth cones (Ch. 9).

Truncal ataxia Inability to maintain the upright position; a feature of midline cerebellar disease (Ch. 25).

Two-point discrimination A test used to assess discriminative touch (Ch. 15).

Ulnar nerve entrapment Compression of the ulnar nerve at the elbow (Ch. 12).

Uncal herniation Displacement of the uncus through the tentorial notch (Ch. 6).

Unconscious proprioception See *Non-conscious proprioception*.

Uncus L. 'hook'. In the anterior temporal lobe (Chs 2, 34).

Unimodal sensory cortex Primary somatic sensory, visual, or auditory cortex (Ch. 29).

Unstable bladder See *Detrusor instability*.

Upper motor neuron Corticonuclear–corticospinal neuron.

Upper motor neuron signs Physical signs indicating presence of upper motor neuron disorder (Ch. 16).

Up-regulation Increase in the number of membrane receptors (Chs 33, 34).

Urinary retention Inability to void urine (Ch. 13).

Uvula L. 'little grape'. A lobule of the cerebellum (Ch. 25).

Vagus L. 'wandering', with reference to the tenth cranial nerve (Ch. 18).

Vallecula L. 'little valley' between the cerebellar hemispheres (Ch. 25).

Ventricle L. 'little belly'.

Verbal paraphrasia In Wernicke aphasia, the use of words of allied meaning (Ch. 32).

Vergence Convergence of gaze for close-up viewing (Ch. 23).

Vermis L. 'worm'. Refers to the segmented appearance of the vermis of the cerebellum (Ch. 25).

Vestibular nystagmus Nystagmus resulting from vestibular disorder (Ch. 19).

Vestibuloocular reflexes Reflexes that maintain the gaze on a selected target despite movements of the head (Ch. 19).

Vibration sense A test of posterior column function, using a tuning fork placed on a bone, e.g. shaft of tibia (Ch. 15).

Visceral referred pain Visceral pain referred to somatic structures innervated from the same segmental levels of the spinal cord (Ch. 13).

Viscerosomatic pain Pain caused by spread of disease from visceral to somatic structures (Ch. 13).

Visual evoked potentials Potentials evoked in the visual cortex when the retina is stimulated by a checkerboard pattern (Ch. 31).

Volume transmission Non-synaptic release of neuropeptides into the extracellular space (Ch. 6).

Wallerian degeneration Orthograde degeneration of a peripheral nerve (Ch. 7).

Warm caloric test A test of kinetic labyrinthine function (Ch. 19).

Wernicke's area Area of the temporal lobe concerned with understanding the spoken word (Ch. 32).

Wind-up phenomenon Sustained state of excitation of central pain-projecting neurons induced by glutamate activation of NMDA receptors (Ch. 34).

Withdrawal reflex Reflex retraction of a limb in response to a noxious stimulus; includes the flexor reflex (Ch. 14).

Working memory Holding relevant memories briefly in mind while performing a task (Ch. 34).

Index

Note: Individual arteries, veins and nerves are listed under the headings Arteries, Veins and Nerves respectively. Page numbers followed by "f" indicate figures, "t" indicate tables, and "b" indicate boxes.

Index